DEDICATION

Th ... and Columbia
U ... and reinforced
cr ...

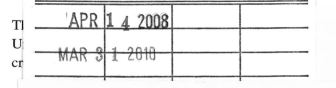

TABLE OF CONTENTS

PREFACE

Educators may have difficulty assisting some of their learners to learn. Nurse educators have the additional difficulty of helping learners to transfer classroom learning to clinical situations.

Why This Book Is Needed

Aiding learners in learning facts and procedures is frequently only part of the task of nurse educators; they must also teach learners aspects of the helping relationship, how to think critically to solve health care problems, and how to translate or transfer that knowledge to the clinical situation. Added to these difficulties is the additional stress of increasing learner to educator ratios, decline in the number of doctorally prepared nursing faculty and decreasing availability of clinical facilities (Berlin and Sechrist, 2002). This situation may result in a cadre of frustrated nurse educators who are dissatisfied with the lecture method of presentation, yet feel it is the only way to deal with large numbers of learners.

This book provides nurse educators with legitimate and evidence-based classroom experiences that engage learners in active, independent learning methods. Not only are active methods of learning more apt to provide greater evidence of learning, they have the potential to promote independent graduates and practitioners who have learned how to be involved in their own learning, how to use problem-solving methods, and how to transfer what they have learned to the clinical arena.

As a nurse educator in several different levels of nursing programs, I found myself forced into the position of having too many learners and not enough instructional skill. Initially, my problems centered around organizing course content into some reasonable style for presentation. Later, my problems focused on finding ways to design humanistic and efficient learning systems.

Many nurse educators face these issues, and I hope this book will assist both new and seasoned nurse educators to design and use effective learning systems where content and evaluation are based on behavioral objectives, and to consider innovative teaching methods as a way of dealing with the dehumanizing effect of increasing learner to educator ratios, decreasing clinical facilities, and the need for critical thinking skills.

Books are available for nurse educators where curriculum theory or educational techniques are presented. No texts are available for either the novice or experienced nurse educator that translate theory into action and provide a repertoire of instructional approaches as well as instructions for how to develop and use them. Consequently, nurse educators have for the most part been socialized into two aspects of their role: appreciation of learner needs, and an ethical sense of dedication to teaching.

A third part of this role, self-image as a confident manager of learning experiences, remains to be developed. Education courses provide theory, but they may neglect to teach the budding nurse educator how to apply theory in an efficient yet humanistic way.

An efficient yet humanistic nurse educator is able to choose from a wide repertoire of techniques based on specific assessments and provide legitimate practice experiences for learners based on a personal philosophy of nursing education. This book focuses on maximizing both the helping elements of the nurse/client relationship and the use of learning resources.

Novice nurse educators are at a high risk to "burn out" quickly because they are usually ill-prepared to deal with the overwhelming organizational demands of teaching. A common solution to this problem is to settle on one method of instruction, frequently the lecture format, as a way of controlling instructor anxiety. Because evidence shows that lecture is not a good way to enhance critical thinking or transfer learning to the clinical area, this book focuses on ways to help learners learn concepts and how to apply them with patients or clients.

Learning styles must also be added to the mix. Learners have different learning styles and a nearly universal need for novelty of presentation and meaningfulness of content. Nurse educators need a wide knowledge of, and expertise in, various learning formats so an appropriate method can be chosen for a particular student or situation.

Even experienced nurse educators may not have large repertoires of educational formats. Some may have settled on one method of instruction and/or may be unaware of some interaction instructional approaches such as simulation gaming, peer supervision, and value clarification.

This book is especially timely now as nursing class sizes are expanding, learner to educator ratios are increasing, educational funds are shrinking, and the Internet is becoming an important learning setting. Nurse educators need to become more skilled in the development and use of their own inexpensive, yet effective, learning tools. This book fills the gap between educational and learning theories and their application to nursing instruction.

Design of the Book

This book is divided into six chapters. At the end of each chapter is a series of exercises designed to assist the nurse educator to help learners apply theory, assessments, and interventions presented in the chapter. Each chapter also presents Nurse Educator Vignettes and Nurse Educator Challenges to help learners understand and apply the material.

Chapter 1 lays the conceptual framework for the other five chapters. It includes a list of proposed nurse educator competencies, the philosophy of nursing education espoused in this book, adult learning principles and theory, critical-thinking skills, transfer of learning, learner-centered environments, and evidence-based teaching strategies. It provides a discussion of how the self-image the nurse educator and learner bring to the classroom can influence learning, as well as teaching dilemmas the nurse educator can face. Correlations between the educator/learner relationship and the nurse/client relationship are described. Ways to assess communication, humanism, and learner preferences and styles are included.

Chapter 2 presents principles of effective learning system design. Included here are ways to identify phases of learning, pinpoint learning system problems, formulate learning objectives, devise evaluation procedures, select and sequence learning content, and identify variables to consider when choosing a teaching method. Because the amount of nurse educator control or responsibility for learning decisions will influence learning system design, a discussion of teaching and learning contracts is also included in this chapter

Chapters 3–6 give in-depth coverage of interactive and innovative teaching methods that evoke critical thinking and are meant to expand the nurse educator's repertoire of classroom skills. **Chapter 3** compares and contrasts role playing, simulation and simulation gaming. Advantages and disadvantages of each method are presented, and detailed suggestions for using each method are included.

Chapter 4 discusses peer learning and other group methods. Basic information about classroom dynamics and group phases is provided. Detailed suggestions for the use of peer learning discussion and support groups, small-group tutorials, and theme-centered groups are offered. A multitude of suggestions are offered to assist nurse educators to enhance critical thinking while working with a large class of students.

Chapter 5 presents some little-known, but highly valuable learning methods that can assist learners to develop self-awareness and integrate learning experiences. These tools include value clarification, perceptual exercises, journal writing, and poetry writing.

Chapter 6 covers issues surrounding individualized learning and examines several approaches to individualization. Methods of learning that are frequently used in the individualized approach are also covered, such as programmed instruction, audiotapes, films and filmstrips, videotapes, videoconferencing, the Internet, distance learning, and computer and television instruction.

Best wishes in your journey,

Carolyn Chambers Clark

ACKNOWLEDGMENTS

I wish to thank Judith Ackerhalt, RN, EdD, and Susan Torreano DiFabio, RN, MS. For many years, we participated in a nursing peer support and education brainstorming group. Many hours of our meetings were devoted to mutual sharing and learning. Their support, critical comments about the manuscript, discussion of their previous educational experience, present philosophies of nursing education, and open sharing of specific instructional skills and exercises have enriched my conceptual horizons as an educator. I am indebted to them for their support and theoretical insight.

I also wish to acknowledge Carole Shea, RN, PhD. We engaged in an ongoing dialogue concerning the essence of nursing education and the difficulties of being a nurse educator and nursing student that has clarified my thinking about these roles.

I gratefully acknowledge Emily Ekle and Jamie Chase, who managed to humanize the editor/author relationship while providing skillful direction.

Part I
Theory and Concepts

ONE

Challenges for the Nurse Educator

■ INSTRUCTIONAL GOALS

Upon completing this chapter and the nurse educator learning experiences, the learner will be able to:

- Write a personal philosophy of nursing education
- Try out a teaching/learning strategy and share results
- Conduct an experiment about finding uniqueness in learners
- Complete an empathy experiment with at least three learners
- Try out an ethics/moral development program
- Produce a written plan for enhancing classroom management skills
- Write in a journal about the process of becoming a nurse educator

The more advanced nurse educator will be able to:

- Debate the importance of learning styles
- Put into action a plan for enhancing the moral development of a group of learners
- Work in concert with a more seasoned nurse educator to build an environment for creative learning

- Test a helping model with three or more learners
- Devise a problem statement for a study of learning challenges for nurse educators or learners
- Take a leadership, legislative, or policy role using feedback principles
- Partner with an advanced doctoral learner from a related discipline to develop a problem statement and research design for transfer of learning

Key Terms

Andragogy	Humanistic classroom
Cognitive complexity	Inquiry model
Constructivist school of learning	Learner-centered environment
Critical thinking	Learning challenges
Dependency/authority processes	Learning role model
Developmental theory of helping	Learning styles
Educator-centered environment	Manager of classroom learning
Educator/learner identification	Mastery through overfamiliarity
Empathy	Moral development
Formative & Summative assessment	Novice educators
Helping model	Philosophy of nursing education
Helping process	Professional self-image
Humanism	Transfer of learning

Introduction

The legendary Florence Nightengale lived out the importance of the teaching role in nursing (Attewell, 1998). Since then, the teaching/learning process has become a top priority for nurses working with clients. Teaching is not inborn—it is a challenge requiring special knowledge and skills. This chapter explores challenges nurse educators must meet and suggests ways to be successful. These challenges are reflected in the instructional goals for this chapter and include developing a philosophy of nursing education, meeting expected nurse educator competencies, examining and intervening in professional self-image, developing teaching materials based on adult learning principles, enhancing critical thinking abilities in learners, creating learner-centered environments, using classroom exercises to encourage transfer of learning to the clinical area, identifying learning challenges and preferences, using self-directed learning, and enhancing cognitive complexity and moral development.

The information in this chapter applies whether the learner plans to function in an academic, staff development, or client* education setting. All of the concepts discussed must be addressed to provide a positive learning experience. In all three settings, a philosophy of nursing education is developed as a beginning step.

A Philosophy of Nursing Education

Part of taking on the role of nurse educator includes developing a **philosophy of nursing education**. The example that follows shows how one novice nurse educator learned about a philosophy of nursing education and its purpose.

> Mary C., a new learner in a masters degree nursing education program, came to class one evening with a question. "I've been asked to develop an infection control program for employees at the hospital where I work on weekends. Where is the best place to start? Should I look up articles or devise an outline?" Mary's instructor told her, "The best starting point is a philosophy of nursing education. A philosophy guides learning objectives and learning strategies. Once you have a philosophy, you will have a direction for developing learning experiences."

Developing a nursing philosophy is an ever-evolving process that grows as nurse educators gain classroom skill and experience. This book espouses one philosophy of nursing education. Within this philosophical framework, learning challenges, the helping relationship, and a humanizing learning

> A philosophy of nursing education is an evolving process that guides learning objectives and learning strategies.

environment are crucial to the development of the professional identity of the nurse educator and the nurse. Classroom experiences will have greater transfer value to client situations when learning is focused on:

- Being free (within the constraints of legitimate structure and classroom experiences),
- Taking responsibility for learning,

---

*Client is used throughout to refer to someone who participates in care and is not just a passive recipient. This is only appropriate because active and interactive learning is proposed in this book.

- Fusing cognitive, affective, and perceptual-motor skills into an integrated whole, and
- Actively examining and practicing helping skills.

This philosophy further espouses the belief that learners can increase cognitive complexity, decrease helping/learning problems, and clarify their values by actively participating in structured classroom experiences. As a testament to this philosophy, structured classroom exercises appear at the end of each chapter.

In accordance with this philosophy, the nurse educator is viewed as a **manager of classroom learning** who assesses learning styles, preferences, and problems, and devises or has at hand a host of learning exercises that can be used, depending on the outcome of the assessment. Being a classroom manager requires a very active presence from the nurse educator. The example below shows some of the dilemmas novice nurse educators may encounter when they consider the idea of being a classroom manager.

> A manager of classroom learning assesses student learning styles, preferences, and problems and from there devises a host of learning exercises to use, sets the climate for learning, and offers explicit goals and directions for classroom behavior.

Josh D., a continuing education instructor, shared his feelings of discomfort with a colleague about being a classroom manager. "I've been using lectures to teach material for so long, I don't want to switch to another method. Might as well just hand out materials and not even show up for class."

■ Nurse Educator Challenge

What answers could Josh receive about being a classroom manager to allay his discomfort?

A classroom manager requires more human contact, not less, than an educator who conducts a lecture or discussion. Lectures and discussions can be taped, and they can be presented without the presence of an instructor. Managing a classroom requires a great deal of preplanning and a high level of assessment and intervention skills. A climate must be set and learners given specific learning goals and explicit limits of behavior in the classroom. Within these limits, creative learning efforts are encouraged. This requires that educators and/or learners plan alternative ways of learning each concept or skill. At least some of these alternatives are chosen to fuse cognitive, affective, and/or perceptual-motor skills into a whole experience.

> A manager of classroom learning creates a climate for learning, sets explicit limits and goals for behavior, fuses cognitive, affective, and perceptual-motor skills into a whole experience, and allows for individualized learning, repetition, and reinforcement of concepts.

Juliana R., a new nurse educator, opened the next class with a short video that ended at a crucial decision point. She invited the class to discuss the best nursing response to the situation and then to break into small groups and role play various reactions. After the role-playing situation, she brought the class back together to discuss what worked, what didn't, and why; what concepts they identified; and how they planned to use what they learned in the clinical area.

■ Nurse Educator Challenge

What evidence is there that Juliana managed the class?

Variety and alternative learning experiences allow for individualized learning as well as repetition and reinforcement of concepts. Variety and wholeness are basic to real-life situations and are used to increase transfer to clinical situations. Neophyte nurse educators struggle with their own anxiety about performing and have not yet developed a strong professional identity as teachers. The best way to increase learner involvement, yet decrease anxiety about losing control of the classroom, is to choose activities that provide built-in control. For example, if the class is divided into small discussion groups, structure needs to be tight and should include specific written directions such as:

- How to proceed,
- Step-by-step actions to be taken to complete the exercise,
- How to discuss the exercise upon its completion, and
- How the group leader can lead the group to keep on task.

Some classroom learning is self-paced when this philosophy is implemented. Learners work at their own rate until they meet a criterion or cutoff point that the nurse educator has set as essential for learning. More about how to do this appears in Chapter 2. Brighter learners are motivated in this criterion-based system by being able to move onto tasks that are continually challenging; the less apt learner is given confidence by attaining success (Valiathan, 2002). Figure 1–1 is a visual representation of the philosophical approach presented in this book. This philosophy in action consists of learners, both free and responsible, whose professional identities are moving toward a fusion of their own unique selves with the problem-solving, technical, and helping skills of a professional nurse. This outcome occurs when freedom and control are in balance; and perceptual-motor, affective, and cognitive learning are available in equal parts.

At first glance, it may appear that the implementation of such a philosophy would require an even smaller educator/learner ratio. Most of the skills and techniques found in Chapters 3–6 can be used even with a large lecture group. Some exercises require more space than others. For example, some of the simulation games and most of the small-group exercises require that chairs be moved and enough moving space or additional rooms are available to enable groups to work without distracting one another.

This philosophy requires that the nurse educator be skilled in designing effective learning systems. Chapter 2 focuses on how to accomplish that. Hand-in-hand with the development of a philosophy, nurse educators must develop knowledge and competencies to help guide educational programs.

Figure 1–1 Development of a professional identify in learners: Nursing philosophy in action

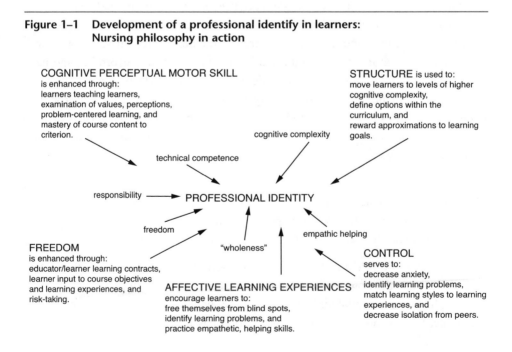

COGNITIVE PERCEPTUAL MOTOR SKILL
is enhanced through:
learners teaching learners,
examination of values, perceptions,
problem-centered learning, and
mastery of course content to
criterion.

STRUCTURE is used to:
move learners to levels of higher
cognitive complexity,
define options within the
curriculum, and
reward approximations to learning
goals.

cognitive complexity

technical competence

responsibility ——▸ PROFESSIONAL IDENTITY

freedom

"wholeness"

empathic helping

FREEDOM
is enhanced through:
educator/learner learning contracts,
learner input to course objectives
and learning experiences, and
risk-taking.

AFFECTIVE LEARNING EXPERIENCES
encourage learners to:
free themselves from blind spots,
identify learning problems, and
practice empathic, helping skills.

CONTROL
serves to:
decrease anxiety,
identify learning problems,
match learning styles to learning
experiences, and
decrease isolation from peers.

Nurse Educator Competencies

As the concern for adequate numbers of well-prepared nurse educators grew, the Council on Collegiate Education in Nursing, an affiliate of the Southern Regional Education Board (SREB), took notice. They selected and charged an ad hoc task force to identify and validate competencies that reflect the knowledge, skills, and abilities needed by nurse educators whether they attain a master's or doctoral degree, and regardless of the settings in which they practiced (Southern Regional Education Council on Collegiate Education in Nursing, 2002; Davis, Stullenbarger, Dearman, and Kelley, 2005).

The task force developed a blended competency model to guide the preparation of the nurse educator at the master's and/or doctoral level using three roles: teacher, scholar, and collaborator. Nurse educator graduate education ideology included:

- Advanced preparation in a field,
- Mastery of a core of knowledge,
- Independent study,
- Active scholarship and research/lifetime inquiry, and
- Critical understanding of issues in the field (Davis et al., 2005).

Core knowledge and skills within the teacher role included:

- Application of learning theories and instructional strategies,
- Use of technology,
- Curriculum and program development,
- Use of evaluation/measurement tools,
- Knowledge of legal standards and cultural influence,
- Mentoring and effective communication skills, and
- Incorporation of professional nursing and nursing education values (Davis et al., 2005).

Graduate nursing education values include leadership, open-mindedness, independence in thinking, accountability, competency, and an interdisciplinary approach. Core knowledge and skills within the scholar role include inquiry and research in education; mentoring; awareness of trends, issues, and needs in nursing education; and using an intuitive, creative, analytical thinking, and caring attitude. The collaborator role for nurse educators includes leadership, communication, negotiation, organization, change theories, problem-solving/decision-making, and legislative/policy development (Davis et al., 2005).

Because educators and learners bring beliefs, habits, and the memory of experiences to the classroom, nurse educators must focus not only on instructional content and strategies, but also on the process of what is occurring in the classroom. One way to begin this learning process is to examine professional self-images.

Professional Self-Image

The **professional self-image** of the novice nurse educator and the professional self-image of the learner develop along parallel lines. Each moves forward to take on a new professional identity and each is confronted with a number of inner processes that may be reflected in outer processes with each other (Cottrell, 2002; Callaghan, 2006; Eckstein and Wallerstein, 1971). Professional identity as a nurse is not synonymous with professional identity as an educator. Great clinicians or researchers are not necessarily great teachers, especially when they tend to teach the way they were taught (Stuart, Hoge, & Tondora, 2004).

> The professional self-image of the nurse educator develops along parallel lines with the learner's self-image, and includes both inner and outer processes.

Novice nurse educators are frequently hired as teachers without being told that there are identifiable learning processes and phases. Nurse educators must expect specific teaching and learning challenges, but realize that they can be overcome. Blending technical and human relationship skills is one way to begin.

Blending Technical and Human Relationship Skills

In the classroom, learning is the goal and the development of the educator is inextricably woven into the development of the learner. One aspect of the process to be mastered through learning is the knowledge and application of technical and human relationship skills.

The novice learner is at first apt to carry out nursing or learning procedures in a mechanical way. The focus is on technical skill and not on how the procedure is affecting the client. Likewise, novice nurse educators are often too busy paying attention to the mechanics of presenting material to learners to pay attention to what effect the information is having on them.

In this early phase, educators and learners often complain that the new skills they are learning seem alien or foreign to them. With practice and with effective feedback, both groups come to understand how to blend technique with self and how to use the skill to enhance the nurse/client or nurse educator/learner relationship. Another process nurse educators must address is the integration of values and rules in the classroom.

Integrating Values and Rules

Another aspect of the professional self-image that needs to be learned involves taking in and integrating the appropriate values and rules of the profession. At first, both learners and novice educators may rebel. Learners may question professional values, avoid taking responsibility for their own actions, or view nurse/client confidentiality as trivial.

Some classroom values, such as humanism, active learning, and structured learning experiences based on learner needs and preferences, may seem difficult to implement and questionable in purpose. The relevance of working out possible solutions, given the constraints of the work environment and of meeting deadlines for class and work, can seem trivial in early phases of professional development. It may just be easier to teach as one was taught, which is often to lecture.

> Bob W., a beginning nurse educator, struggled with the content of his first classroom teaching experience. He had planned to allow for class participation, but he felt pressured to provide a large amount of material, and that left no time for class discussion. He ended up lecturing the whole time and felt frustrated that he hadn't been able to cover everything that was in the textbook.

■ **Nurse Educator Challenge**

What phase of professional development has Bob reached?

When professional values and rules are internalized, there is a deeper understanding of the meaning and purpose of values and rules for conduct. The next example demonstrates an internalization of professional nurse educator values and rules.

> Julie X., a seasoned nurse educator, subscribed to the philosophy espoused in this book. She felt the same pressures to provide content, but reminded herself that learners had an excellent textbook and must begin to take responsibility for their own learning by reading the book. Julie planned her classroom activities so they always included at least one interactive activity and allowed time for a debriefing

period so learners could identify the concepts they'd learned and discuss how to use them with clients. At the end of class, Julie felt invigorated and several learners stayed after class to tell her how much they'd learned from the interactive exercise.

A third, perhaps overriding, aspect of professional self-image is the development and use of a conceptual framework when working with clients.

Developing a Conceptual Framework

Learners must know the client with whom they are dealing. A conceptual framework can guide this journey. Some conceptual frameworks to use include:

- Personality theory,
- Illness/wellness concepts,
- Cultural differences,
- Learning styles, and
- Nursing process.

Without a conceptual framework within which to view the process of helping clients, procedures and techniques remain mechanical. The nurse educator too must have a conceptual framework within which to view the process of how learners grow and become self-directed. Such a framework enables the educator to prepare effective learning experiences and adapt them based on learning needs, styles, and preferences, not on educator preferences.

As conceptual frameworks are developed, professional self-images become clearer, teaching/learning problems often decrease, and learners and educators begin to see that teaching or helping consists neither of forcing the other to comply nor of leaving the other alone without direction as to how to proceed to attain the goal. As the conceptual framework deepens and becomes enriched, interrelated patterns and processes take on added meaning. While working on this challenge, the nurse educator must also observe for any sign of homogenizing the class, clients, or staff.

Moving Past Homogenization

In early phases of professional development, both learners and educators tend to categorize or homogenize target populations based on (ideal) textbook descriptions, on their anxiety about their own roles, or on their earlier interpersonal learning. Examples of homogenization include learner statements such as, "The clients...such and such," or "The staff...such and such," or "The learners...such and such." Nurse educator statements to use to help learners move beyond the homogenization stage include:

- "Tell me about one client who..."
- "Tell me about one staff member who..."
- "Tell me what you need to know to work with this client."

Homogenization can also occur when nurse educators speak to the entire class as if it is not composed of individuals with different learning styles and preferences. It may be easier for educators to read from notes or present slides to learners than to think about how to lead learners to identify and use concepts, solve problems, and come to their own conclusions about data so they can apply it in the clinical area.

According to one study, classroom experiences that engage learners in active learning is precisely what is needed. In fact, it may be the only way to help learners develop critical thinking skills (Sharif and Masoumi, 2005).

Sharif and Masoumi (2005) used focus groups (an organized discussion) to obtain baccalaureate nursing learner opinion and experiences about their clinical practice. They identified the following themes: the theory-practice gap, clinical supervision, professional role, and clinical anxiety. Learners reported seeing their instructor's role as an evaluative person, not a helping educator. Nearly all learners reported the lack of integration of theory into clinical practice.

Neglecting active engagement of learners in learning can lead to more learning problems, increased educator and learner frustration and apathy, and decreased attainment of learning goals. However, not all learners need the same amount of structure to make the connection between theory and practice. For example, if the nurse educator expects all learners to be self-directing, frustration may result with some learners. These feelings are most likely to occur when the educator homogenizes the class and refuses to see that some learners need structure and assistance to learn how to be self-directing.

Sara J., a new nurse educator, immersed herself in her lecture notes and when learners started to nod off in class, or whisper to each other, she just talked louder. When Sara gave them an assignment to interview three people before the next class, she heard a lot of grumbling. She thought to herself, "They're just unmotivated. I have to talk to them after class and see if they're not understanding me."

When the need for structure and assistance is not diagnosed, it is easy to become angry with learners, to view them as spiteful or unmotivated, or to assume that if only the nurse educator's communication were clearer, difficulties would disappear. The educator may then focus on clarifying general communication rather than on assessing and intervening in individual learning problems.

The novice nurse educator must begin to identify learner issues so that their professional self continues to be developed and organized. Lack of professional self-development will inevitably interfere with attempts to be helpful to clients.

■ Nurse Educator Challenge

Explain how lack of professional self-development could interfere with attempts to help clients. Give specific examples and a rationale for your answer. *Hint:* Study the reactions of Sara in the previous vignette for clues.

Developing each of these components is best viewed by the nurse educator as an interrelated and ever-evolving process. The ideal is never completely attained and challenges in helping, teaching, and learning require continual vigilance and attention. Lack of progress in the development of these aspects signals that assistance from more skilled educators is needed. At the same time, nurse educators can begin to keep a classroom diary of events. The diary can help the nurse educator begin to identify classroom situations that can or should be remedied. See the following example of one nurse educator's entry in her diary.

Today a couple of learner questions got lost in the shuffle and I didn't get to answer them. I've got to remember to allow time for classroom discussion. For now, I'll just bring up the questions at the next class and see how that works.

While examining classroom process, the nurse educator will grow in the ability to diagnose and intervene in problematic situations. Tuning into the nurse educator/learner process is an important step.

Tuning into the Nurse Educator/Learner Process

One factor that prevents nurse educators (and learners) from being more free to develop creative learning environments is the incorporation of undeveloped aspects of the professional self, including unorganized and undeveloped potentials. These aspects of self have an effect on the helping relationship.

People both need and fear others. One of the manifestations of these mixed reactions to others is that while participants in interactions sense each other on many levels, they acknowledge only a limited range of what they send or perceive. This tuning-out process is apt to occur in neophyte educators who are deeply immersed in thinking about what they will say or do next and how it will be received by the class, rather than concentrating on learner feedback and learner needs and challenges (Cashwell, 1994; Kagan, 1975).

Both nurse educators and learners develop their professional selves and demonstrate the use of technical and human competence within a consistent conceptual framework. Over the years, educators and learners, as human beings, have developed characteristic patterns of relating to others and of learning in social environments. These affective components of the learning process can be assessed and intervened in to achieve a development in the professional self of both educator and learner. Yancey (2004) described the use of Dr. Rosemarie Rizzo Parse's teaching-learning processes to provide a framework for identifying and changing learner processes. Journal writing, reflection, and participation in dialogue helped nursing learners discover new meaning for themselves. While the nurse educator continues to write in a classroom diary, learners can be assigned a similar task of journaling daily to identify successful and not so successful teaching/learning processes. The result can be kept private for reflection, discussed in class, or become the basis of an assigned paper on one of the concepts identified.

Leenerts (2003) described the use of knowing self with nursing learners. Personal knowledge or awareness of self was conceptualized as a fundamental pattern of knowing in nursing. Personal knowledge is essential for learning the artful use of self in nurse/client and educator/learner relationships. The caring relationship is based on the nurse's therapeutic use of self to help clients fully use their potentials in physical, psychological, spiritual, and social challenges.

The reason this is such a pivotal concept is that unknown aspects of self can interfere in learner ability to be caring. The example that follows demonstrates how one nurse educator tuned into learner feelings and used them to be a role model for the class.

> When the nurse educator showed a short video on hospice care, Jennifer B., a nursing learner, told the class that she'd been unable to talk to a dying client in the nursing home clinical the previous day. "I don't know what happened to me. I just started crying and ran out of the room." With assistance from the educator

and her peers, Jennifer was able to see the connection between her mother's death six months ago and her inability to help the dying client. With classroom support, Jennifer began to problem solve about how to handle the situation. The next day, Jennifer went back to see her client and was able to hold his hand and sit with him. She also apologized for leaving so abruptly the previous day and told him her leaving had nothing to do with him.

Learning or relational challenges that occur in the nurse/client relationship are frequently mirrored in the educator/learner relationship. Common learning problems that nurse educators can begin to identify include:

> Learning challenges include dependency/authority processes, educator/learning identifications, and mastery through overfamiliarity.

- Dependency/authority processes,
- Educator/learner identifications, and
- Mastery through overfamiliarity.

Dependency/Authority Processes

Learners are dependent on nurse educators just as educators are dependent on learners as participants in developing a teaching/learning process. Both may try to appear competent and expert as a way of covering their insecurity about their capabilities. As professional identity grows, there may be less need for this process. The learner example below focuses on **dependency/authority** issues.

> Without intervention, dependency/authoritarian processes can lead to under- or overstructuring class activities.

Sally Z. often cut class and made derogatory comments about the nurse educator. When the nurse educator reminded Sally that her assignment was handed in late, she reported the nurse educator to the administration, claiming she'd been treated unfairly.

Learners who resist regulations, refuse to accept the learner role, do not attend class, or compete with the nurse educator are all exemplifying challenges related to legitimate limits of authority. This process can also be played out by nurse educators.

Dr. Evans, a new nurse educator who just obtained her doctorate, wanted to establish rapport with learners so she spoke extemporaneously to the class, and shared personal information about herself with learners.

Nurse educators who plan to speak extemporaneously or spend the class speaking informally with learners, exemplify a need to set legitimate limits of authority.

> Ms. Debussy, a nurse educator, insisted learners remain quiet in class and quaffed discussions when learners tried to bring up points they needed to be clarified. Whenever learners showed evidence of spontaneity or creativity, the nurse educator reminded them she had a lot of information to cover that day and suggested perhaps they could discuss their questions among themselves or come to her office during office hours.

Educators who allow for no interaction between themselves and learners, and between learners and other learners, or who do not encourage spontaneity or creativity in the classroom, may need assistance in how to share authority, responsibility, and control for learning.

It's not unusual for inexperienced nurse educators to vacillate between insufficient classroom structure and direction on the one hand, and authoritarian dictums on the other. With experience and requisite skills, nurse educators can provide adequately balanced amounts of structure and freedom in classrooms. The more time spent in developing classroom exercises, in planning for different ways of reinforcing the concepts for that class period, and in thinking through how to anticipate and handle classroom happenings, the more time will be available to allow for freedom and flexibility during the actual class period.

It is often the educator's uncertainty and anxiety about how things will progress during a class period that leads to vacillation between insufficient classroom structure and authoritarian control. Just as learners need structure to decrease their anxiety about learning, so do nurse educators.

Nurse educators must learn how to structure learning experiences not only for the sake of learners, but also in order to allay their own anxiety. Without adequate structure in the classroom, novice educators may label learners as unwilling to learn, unable to relate to authority, or unable to receive help.

Upon examination of their professional selves, nurse educators may believe that they can maintain authority only through authoritarian devices or when receiving support and assistance from administrators. The other side of the coin of authoritarianism is dependency. Educators or learners who have unrealistic expectations of being taken care of or being loved by others are carrying around undeveloped professional selves. Another version of the dependency issue is exemplified by learners who pretend that the classroom does not fit within the larger school system, where administrative rules and limitations add constraints. These learners are apt to be disappointed when they find the educator is not omnipotent and cannot change administrative policies.

The educator's version of this struggle is to react with guilt and overexplanation when learners point out this lack of omnipotence. In either case, refusal to acknowledge larger system constraints results in teaching and learning difficulties. A variation of this theme occurs when educators join forces with learners against the administration. Such an action may be based on a need to be liked by the learners or to be their friend. The result is not unlike the disorganization that occurs in families when one parent crosses generation lines and sides with the children against the other parent. For stability to resume, authority lines must be maintained. The example below exemplifies this issue.

> Jacob, a baccalaureate nursing learner, frequently complained to a nurse educator about the hospital administration and tried to convince her to sign a petition he'd generated in support of changes to make the work environment more healthy. The nurse educator told him she understood his position but she doubted a petition would work. She suggested they brainstorm ways Jacob could achieve his goal. Together, they came up with a plan to have Jacob research possible actions he could take that might bring about change.

■ Nurse Educator Challenge

Come up with at least three actions Jacob could take to achieve his goal.

As shown in the example above, one solution to this dilemma is for the educator to refuse to work against the hospital administration, and to find ways to work together with learners within the existing framework to solve a problem. This solution allows learners to take more responsibility for their own learning and shows cooperation, not confrontation, is more apt to get a positive response. When a problem is structured in this way, learners can view it as solvable rather than as external and unsolvable.

Other examples of dependency by learners are: "I'm helpless, spoon feed me," or "I need therapy, not learning." The parallel experience that occurs between nursing learners and their clients becomes apparent through such statements as "I can't help this client because I'm too much like her," and "I had to take total care of the client because he's not able to do anything by himself." Educator/learner identification is a process of importance to nurse educators. Sometimes it's a healthy process that can enhance learner growth. When the process goes awry, the nurse educator intervenes.

Educator/Learner Identification

Developing **identification** is a process that can benefit both nurse educators and learners. Educators can receive a deep sense of gratification when they feel that they have taught successfully. Learners can be helped to develop independent thought and action and to grow to be coworkers with nurse educators. When the identification process is used this way, nurse educators are eternal learners who help their learners to identify with the process of continual learning rather than with static ideas or theories (Callaghan, 2006; Cashwell, 1994; Ekstein and Wallerstein, 1971).

> Educator/learner identification is probably operating when students become attached to and take on the qualities of the nurse educator.

Nurse educators are learners too. The obvious example of this is shown by how much educators learn about a topic when they are asked to teach a course. Being able to assimilate content and convey it in an understandable way to learners requires a much deeper level of familiarity than is achieved by taking a course in the subject. Learners can provide valuable learning for nurse educators who must be ready to receive the information. When an educator is open to suggestions and cues from learners, much learning on both sides can occur. When the identification process goes awry for the nurse educator, learners may be viewed as extensions of nurse educators and as proof of their competence.

Learner identification processes can also go awry. Learners who idealize educators may come to devalue them once their own professional competency increases, almost as if they were thinking, "If I can achieve this, it must be valueless." Other learners, who mystify the learning process, may feel they cannot learn because to do so would be trampling on forbidden ground. Learners who place educators on a pedestal are more likely to dominate clients. To them, relationships may be conceptualized as hierarchical, with the educator at the top, the learner next, and the client at the bottom. This learner domination may be noted in behaviors such as giving advice prior to properly understanding the situation, doing "for" client, and being unable to acknowledge the healthy, independent characteristics of the client.

Nurse educators can help learners use healthy identification by praising their attempts to operate in a professional manner. Nurse educators can intervene in unhealthy identification processes by asking learners to brainstorm ways to work in the classroom and with clients in egalitarian relationships. **Mastery through overfamiliarity** is another process that can impede learning.

Mastery through Overfamiliarity

The new and different creates anxiety in everyone, including both educators and learners. Both may seek to master new teaching and learning situations by casting the new in the mold of older situations (Callaghan, 2006; Cashwell, 1994; Ekstein and Wallerstein, 1971). Beginning where the learner is and progressing from simple to complex, or from known to unknown, learning situations are examples of constructive use of past experiences.

When educators or learners underreact to new learning situations by pretending that "there is nothing new here," this is a signal that self-image is underdeveloped. For example, nursing learners who have worked as nursing aides frequently complain that relearning the taking of vital signs is unnecessary because they are already familiar with it. Upon investigation, it often becomes evident that their skills or theoretical knowledge is shaky, yet to cover their fear of being exposed as inadequate, they seem outwardly blasé. Educators who do not read this learning challenge correctly may be intimidated by learners and tend to wonder, "Maybe they are right, and I am wrong. Maybe I have underestimated them."

> Mastery through over-familiarity is covering a fear of being inadequate by underreacting to learning situations and claiming there is nothing new.

The educator's version of this situation is exemplified most clearly by neophyte teachers who prepare classroom materials at or above the educational level at which they were taught. Frequently educators have one degree more than their learners; thus, teachers with master's degrees may teach at that level to baccalaureate learners. Because their latest learning experience is most familiar, nurse educators may assume that because they know the material, they can breeze through it and get on to more difficult material. This results in the educator assuming learners are more knowledgeable or sophisticated than they actually are.

Some educators even prepare material above the level at which they were taught in an effort to decrease their anxiety about being inadequately prepared to teach. Such reactions are probably due to an undeveloped self-image as educator as well as to an error in confusing inadequate content knowledge with inadequate teaching skill. Part of the difficulty may even be a lack of conceptual framework for working with adult learners. Juanita exemplifies a nursing learner who needed additional learning experiences.

> Juanita, a new RN-to-BSN learner had many ideas to contribute to classroom discussion. When asked for a conceptual framework, she was unable to provide one. She also asked the nurse educator to coffee or lunch several days in a row, and neglected to turn an assignment in on the required date, claiming she needed more time.

■ Nurse Educator Challenge

How would you handle Juanita's behavior? Give a rationale for your answer.

Nurse Educator Tips

Use these questions to help identify learners who may need additional learning experiences.

Does the learner:
- Neglect to use a conceptual framework?
- Ask for or imply the need to be a friend, child, or foe?
- Need more structure to be self-directing?
- Need more freedom to be self-directing?
- Resist regulations and class rules or other appropriate limits?
- Devalue the content or learning process?
- Place the nurse educator on a pedestal?

Use these questions to identify areas that require change in classroom structure.

Do I . . .
- "Feed" learners by always lecturing?
- Talk informally with learners rather than set adequate amounts of classroom structure and freedom?
- See some learners as spiteful and unmotivated?
- Join forces with learners against administration?
- Let some learners "off the hook" from meeting classroom rules?
- Prepare learning materials that are either too easy or too advanced for learners?

Adult Learning Theory and Principles

Teaching nursing learners involves teaching adults. Teaching methods must be appropriate for adult learning. As Stuart, Hoge, and Tondora (2004) remind us, teaching is not the same thing as learning. Following adult learning principles means structuring learning that must:

- Be active, not passive,
- Be driven by the need to know,
- Take place in the context of solving a problem or in daily activities and is immediately relevant to the learner,
- Activate prior knowledge and experience,
- Have an element of self-direction and self-responsibility,
- Provide a bridge and/or support to help learners develop independent problem-solving skills, and
- Be an egalitarian, two-way process between educator and learner and not a "handing down of knowledge" by the educator (Davies, 2000; Knowles, Holton, and Swanson, 1998; Knowles, 1990).

A school of learning that may be most apropos for educating nursing learners is the constructivist approach.

Constructivist School of Learning

The **constructivist school of learning** holds that knowledge is best remembered in the context in which it is learned, uses problem solving to find a solution to a situation that is relevant to the needs of the learner, is self-directed yet interactive, and is a negotiated process between educator and learner (Stuart, Hoge, and Tondora, 2004).

> The constructivist school of learning holds that knowledge is best remembered in the context in which it's learned, uses problem solving in a relevant situation, is self-directed, interactive, and negotiated.

Knowles is another theorist whose work is very applicable to nurse educators who work with adult learners.

Andragogy Learning Theory

Knowles (1990, 1998) used the term **andragogy** to describe his adult learning theory. He contended that what drives adult learning are: learner readiness, the need to know, what the learner brings to the learning situation, and a problem-based approach in an atmosphere of mutual support and respect. The main motivation of adult learners is to learn something they can apply in an immediate situation.

Nursing learners attend class so they can learn something they can apply in the clinical situation. If the information presented is not relevant to the clinical situation, motivation to learn may be low. Because nursing learners are adults, they may question the benefit they will derive from the subject being taught.

Novice nurse educators may struggle to deal effectively when learners try to have input into their learning. A common solution is to quell classroom discussion and try to maintain a steady stream of one-way information giving. Adult learners must be active in other ways. They need to participate in diagnosing their own needs, formulating learning objectives that are relevant to their needs, and evaluating their own learning. To enhance learning, nurse educators should:

> Andragogy theory includes Knowles' belief that learner readiness, need to know, learner characteristics, and a problem-based approach in an atmosphere of mutual respect drive adult learning.

- Find ways to evaluate learner readiness and build on previous learning,
- Actively engage learners in the learning process,
- Provide information that has meaning to learners, and
- Help learners integrate information in an understandable way.

Learning domains can guide nurse educators in constructing learning objectives to engage learners.

Learning Domains

Bloom created a learning taxonomy in 1956 that was revised by Anderson and Krathwohl in 2001. According to this theory, all learning can be classified into one of three broad categories or **domains**.

- The cognitive domain is known as the "thinking" domain. Learning in this category involves acquiring information. Learning strategies used to stimulate learning in this domain include lecture, computer-assisted instruction, and one-to-one instruction.
- The affective domain is also called the "feeling" domain. Learning in this domain enhances the internalization or commitment to feelings expressed as attitudes, emotions, values, and/or beliefs. Learning strategies that are believed

to enhance learning in this domain include role-playing, case studies, simulation, games, and group discussion.

- The psychomotor domain is known as the "skills" domain. Learning in this category involves acquiring motor abilities and capabilities to perform nursing procedures. Learning strategies most often used to enhance learning in this domain include demonstration, return demonstration, and practice. (Forehand, 2005; Su, Osisec, and Starnes, 2004, 2005; Stuart, Hoge, and Tondora, 2004; Anderson and Krathwohl, 2001).

This taxonomy can help nurse educators develop learning objectives. Chapter 2 provides more specifics on how to use learning domains to make sure learning systems are effective.

The cognitive domain is prominent in most classrooms, as educators may be more confident giving information than focusing on feeling or skill-building. This is true despite the fact that affective learning is most important when developing a value system and evaluating ethical issues in health care situations (Ginsburg, 2004).

Learning domains are categories of learning that include cognitive, affective, and psychomotor behaviors.

In addition to using learning theory and principles and learning domains, nurse educators must enhance learner critical thinking skills.

Critical Thinking Skills

Sometime in the late 1980s, interest in education shifted from evaluating curriculum processes to evaluating learner outcomes (Walsh and Seldomridge, 2006). The focus of evaluation shifted from what was being taught to what learners were learning when the National League for Nursing Accrediting Commission (1997) and the American Association of Colleges of Nursing (1998) identified **critical thinking** as an expected program outcome. Faculty and administration of nursing programs, anxious to be accredited, hastened to find reliable and valid ways to demonstrate an increase in critical thinking in their learners as a result of their teaching. Nurses must learn to use critical thinking by:

- Conceptualizing,
- Applying,
- Analyzing,
- Synthesizing, and/or
- Evaluating information to guide their action.

Mere acquisition of information or possession of a set of skills alone is not enough to qualify as critical thinking.

Why is critical thinking important? Nurses must not use biased, distorted, partial, uninformed, or prejudicial thinking in their approach, which is why learning to think critically is mandatory for all nursing learners. Noncritical thinking is costly in money and in quality of life. Scriven & Paul (2004) propose that a critical thinker:

> Critical thinking is the process of actively conceptualizing, applying, analyzing, synthesizing, and/or evaluating information to guide action.

- Raises vital questions and problems in a clear and precise manner;
- Gathers relevant information and comes to well-reasoned conclusions and solutions by testing them against relevant criteria and standards;
- Assesses assumptions, implications, and practical consequences; and
- Communicates effectively with others to figure out solutions to complex problems.

Measures of Critical Thinking

Two instruments widely accepted for measuring critical thinking skills are available. They were selected by the task force at one northeastern university because of their wide acceptance and use as sound psychometric measures (Walsh and Seldomridge, 2006). They focus on the ability to infer, recognize assumptions, deduce, interpret, and evaluate arguments, and as a result allow for comparison across settings. Both are relatively inexpensive, can be scored by hand, and take less than an hour to administer.

The first instrument is the Watson-Glaser Critical Thinking Appraisal, Form S (WGCTA) (Watson and Glaser 1994). This instrument was selected for its ability to evaluate critical thinking dispositions such as open-mindedness, truth-seeking, systematicity, confidence, analyticity, inquisitiveness, and maturity. The other instrument is the California Critical Thinking Dispositions Inventory (CCTDI) (Facione, 1992).

Several researchers have used one or the other instruments in their work. Walsh and Seldomridge (2006) found only modest gains in critical thinking in their population of undergraduate learners as they progressed over the years of their nursing studies. This led the authors to question their definition of critical thinking (knowing what to believe or do) and the usefulness of standardized measuring instruments.

Other researchers also had inconsistent results measuring critical thinking abilities probably due to lack of standardization of dependent measures and failure to clearly identify the critical thinking skill that would be improved due to the intervention

(Rosignol, 1997; Beckie, Lowry, and Barnett, 2001; Spelic et al., 2001; Profetto-McGrath, 2003; McCarthy, Schuster, Zehr, and McDougal, 1999; Stone, Davidson, Evans, and Hansen, 2001). Because the research findings have been inconsistent, Walsh and Seldomridge (2006) concluded it is time to rethink the problem.

> ### ■ Nurse Educator Challenge
>
> What would you do to improve critical thinking in learners in your classroom? Give a rationale for your answer.

Insights Gained About Critical Thinking

Many years of research and discussion about critical thinking have led to some insights, including:

- Understanding what facilitates and stifles critical thinking may be a more apt focus. Several nurse educators concluded learners need to be taught how to think critically (Allen, Rubenfeld, and Scheffer, 2004), while Diekelmann (2002), Valiga (2003), and Ironside (2004) claimed faculties should debate *how* to teach content, not *what* should be taught.
- Resistances and barriers work together to keep the status quo of lecture as the main approach in many nursing programs. Learner resistance to active learning, inadequate class time, the need to cover content, and insufficient time to prepare critical thinking activities mediate against integrating critical thinking activities into the curriculum (Shell, 2001).
- Other classroom activities work against critical thinking, including the use of multiple-choice questions to prepare learners for licensure exams, which are still graded as correct or incorrect (National Council of State Boards of Nursing, 2006).
- Class size may also dictate against interactive learning, but there are ways to work creatively with large classes. Chapter 4 provides ideas for interactive learning with larger classes.

Yancy, a BSN learner, was shocked to find she failed her last test. When she made an appointment to speak with her instructor, she said, "I can't believe my grade. Are you sure you didn't make a mistake? I studied hard for hours on end."

"How were you studying?" asked the instructor. "It's possible to memorize the material and still not do well on a test. To do well, you need to understand the concepts, not just memorize them."

The research on critical thinking in nursing may help explain what's lacking in some nursing classrooms.

Critical Thinking Research

Attempts to show which classroom strategies have a positive effect on critical thinking have been mostly inconclusive. Walsh and Seldomridge (2006) state that these findings may be due to lack of standardization of dependent measures and failure to clearly identify the critical thinking skill that would be improved due to the intervention.

Web-based interventions have demonstrated that learners learned as well as or better than learners receiving traditional instruction, but critical thinking skills were not examined (Anderson and Mercer, 2004; Billings, Connors, and Skiba, 2001; Kearns, Shoaf, and Summey, 2004; Leasure, Davis, and Thievon, 2000).

Kautz and associates (2005) evaluated the development of clinical reasoning skills among nursing learners enrolled in a medical-surgical course. They used teaching-learning strategies associated with self-regulated learning and the application of the Outcome Present State Test (OPT) Model of Clinical Reasoning to structure learning with junior-level baccalaureate learners. Learners made gains in learning associated with the OPT model. Qualitative analysis of self-regulated learning journal data showed learners made significant gains in self-observation, self-judgment, knowledge, and use of health care resources.

Shin and colleagues (2006) found that senior nursing learners in baccalaureate programs scored statistically higher in critical thinking skills as measured by the California Critical Thinking Disposition Inventory (CCTDI) than learners in the RN-to-BSN group. The learners who scored the lowest on the CCTDI belonged to the associate degree learner group. The senior baccalaureate learners scored significantly higher on critical thinking, especially truth-seeking, open-mindedness, self-confidence, and maturity of judgment, analysis, evaluation, inference, deductive reasoning, and inductive reasoning. The nurse educators for the baccalaureate program must have been doing something right when teaching critical thinking skills.

Teaching Critical Thinking Skills

Wanda was teaching a class of master's degree learners using classroom case studies. She separated the class into dyads: one assumed the role of the client and received a full client chart, including history, physical examination information, results, and laboratory data. The other learner in each dyad assumed the role of the nurse and was given 20 minutes to gather client data, analyze it, make a diagnosis, and come up with treatments. The "clients" were advised only to divulge the information specifically accessed. Wanda used the last ten minutes of the class to synthesize what was learned, discuss any issues uncovered, and generally debrief the participants.

Oral questioning shows promise as a way to teach learners critical thinking, but only if higher-level questions are used (Sellappah, Hussey, Blackmore, and McMurray, 1998). Logic client concept maps and models that contain an account of an illness or health issue can lead to using inductive and deductive thinking to examine alternate actions nurses should take. A qualitative analysis of learner reactions to logic models provided evidence that learners found them helpful in making decisions about client care, predicting outcomes of their interventions, and thinking critically (Ellermann, Kataoka-Yahiro, and Wong, 2006).

Many methods can promote learners' critical thinking, including written or simulated case studies, concept mapping, journal reading, and role play/simulation (Ellermann, Kataoka-Yahiro, and Wong, 2005; Baumberger-Henry, 2005; Reising, 2004; Tomey, 2003; Cote-Arsenault, 2004; Jeffries, 2005; Phillips, 2005; Akinsanya and Williams, 2004; Luckowski, 2003; Staib, 2003; Ibarreta and McLeod, 2004; Wagner and Ash, 1998). For specific uses of these approaches with large classes, see Chapter 4.

Although lecturing may be the most comfortable for many nurse educators, does it enhance critical thinking?

Dilemmas Related to Teaching Critical Thinking

Packaged lectures produced via computer software may give learners the idea they are in class to be entertained and that they should sit back and not participate. Walsh and Seldomridge (2006) cautioned that packaged lectures leave little room for learners to take active roles in classroom activities and reinforce passive learning. Although such approaches may be urged by administrators, feeding learners with facts will not help learners to think critically or retain information. For example, in a typical 50-minute lecture class, learners retain 70% of what is conveyed in the first 10 minutes, but only 20% for the last ten minutes (Montgomery and Groat, 1998).

Because critical thinking has not been adequately defined to date, it may be wise for educators to decide which kinds of critical thinking to promote, and then define and operationalize them for various learner levels. For example:

- Problem-solving allows learners to transfer theory into practice;
- Decision-making helps learners anticipate potential problems;
- Diagnostic reasoning helps learners settle on a client's condition by ruling out improbable conclusions (Walsh and Seldomridge, 2006).

■ **Nurse Educator Challenge**

Decide on one kind of critical thinking and suggest ways to operationalize a teaching program for that aspect.

Nurse Educator Tips

Walsh and Seldomridge (2006) suggest ways to promote critical thinking in the classroom:

- Change a "content coverage" philosophy; total coverage of a content area is the job of a textbook, not a nurse educator.
- Avoid spoon-feeding facts; instead, provide or demonstrate principles that will assist learners to develop critical thinking habits.

For more ideas about ways to enhance critical thinking, see Chapters 3–6 in this book. In addition to enhancing critical thinking, nurse educators put emphasis on learner-centered environments and curricula.

Learner-Centered Environments and Curricula

Educator-centered environments focus on a one-way transmission of knowledge. Most nursing curricula are content-heavy. To become learner-centered means deleting, not adding, content (Candela, Dalley, and Benzel-Lindley, 2006).

> Educator-centered environments include lectures and other one-way transmissions of information.

Learner-centered environments pay careful attention to the knowledge, skills, attitudes and beliefs that learners bring with them into the classroom. Learner-centered environments are culturally appropriate, culturally compatible, and culturally relevant.

Carlos, a learner in the master's degree nursing education specialty, planned to teach in the continuing education department of a nearby hospital once he got his degree. He brought many ideas to class about how to adapt learning materials for the Hispanic-speaking population they served.

His professor, a devotee of learner-centered environments and curricula, encouraged his efforts and suggested he write a paper detailing his ideas. When Carlos finished his paper, he decided to use the materials in his thesis research.

Educators who used learner-centered environments and curricula focus on using knowledge to address problems in real-life contexts. To be learner-centered, educators must focus on what learners need to know and be able to do in order to be effective. This requires using multiple assessment strategies in the classroom and clinical setting (Candela, Dalley, and Benzel-Lindley, 2006).

■ **Nurse Educator Challenge**

Come up with three ways Carlos's professor could use to assess his knowledge of three common clinical nursing situations using multiple assessment strategies.

> Learner-centered environments build bridges between the subject matter and the learners, use informal ideas learners bring to the classroom, and help develop alternate viewpoints.

An educator must find an appropriate balance between activities designed to promote understanding and those designed to promote skills necessary to function in the clinical area. Feedback from nurse educators, peers, and self should occur continuously, but not intrusively, as part of instruction.

Research on Learner Preferences

Walker and colleagues (2004) examined the different expressed learning preferences for 134 junior and senior nursing learners enrolled in a 4-year baccalaureate-nursing program. Twenty-five subjects represented Generation X (born between 1965 and 1976, highly independent, willing to challenge authority and the status quo, multi-taskers with parallel thinking processes, technologically-literate, concrete thinkers) and 105 represented Generation Y (born since 1982; most culturally diverse generation of all times, with 36% being non-white or Hispanic; self-reliant; questioning; technologically advanced beyond any other age group; linear thinking analytical ability and addicted to visual media.)

The researchers used a descriptive survey design to compare the generational differences among nursing learners to their perceived preferences in teaching methods. The reliability coefficient for the survey, Cronbach's alpha, was .82. Other statistical tests used included the Whitney Mann U, Chi-Square, the Pearson Product Correlation, and the ANOVA. Findings included:

- 85% preferred skill demonstration and return demonstration rather than lecture before skill performance in the clinical area.
- The majority of both age groups indicated a stronger preference for case study or group work when they encountered difficult to understand material.
- 90% preferred to have at least some class meetings, not a totally web-based method of study.
- 71% of both age groups indicated an interest in hearing stories from faculty of actual clinical events.
- 96% indicated strong preference for handouts that followed along with the lecture material and coincided with visual screen or overhead.
- 100% indicated they always wanted to know why they were learning the material.

■ Nurse Educator Challenge

Based on these findings, what kind of teaching strategies would you use for a class of primarily Generation X learners? Generation Y learners?

Bear in mind the findings of the Walker and colleagues study may only pertain to the population under study.

Nurse Educator Tips

Some ways to decide on appropriate content and allow for a move toward learner-centered environments are:

- Study the literature for the latest information on essential concepts and skills needed by nurses in current and future practice settings—for example, current publications of the American Association of Colleges of Nursing and the Pew Health Professions Commission.
- Decide if nursing learners will use this information in general practice with a majority of clients; if not, delete it.
- Question a tendency to include content because it is favored; it may not be necessary.

Deciding on content is only half of the struggle. Other barriers to moving from educator-centered to learner-centered environments may arise, including administrative and self-imposed restrictions. Fear of losing academic rigor may rear its head. When entire faculties agree to move in the direction of learner-centered environments, faculty development programs must be in place to support and encourage educators who may be learning new strategies (Candela, Dalley, and Benzel-Lindley, 2006). An important procedure for learner-centered advocates is formative assessment.

Formative and Summative Learner Assessment

Dr. Carter, a professor in the doctoral nursing education program, and a master's degree learner in another specialty area were completing research on formative assessment. Several of her doctoral learners also collected and helped analyze data. They compared learning outcomes for learners who wrote a final paper for a grade versus learners who took a series of mini-written and hands-on exams throughout the semester. They also collected data on learner reactions to the two methods of assessment. The learners who participated in mini-tests claimed they learned more from their mistakes on some mini-tests than from attaining higher grades.

Formative assessment is evaluation that occurs throughout the course.

Formative assessment (throughout the course) is preferred to **summative assessment** (a paper or test at the end of the course). Formative assessment offers opportunities for learners to revise their thinking and behavior before the final grade. Learner-centered environments build in the expectation that everyone, including the nurse educator, is there to learn and everyone can learn from mistakes (Bransford, Brown,

> Summative assessment occurs only at the end of a course.

and Cocking, 1999). For specific examples of how to provide a learner-centered environment, even with large classrooms, see Chapter 4.

Because nurse learners must be able to provide care for clients or lead other nurses, transfer of learning from the classroom to the clinical area is mandatory.

Transfer of Learning

Transfer of learning is the ability to apply knowledge or procedures learned in one context to another setting (National Science Foundation 2003). Transfer is one of the major criteria used to assess the relative effectiveness of different instructional procedures. Nurse educators are concerned with the correlation between practice of classroom exercises and their effect upon performance of those tasks in the nursing learner/client relationship. Educator/learner interactions and specific classroom exercises practice, learners can come up with novel solutions to problems (Mester, 2003).

> Transfer of learning occurs when nursing learners apply knowledge or procedures they learned in the classroom to clinical practice.

The study of transfer in nursing education is an important goal. Findings from the National Science Foundation may be of benefit (Mester, 2003).

Research Findings about Transfer

Research findings about transfer that can drive future nurse educator research include the following:

- Transfer is enhanced when the learner abstracts the deep principles underlying the knowledge being learned; and that abstraction is facilitated by opportunities to experience concepts and principles in multiple contexts.
- To facilitate transfer, instruction may need to be structured in ways counterintuitive to both educator and learner.
- When learners are asked which method of practice is better for their own learning, they often have erroneous perceptions.
- Transfer is more apt to occur when learners must provide a significant amount of active processing of materials. (Mester, 2003).

Transfer explains the use of school nursing laboratories, where learners practice making hospital-style beds, giving bed baths to manikins or fellow learners, and so on. Through this kind of simulated situation, learners practice skills they will use in the future with real-life clients. A spin-off effect of learning through this practice seems to occur concurrently with the development of skills, strategies, or problem-solving modes. Learners can test various approaches; this decreases trial-and-error learning in the real situation and enhances learner confidence. The more lifelike the practice situation is, the more tendency there is for transfer to occur. Transfer is also more apt to occur when there is practice on a variety of related problems and when there is sufficient time to practice. Concepts and principles lend themselves more easily to transfer than does specific information (see Box 1–1).

This may be why learners whose training in how to act in the clinical situation is mostly based on lectures may perform quite poorly with clients. The first place to practice transfer of learning is in the classroom (Clark, 2000). For transfer to occur, learning tasks need to be carefully selected, and learners need to be guided during initial learning. They should also be expected to have read assigned texts prior to coming to class.

Box 1–1 Research Questions Regarding Transfer

Research questions suggested by a recent National Science Foundation conference (Mester, 2003) that could fuel research by nurse educators include:

- What remains invariant from the learning context to the transfer context?
- What are the cues and strategies that trigger appropriate knowledge to be applied in a referent (clinical) situation?
- How important are learner expectations during original learning and transfer?
- To what extent do future employers want nurses with narrowly defined skills as compared to broad abilities to solve problems and learn new skills?
- What are the contextual factors (especially socio-cultural factors) that shape attitudes when entering new contexts that involve transfer?
- Teaching to test is a common educational technique, but how can tests be devised that assess transfer to clinical situations so that nurse educators prepare excellent practitioners?
- What is the relationship between learner behavior in in-class simulations or simulation games and real-world action in a clinical area?

Nurse Educator Tips

To enhance transfer from classroom to clinical area:

- Teach by concept, not content.
- Assist learners to identify concepts by becoming immersed in a situation similar to the clinical situation by using role playing, simulation, and simulation gaming.
- Allow time for learners to feel confident by testing various approaches.
- Note there is a brief slowdown in the learning curve when a new approach is introduced; overlook the confusion some learners may show and watch for the strengthening of previously acquired skills and knowledge.
- Make classroom activities lifelike to enhance transfer to the clinical situation—for example, what if the concept for today is infection control? Instead of learners walking into a classroom with all the chairs facing the front, they found chairs in small groups with signs such as ICU, nurses' station, treatment room, infection control, and so on, and learners were given a situation straight out of the television show *ER* to deal with?
- Instead of identifying the concept for the day, ask the learners at the end of the activity, "What concept did you learn today?" This approach will promote even more transfer.

Teaching Dilemmas

Corrine, a new member of the education department at Everest Medical Center, came to work with high expectations about what she planned to accomplish. She soon became caught up in the bureaucratic and political climate. Without a mentor to guide her, she began to lose her excitement and focus. Every evening she went home feeling depressed and fatigued, unable to feel good about the little she'd accomplished. When she saw an article in the medical center's newsletter about a mentoring program for new employees, she signed up. She was paired with an experienced nurse educator who took her to lunch and explained some of the ways to work through or around bureaucratic and political structures. Corrine started to feel better about her job and herself. She had an ally and a friend whom she could turn to for wisdom and support. Her work productivity increased and she eventually became a mentor for a new nurse educator who joined the staff.

Corrine could just as well have been a nurse educator in an academic setting. No matter the setting, novice nurse educators are faced with a complicating factor in their professional identity: there may be minimal assistance available for the new teacher from seasoned educators (Foley, et al., 2001). Experienced faculty are involved in designing their own course content or meeting administration requests. They may not be available as role models for ways of structuring and conducting classroom activities to achieve a balance between structure and freedom and a fusion of cognitive, affective, and perceptual-motor learning.

Acquiring high-level, complex classroom skill is no easy task even with support, direction, and demonstration. When no systematic attempt is made to assist novice nurse educators in evaluating their teaching strengths and weaknesses and to provide remedial experiences at the point of entry into a teaching/learning system, teaching dilemmas can result.

Anxious and confused **novice educators** may feel that they should be experts. This, in turn, may result in grandiose thinking, in feelings of guilt, or in mental self-punishment for not being more successful with learners. The latter defense may at first result in frantic attempts to please learners or to be approved of by administrators, and may eventually result in apathy, just as Corrine had experienced. The young educator, emotionally and physically drained by the position, may leave. Some fortunate nurse educators like Corrine may find a mentoring program by chance, enroll, and learn new skills. Other nurse educators may seek out a nurse educator they admire and request a mentoring relationship. Still others may revert to the comfort of teaching by the method that they were taught—usually the lecture method—or to blaming learners for their lack of motivation.

> Common teaching dilemmas can include a situation where novice nurse educators may experience anxiety and guilt if they're unable to maneuver the complex and difficult waters of the classroom without an adequate role model in place.

Even though the philosophy of this book runs counter to the lecture method of teaching, it is important to discuss situations for which it may be appropriate.

Lecturing

Lecture is a method of transmitting information that is meant to serve specified purposes. It not meant to be used to repeat facts or to restate what other authors (textbooks, journal articles, and so on) have already stated. Lectures are meant to present:

- A synthesis of information,
- The lecturer's view of the topic,
- Special material that has not been published,
- Motivation or inspiration for learners, and
- Expected learning outcomes.

Box 1–2   Disadvantages of the Lecture Method

1. *Because of educator inabilities, the learner may experience boredom and inattention* —many learners do not have the requisite knowledge to benefit from the prompts and guidance the lecturer hopes to provide. With no active part other than note-taking, many learners become bored or inattentive. On the educator side, it is the rare lecturer who is entertaining or interpersonally effective enough not to feel frustrated with the lecture method.
2. *Inability to develop complex cognitive and creative skills*—the lecture may not provide for the development of complex cognitive and creative skills of learners. Greater flexibility of thought, breadth of perspective, openness to experience, autonomy and integrity do not necessarily follow because the learner hears in a lecture that these are important attributes. As with other skills, complex thinking and creative ability are learned in a sequential way through *practice.*
3. *Likelihood of learner distortion*—learners may distort what the educator is saying during a lecture. The lecturer may talk on without checking to ensure that information has been understood, and possible distortions in information sent and received will not be corrected. Because learners usually are given reading assignments in addition to lecture material, these distortions may be either rectified or compounded.
4. *Misunderstanding and decreased self-esteem*—an even thornier problem occurs in the lecture situation, and one or more learners present their discordant views to what has been verbalized. From the learner perspective, the expression of their ideas is a creative effort. From the educator perspective, discordant views may be interpreted as misunderstanding, interruption in the flow of the lecture, or even attack. Because the traditional lecture method does not lend itself to feedback from learners about how messages are being heard and understood, frustration and decreased self-esteem can result on both sides.

The lecture is meant to be a novel presentation and must be organized to meet clear end goals, or it will most probably end in failure. Unfortunately, many nurse educators may not be interesting lecturers, and may end up stating textbooks verbatim; this is a waste of instructor time. Even when lectures can be presented clearly and as a synthesis of information, they have several disadvantages (see Box 1–2).

One way that offers the potential for novice educators to get a grip on learning needs is an assessment of learning challenges.

Learning Challenges: Assessment and Interventions

Box 1–3 shows an assessment tool nurse educators can use to assess learning challenges. For best results, nurse educators fill out the tool prior to administering it to learners. It is important to provide sufficient time for nurse educators to identify their own challenges and plan interventions.

The first class period is a critical time to use this assessment with learners, because it can reveal how they will both learn and oppose learning. Once nurse educators can identify their own learning challenges and those of their learners, problem-solving efforts can be used to rectify them. If a learning challenge is the nurse educator's, it is

Box 1–3 Assessment of Learning Challenges

Directions: Novice nurse educators and learners will most surely have a number of different learning challenges; some are more likely to occur at particular phases in the teaching/learning process. Learning challenges can be thought of as potential growth experiences if educator and student are open to their examination. Look at each item below and its examples.

Check those that apply to you, and make a note to yourself to begin work to overcome them. It is suggested that you use this guide to assess your learning challenges at the beginning, middle, and end of each semester. Note where growth has occurred and where you wish to improve. It may help to ask a trusted colleague to sit in on your class to give you feedback on the impression you give, since it is not unusual for people to be unaware of some of their learning challenges.

(continues)

Box 1–3　Assessment of Learning Challenges (continued)

❏　1.　I find myself trying to prove that the educator/learner/client is wrong, and I am right/expert.

Examples:
- I get caught up in how people say things or in the words they choose, rather than in the issues.
- I feel the educator/learner/client can't teach me anything.
- I feel very stubborn about changing my mind on issues.
- I am reluctant to admit that I don't have all the answers.

❏　2.　I have difficulty setting/accepting legitimate limits of authority.

Examples:
- I have difficulty deciding when to remain firm on a standard and when to be flexible in the means of reaching it.
- I allow too many people to interrupt me.
- I can't say "no" when it is helpful to do so.
- I don't start or end/attend class on time or structure/focus on learning tasks.
- I am unable to give supportive negative feedback for fear of hurting others' feelings.
- I do not allow others who have authority or knowledge to teach me.

❏　3.　I tend to overly expose or overapologize for my limitations.

Examples:
- I find myself beginning statements with phrases such as, "I may be wrong, but..."
- I tell people about my weaknesses or problems when I first meet them.
- I always take the blame when something goes wrong.
- I punish myself for not being perfect.

❏　4.　I expect that others will take total responsibility for learning.

Examples:
- I assume that all students know their strengths and limitations and how to structure their own learning experiences.
- I find that I refuse to think of ways in which I can participate in learning, such as finding out what learning resources are available or trying out new situations or solutions.
- I wait for others to take the lead.
- I do not think of myself as a self-directed learner.

(continues)

Box 1–3   Assessment of Learning Challenges (continued)

❑   5. I tend to be uninvolved, devaluing, or avoiding in relation to a course/ learner/educator/a client.

Examples:
- I tend to smooth over disagreements or conflicts without teaching/learning how to resolve them constructively.
- I don't complete assignments/class presentations until the last minute.
- I daydream in the class a lot.
- I tend to neglect the updating of course materials/learning needs.

❑   6. I am overinvolved or overinvested in learners/grades/educator/client.

Examples:
- I feel that my personal esteem rises and falls according to others' evaluation or their ability to perform effectively.
- I tend to check up on others too frequently, and I am overly critical of them.
- I am more concerned about grades than about learning.
- In my spare time I think about or spend time helping educators/ learners/clients.

❑   7. I may confuse knowledge of course content with knowing how to apply or implement it.

Examples:
- I grasp theory and concepts, but I don't notice when I'm not using them with learners/clients.
- I tend to assume that if I know something, I should magically be able to teach it to others.
- I spend minimal time planning how to apply or implement concepts in class/clinical settings or in seeking out ways of evaluating what I need to know about teaching/learning.
- I tend to believe that educators and great nurses are born, not made.
- I hesitate to use questions that evoke critical thinking processes.

❑   8. I am overly skeptical and/or question the use of this class/ material/experience.

Examples:
- I question the relevance of this course.
- There is nothing in this course that will contribute to my career or personal objectives.
- I doubt whether this class can provide meaningful information.

Box 1–3   Assessment of Learning Challenges (continued)

❑   9. I try to get learners/educators/clients to take care of me.

Examples:
- I continually look for reassurance, understanding, or thanks.
- I like others to become involved in my personal problems.
- I expect exceptions to the rules to be made for me when I'm not feeling well or because of my personal difficulties.
- I assume I can't do anything on my own.

❑ 10. I idealize or overidentify with the educator/learner/client.

Examples:
- I feel very inadequate when I compare myself with others.
- I assume that designated authorities or peers know more than I do.
- I overquote "experts" and make extensive use of quotes rather than paraphrasing or adding my own ideas.
- I accept everything others say or do without questioning it.
- I am preoccupied with the person rather than with the learning or helping process.

❑ 11. I automatically assume the role of well-intentioned, controlling, wise parent with others.

Examples:
- I quickly give advice.
- I do "for" rather than "with" others.
- I interpret things without understanding the facts.
- I assume I always know what's best for others.

❑ 12. I have difficulty accepting criticism or views that are different from mine.

Examples:
- I feel hurt, depressed, embarrassed, angry, or ashamed when others point out my limitations.
- I cannot own up to my mistakes and tend to make excuses.
- I take the offense and attack or blame others before they can criticize me.
- Theories or learning experiences that are new to me often seem to be far-fetched or impractical.

(continues)

Box 1–3   Assessment of Learning Challenges (continued)

☐ 13. I wait until situations reach crisis proportions before seeking assistance or collaborating on a solution.

Examples:
- I pretend I have no learning problems even though I know everyone does.
- I avoid setting learning objectives for myself.
- I expect others to read my mind and know when I need help.
- I tend to hope problems will go away or I wait for someone else to step in and deal with them.

☐ 14. I homogenize the class/client/group and treat everyone the same.

Examples:
- I refuse to structure/fully immerse myself in different learning experiences for learners/clients based on their differences in learning styles.
- My attitude is: all educators/learners/clients are the same and should be treated as such.
- I find myself referring to "the class" or "the clients" rather than to individuals with unique characteristics.

Developed in collaboration with Susan DiFabio and Judith Ackerhalt.

Nurse Educator Tip

Learners fill out the learning challenges assessment and hand it back to the nurse educator for analysis. Having a composite picture of learner challenges can provide clues to structuring class materials and activities to help learners overcome their self-identified learning issues.

his or her responsibility to rectify it. For example, nurse educators who have difficulty conveying enthusiasm or using nonverbal communication can take an assertiveness training course or a course using video replay to help participants learn a more useful presentation of self in a group.

Dr. Gonzalez, a new nurse educator in the master's degree nursing program, filled out the Learning Challenges Assessment. Although she'd never thought much about it before, she realized that she had difficulty setting legitimate limits of authority because the learners were so close in age to her. She also apologized frequently, making her think that maybe she overapologized. Those were the only learning challenges she identified for herself, but she remembered several situations where learners had difficulty accepting peer criticism or tended to wait until situations reached a crisis point before seeking assistance.

If the learning challenge is the learner's, it is the educator's responsibility to help the learner identify and accept it. Such an approach to learning responsibility is in line with Ekstein and Wallerstein's classic definition of learning: "a growth that finally becomes self-initiated by learners and is not left to immature devices of indoctrination or the chance of running into a teacher to whom one happens to take" (1971, p. 99).

Nurse educators must continuously and systematically examine, modify, and create educational practices to increase certain kinds of learning. Such an approach leaves the choice of how and when to use specific educational strategies up to the individual educator. It presumes a particular technique or strategy will be used only after having systematically evaluated its use.

Nurse Educator Tip

Examine discrepancies between intentions and actual practices.

1. Explicitly state the kinds of learning to be cultivated—for example, increasing learner helping skills or developing learner problem-solving skills.
2. Videotape a classroom segment.
3. Critically analyze the videotape to identify those aspects of educator/learner interaction that inhibit achievement of the goal.
4. Learn alternate strategies or techniques to attain the learning goal.
5. Anticipate the consequences of each strategy or technique.
6. Choose and test the strategy or technique that is most useful in attaining the learning goal via a simulated classroom or actual work with learners.
7. Re-analyze the Learner Challenges Assessment to find potential nurse educator issues that haven't been resolved.

The Helping Relationship and Humanism

The nurse/client relationship is a helping relationship; so is the nurse educator/learner relationship. Being helpful, seeking help, and accepting help are all components of the **helping process**. One way for learners to enhance their helping ability is to develop appropriate help-seeking and help-accepting behaviors in relation to nurse educators. When there are problems in learning the helping relationship, they are evident in both the nurse/client relationship and in the educator/learner relationship.

> The helping process is important to both nurse educator and nursing learner and includes being helpful, seeking help, and accepting help.

Research has shown that, overall, nursing faculty tend to be teacher-centered. Associate degree faculty may be more teacher-centered than baccalaureate and higher degree faculty, who, in turn, split between teacher-centered and learner-centered instruction (Papes, 1998).

■ **Nurse Educator Challenge**

What one thing should be done to make learning more learner-centered? Give a rationale for your answer.

Learning methods based purely on the transmission of technical knowledge (teacher-centered) will obscure learning problems. Such methods will prevent the nurse educator from substantially affecting the helping aspects of learners in their relationships with clients. Since neither educators nor learners can hope to be fully actualized, both must attune themselves to aspects of themselves that may interfere with positive learning (see Box 1–3). Nurse educators must begin to focus more attention on learning challenges, because if they do not, these aspects of behavior will be replicated in learner relationships with clients.

Helping Models

Ekstein and Wallerstein (1971) developed a helping model by studying the helping relationship between supervisor and psychotherapist. In 2006, Callaghan revisited the earlier model. He agreed that help does not consist of taking over the problem and dealing with it by giving advice or doing for the client, but of intervening in one's own helping weaknesses and strengthening others so they can learn to cope with the problem.

This model has relevance for nurse educators, especially when presenting theory and concepts. It is important not to assume nursing learners will be able to make the gigantic leap from theoretical conceptualization to clinical application. It is in this bridging period between providing theory and showing learners how to apply theory to practice that nurse educators can provide helpful assistance. It is also a truism that the nurse educator/learner relationship is a relationship and as such, has characteristics of other communicational systems, which include the following:

- The need to communicate,
- All messages are potentially ambiguous and different learners will derive different meanings from the same message,
- All communication refers both to the content and to the relationships between participants,
- Punctuation is arbitrary, adopt the other's point of view to increase empathy and understanding,
- It is important to be aware of and respond to both content and relationship messages,
- Noise is the inevitable physical, physiological, psychological, and semantic interference that distorts a message,
- Competence is the knowledge and ability to use your own communication system, and
- Messages can quickly overload channels making meaningful interaction impossible (DeVito, 2005).

■ Nurse Educator Challenge

Consider each of the communication tenets above and tell how each affects the nurse educator role. Give examples.

Stock-Ward and Javorek (2003) developed a **development theory of helping** that can also be beneficial to nurse educators. At level one of Stock-Ward and Javorek's developmental model, learners have limited experience with their role and experience confusion about rules and procedures. They want to know, "Am I

Developmental theory of helping includes three levels of help nurse educators can provide depending on learner level of professional development.

doing this right?" They want to be liked and may be quite dependent on supervisors, for structure, information, and support. They try to find the "one right way" to do things. They show high motivation and appear eager to learn, but also have low self-confidence and can be easily discouraged.

Sherry, a beginning BSN learner, frequently came to class looking anxious and overwhelmed. "I don't know if I took care of all the client's needs," she might say to the course instructor, or "I hope I did everything right."

At level two of the developmental model, learners shift their focus from themselves to focus on colleagues. They show more empathy and understanding of others, but may be "sucked in by" colleague problems. They vacillate between being autonomous and asking for assistance.

Tom, a new graduate of the master's degree learner program in the nurse educator specialty, came to work one day and explained that he hadn't been able to sleep. "I kept worrying about my new learners and whether they'd be all right," he confessed over coffee to more seasoned nurse educators. "The learners had their first experience on the unit and I remember how harrowing that can be. Did you feel that way at first?"

At level three of the developmental model, learners become comfortable in their roles, balance their focus on self with focus on others, and appear more self-confident. They accept their professional strengths and weaknesses and begin to trust themselves more, but still seek consultation when needed.

■ **Nurse Educator Challenge**

What level of development are Tom and Sherry demonstrating?

Some situations that are crucial to applying theory to practice occur when requesting learners to:

- Initiate interaction with others,
- Request assistance from others, or
- Work out conflicts with others.

When using this helping model, nurse educators provide specific guidance, helping learners to think through the situation prior to facing the clinical, social, or administrative situation involved. The BSN nursing learner may be thought of as level one, the master's learner as level two, and the doctoral learner as level three. These levels may not always hold as there are exceptional learners at all three levels of education.

For learners at level one, nurse educators take a prescriptive role and:

- Review direct samples of learners' work,
- Provide direct and specific feedback,
- Discuss potential courses of action,
- Set up role-playing situations,
- Provide opportunities to observe staff perform the duties of the job, and
- Talk learners through action step-by-step (Stock-Ward and Javorek, 2003).

For learners at level two, nurse educators step back a bit and work in a more collaborative role and:

- Generate possible alternatives with the learner by brain storming ("What are some other ways to deal with this?"),
- Explore values and personal reactions that may be interfering with competent practice ("You handled this fine yesterday, but today you seem to be having difficulty."),
- Clarify issues of human diversity by providing support, empathy, and encouragement and to normalize concerns ("Yes, many learners feel that way,"),
- Prime learners to think through the situation ("What would happen if you do that?"), and
- Gently confront learners who are avoiding tasks ("I noticed you aren't taking action; let's discuss what's preventing you.") (Stock-Ward and Javorek, 2003)

For learners at level three, nurse educators use a collegial model that implies:

- Confronting more freely because the learner has a solid foundation of skills and confidence,
- Using self-disclosure to facilitate modeling and mentoring,
- Allowing the learner to participate in setting structure for the relationship,
- Avoiding the thought that the learner is so advanced the nurse educator has nothing to offer, and
- Continuing to provide sufficient stimulation and challenge to facilitate professional growth. (Stock-Ward and Javorek, 2003)

> ### ■ Nurse Educator Challenge
>
> Describe three ways to help learners by strengthening them. Provide specific, real, or hypothetical situations.

Elements of helping and influencing are important to the nurse and are crucial to the nurse educator. In teaching, there can be no escape into procedures, no hiding behind equipment.

> The helping model focuses on strengthening others so they can learn to cope with the problem.

Learners will often force the issue to provide help for their learning challenges. They will confront the nurse educator again and again with comments that require helpful responses if the learner is to understand how to deal with the problem. By receiving helpful responses, the learner learns (though modeling) how to help clients.

> Jeff, a nursing learner in the master's teaching specialty program, constantly raised his hand to correct the nurse educator or other learner's comments. Even when data was presented to back up their statements, he refused to change his mind. Dr. Kneff, the instructor in the course, smiled bravely and tried to overlook Jeff's comments, and continued on with her lecture.
>
> After class, Dr. Kneff referred to the Learning Challenges Assessment and that alerted her to the fact that Jeff exhibited the first challenge, "I find myself trying to prove that the educator/learner/client is wrong, and I am right/expert." She made a note to check Jeff's assessment and see if he had self-identified the issue. When she found he hadn't, she decided to speak to him after class the next day and bring up the issue, providing the data of her observations in class. She also reminded herself that Jeff might not be aware of how he was presenting himself in class. She decided to suggest he run a little experiment and keep track of the comments he made in future classes, analyze them, and see which of the learning challenges they best described. It took Jeff a few weeks to identify the dynamics of his behavior. At that point he sought out Dr. Kneff. Together they came up with a plan to rephrase his statements, using the same ideas he'd expressed, but removing the challenging quality of his words. Jeff eventually changed his behavior in class with the help and encouragement of Dr. Kneff, and decided to use the learning challenges format as the basis for his master's research project with clients.

Nurse educators must listen to the problem as verbalized or watch for them to be acted out by the learner, without becoming caught up in only providing information. When nurse educators pay attention to verbal and nonverbal learner requests, their behavior indicates the issue is valid. The next step is to assist in delineating the problem, gathering information about it, and formulating and testing out alternative solutions to the problem. This demonstrates how the helping relationship is a joint problem-solving endeavor. Box 1–4 illustrates some helpful and unhelpful responses to learner comments.

Box 1–4   Helpful and Unhelpful Responses to Student Comments About Problems

Student comments	Nurse educator responses	
	Helpful	Non-helpful
Staff practices poor nursing care.	I guess you're beginning to notice that ideals are rarely met in practice; let's take a look at minimum standards for practice. What staff practices have you noticed that are not up to standard? What ideas do you have?	Things are more complex than you know. You're very critical of nurses. Maybe they're fed up with the system.
I'm afraid of that client.	What is fearful for you? What ways have you overcome your fear before? What have you read about how to deal with clients who frighten the nurse?	You can do it; go on. I'm afraid too, but there's nothing to be afraid of.

(continues)

Box 1–4   Helpful and Unhelpful Responses to Student Comments About Problems
(continued)

| Student comments | Nurse educator responses | |
	Helpful	Non-helpful
I gave the wrong medication to Mr. Smith	What did you give? When did you give it? Sit down with me and we can decide what to do.	What? Oh, no. You should have checked with me before you gave it. He might die because of you.
I don't think I want to be a nurse, anyway.	Has something happened to change your mind? How come?	Why not? Nursing is a good profession. With your performance, you might not make it anyway.
I think I'm the only one who cares about my client.	What's been happening in your relationship with your client? Let's discuss what you mean by caring.	We all feel that way sometimes. You probably are; that unit is so understaffed.
I don't know how to handle the family; they're always asking questions.	What questions are they asking? Which questions are hard for you to answer? Let's role play some questions and try out alternate responses.	Families can be a bother. Just answer their questions and they'll leave you alone.
I don't think you graded me/ evaluated me fairly.	In what way do you think I'm unfair? You could be right; what is your evaluation of your learning?	You're not meeting the course objectives. You're probably right; I often jump to conclusions. That's the way things are.

Box 1–4   Helpful and Unhelpful Responses to Student Comments About Problems (continued)

Student comments	Nurse educator responses	
	Helpful	Non-helpful
My other instructors didn't make me do that.	What is your reaction to being asked to do things differently? I'd like to work this out with you; in what way are my requirements different?	This is a different course. I run things my way. They didn't?

Some of the ways to strengthen learner ability to cope with clients are humanizing the classroom, demonstrating creativity and problem-solving skills, risking failure, timing increases in freedom and responsibility, giving appropriate feedback, and teaching respect for others.

The qualities of caring must be part of the educational climate in which nurses learn. Since nursing is a helping profession, the educational climate needs to be a humanizing one; learners cannot be expected to be human with clients without role models for the helping relationship. The humanistic philosophy and its use in the classroom is explored next.

Humanistic Approach

As a philosophy, **humanism** recognizes the uniqueness and individuality of people (Hesook and Kollak, 2005). This implies that when a humanistic approach is used, educators work to evoke creativity, spontaneity, and distinctiveness of learning style in individual learners. It also suggests that nurse educators themselves demonstrate these same qualities in the classroom.

> Humanism is a philosophy that recognizes the uniqueness and individuality of each person.

■ **Nurse Educator Challenge**

Name three ways to bring humanism to the classroom. Give specific examples.

Nurse Educators as Role Models

Another way educators can create a more humanistic learning environment in addition to becoming role models for learners is by demonstrating their own cognitive, perceptual-motor, and affective nursing skills. By doing so, they take a risk that criticism will be forthcoming from learners. By serving as a **learning role model**, the educator conveys indirectly to learners that it is all right to try, that the environment is safe, and that even expert educators can benefit from skill practice and feedback.

> Being a learning role model means nurse educators demonstrate their own skills, or lack thereof.

Errors in skill demonstration may be especially helpful in the humanization of the classroom. In fact, when nurse educators are able to present themselves as less than perfect, their humanism emerges.

■ **Nurse Educator Challenge**

What words might nurse educators use to convey that they may need additional skill practice?

Another way to role model appropriate nurse educator behaviors is to use an inquiry model of instruction.

Inquiry Model of Instruction

Educators can provide indirect practice in problem-solving for learners by using an **inquiry model** about their own classroom instruction. An inquiry model is one in which nurse educators ask for feedback from learners. Educators can tell learners

> An inquiry model in the classroom includes a willingness and interest in trying alternate solutions and benefiting from input.

they are struggling to improve their own skills, and may be enlisted in the process. Such an approach conveys to learners a willingness and interest to try alternate solutions, and to learn and benefit from input. This provides a strong role-model message that even educators can learn and benefit from. One way to implement an inquiry model of instruction is to ask for feedback from learners. A simple way is to develop a form that contains important feedback questions such as:

- What did you like about class today?
- What did you dislike about class today?
- How could the instructor be more helpful to learners?
- What else would you like your instructor to know about the class today?

The forms are filled out anonymously, providing a greater likelihood of truthful responses. Nurse educators can analyze responses and modify classroom procedures based on learner input. This is not only useful information for previous and future classroom activities, but by asking for feedback, the nurse educator role models effective nurse educator/learner behavior.

Taking Risks

Much of nursing education focuses on doing things correctly and not allowing for failure. Such a focus tends to reinforce stereotypes rather than creative thought and practice. Since everyone makes mistakes, by being willing to risk failure in front of learners, nurse educators can teach them that omnipotence is unrealistic; they also demonstrate how to own up to one's mistakes.

For example, while a new teaching strategy is being tried in class, it may become clear that the method is not working. In this case, nurse educators can use a number of alternative ways to teach learners about how to take advantage of seemingly negative or failure experiences. A humanistic way is to proceed with the strategy but then to lead a discussion, encouraging learners to evaluate the difficulties they encountered and to suggest ways in which the strategy might be made more effective.

> Professor Allenway decided to take a risk in class. She stopped a learning activity midpoint and said, "I don't think this exercise is working; I'd like your help brainstorming about how to use what we've learned from this experience." She paused. "Did you see what I just did? I just pointed out what I did wasn't working? That's something you can do when you're working with learners and either of you notices it's not working."

Taking risks is just one of the many procedures nurse educators can use in a humanistic classroom. Timing changes is another approach that may be especially important when learners are resistant to change.

Timing

Timing may be crucial to the humanistic classroom. When learners have had years of passive, cognitively-oriented learning experiences, there may be initial resistance and unrest when they are offered a freer atmosphere. It is important to reduce classroom structure gradually in order to decrease learner anxiety about increased freedom. Steps to take for a slowed introduction of a humanistic model include:

- Give specific information about how the group will proceed.
- Repeat directions until the class is able to verbalize congruent understanding.
- Give feedback that moves learners to a level at which they can become more effectively involved in learning.

Nurse Educator Tip

Feedback is effective when the following principles are used:

1. Messages are clear, concise, and focused on observed behaviors, not on learner motivations; for example, "I noticed you omitted Step 2 in the procedure."
2. Lack of understanding is clearly expressed at the time information is given; for example, "Before you go on, I'd like to clarify what you meant by . . ."
3. Value or moral judgments are avoided; for example, there is no attempt to shame, threaten, or make the learner feel guilty.
4. Focus is on the present and future. Behavior over which the person has no control is avoided.
5. At least one strength is identified when weaknesses are discussed; for example, "I liked what you said, but let Ginny finish her comment before you talk."
6. Feedback can be verbal or audiovisual; skills that are videotaped during practice can be used to provide feedback to learners that verbal statements cannot.

Nurse educators must focus intensely on role modeling effective feedback to teach learners appropriate ways of giving feedback to clients. Providing feedback is a crucial skill in the helping relationship and one that must become part of the professional identity of nursing learners. Structuring a humanistic classroom is another way to help nursing learners grow into self-directed learners.

Self-Directed Learning

A **humanistic classroom** is a place where learners are trusted as self-directing individuals, divergent ideas are accepted, and individual differences and means toward goals are encouraged. The classroom is a safe place where nursing learners not only learn the facts, but also learn about each other and the implications of the facts they've learned. Learners must feel free to explore and grow in living communion with the subjects they study (Marino, 2000)

In the humanistic classroom, nurse educators feel secure enough to reveal themselves as people, autonomy and freedom are encouraged, feedback is honest, the process (rather than the product) of learning is important, empathy is conveyed, and learners are not discouraged from expressing their feelings and perceptions.

> A humanistic classroom encourages self-directed learning, honest feedback, empathy, and feeling expression.

■ Nurse Educator Challenge

What one thing would you do to make your classrooms more humanistic? Give a rationale for your answer. If possible, decide on a date to implement your goal.

Setting Legitimate Limits

A useful humanistic setting is not a chaotic one. Nurse educators convey respect for learner thoughts, feelings, and perceptions. It is important to convey that displaying humanism is not a one-way process but requires contributions from learners and educators alike.

In the humanistic classroom, learners are expected to demonstrate respect for the educators. Learners are provided with feedback about unrealistic demands or lack of respect for nurse educators. Some examples of humanistic statements that convey limits and the need for respecting others are:

"I hear you saying that you're angry, and I can accept that, but the agreed contract between us was . . ."

"I listened to you, and I expect you to listen to me."

"The syllabus, our contract, says the report was due yesterday. Yours is late and points will be subtracted as per the syllabus."

The humanistic classroom creates a positive learning environment by setting legitimate limits. Once limits are set, the nurse educator can focus on creating other aspects of a positive learning environment.

Creating an Environment for Learning

Nurse educators who create a humanizing classroom environment will probably evoke creative responses in nursing learners. Some conditions that are more likely to lead to creative learning (and that are similar to humanizing factors) are:

- The absence of serious threat to the self,
- The encouragement of appropriate risk-taking,
- The effort to put learners in touch with their feelings,
- The reward of diverse contributions,
- The reduction of isolation from peers,
- Practice in coping with anxiety, fear, frustration, and failure,
- The freeing of learners from their "blind spots" or inability to see alternatives,
- The development of values and purpose, and
- The identification of lack of minimal skill level. (Torrance, 1962)

Once creative learning is an aspect of the learning environment, the nurse educator focuses on other elements of the helping relationship. Chief among these is empathy.

Empathy

A crucial helping skill for both the nurse educator and nursing learner is **empathy**. It is the basis of the helping relationship and an important part of the humanistic classroom.

> Empathy is the basis of a helping relationship and includes communicating the feeling and meaning of the other person.

Carkhuff (1969) is the most well-known proponent of empathy. He developed scales for the assessment of empathic understanding that included five levels.

Level one empathy implies a total lack of listening skills. The verbal and nonverbal behavior of the educator or learner does not attend to or actually detracts significantly from the other's message. Level one behavior might be exemplified by the nurse educator who avoids or fails to notice learner anxiety, joy, fear, or other strong feeling, or the nursing learner who changes the subject when the client talks about dying.

At **level two** empathy, the feeling aspect of a response is diminished. For example, the educator or learner subtracts noticeable affect (feeling) from the communications of the other. Level two behavior may be demonstrated by the nursing learner who tells an angry client, "You're a little upset, but you'll soon feel better," and the educator who smiles and downplays the angry expressions of a learner.

At **levels three through five**, the educator or learner respond in such a way as to communicate the feeling and meaning of the other person. Only at level three and above is communication facilitated and empathy demonstrated. An example of level three empathy is:

> Learner: "I disagree with that and I think . . ."
>
> Nurse educator: "I see that you feel very strongly about that, and if I understand you, your point was . . ."

Empathy is important in the humanizing classroom because the nurse educator role models listening skills and provides practice experiences in constructing empathic responses. The nurse educator also instructs learners about how to use empathic skills with clients. In addition to ensuring that empathy reigns in the classroom, there are other steps the nurse educator can take to humanize the setting.

Nurse Educator's Humanism

Before nurse educators can teach learners empathy skills, educators must ensure they have the needed skills. An early step in humanizing the classroom is an assessment of the educator's humanistic trends and empathic skill (see Box 1–5).

Box 1–5　Nurse Educator's Humanism

Rate yourself on the following questions. A "yes" answer to all 12 questions indicates a high level of humanism. It is probably advisable to ask students for feedback on questions 5, 7, 8, 9, 10, 11, and 12.

1. Do I trust learners to be self-directing?
2. Do I find rewards in facilitating the development of learners (as opposed to receiving approval from students or administrators)?
3. Am I able to move beyond believing that mine is the final and best way to educate or to solve problems?
4. Can I maintain my humanism despite any dehumanizing aspects of my school system?
5. Do I give I learners access to me as a person?

(continues)

Box 1–5   Nurse Educator's Humanism (continued)

---

6. Do I suggest alternative learning experiences?
7. Do I respect learner autonomy and freedom?
8. Do I give honest feedback to learners?
9. Do I share responsibility for learning with learners?
10. Do I foster the process of learning?
11. Do I respond to students so as to reflect accurately their thoughts and feelings?
12. Do I act consistently with the idea that people are the best authority on how they feel and experience situations?

Knowledge of learner learning styles and preferences can help nurse educators respond appropriately to a diverse class, facilitate dialogue between educators and learners, and help educators communicate in the most efficient and effective way.

Learning Preferences, Cognitive Complexity, and Moral Development

There are three other important concepts for nurse educators to evaluate and take action when appropriate are: learner styles and preferences, cognitive complexity, and moral development.

Learning Styles and Preferences

Nurse educators must understand learning styles and preferences because:

- Research on learning suggests dialogue and educator/learner interaction is more appropriate than lecture. To accomplish an effective dialogue, educators must get to know learners.
- Classrooms are increasingly diverse, not only in terms of ethnicity and gender, but also by age, nationality, cultural background, and more. This diversity can affect learning. For example, older learners can draw on a lifetime of experience and are more apt to be independent, while women, in general, approach learning in more connected, empathic, collaborative ways;

African-American and Mexican-American learners may prefer working with others to achieve common goals.

- By making an effort to consider learner preferences, educators may reinvigorate teaching practices (Montgomery & Groat, 1998).

- Individuals learn in different ways and at different rates. Nurse educators must be aware of variations in learner interests, needs, abilities, and previous learning in order to choose appropriate education strategies (Wetzig, 2004).

James and Gardner (1995) defined **learning styles** as the most effective manner learners perceive, process, store, and recall material they learn.

Amy, a learner in a RN-to-BSN program, learned best with flash cards and by reading articles. John, another learner in the class, learned best by watching videos and following an RN around as she worked with clients. Debby, another learner in the class, learned best by reading case studies and discussing them.

> Learning style indicates the most effective way learners perceive, process, store, and recall information.

Learning Style Models

This book presents four learning style models: The Myers-Briggs Type Indicator, the Kolb/McCarthy Learning Circle, Felder-Silyerman Learning Styles Model, and Gasha-Reichmann Learning Styles. Each raises one or more important issues.

Myers-Briggs Type Indicator

The Myers-Briggs Type Indicator is based on Carl Jung's concept of archetypes and was developed by two women: Isabel Briggs Myers and Katherine Cooks Briggs. A profile is identified along four dimensions: orientation to life (extroverted/introverted), perception (sensing/intuitive), decision-making (thinking/feeling), and attitude toward the outer world (judgment/perception). A learner who is extroverted, prefers sensing, feeling and perception, is called an ESFP (the first letter of extroverted, sensing, feeling, and perception), while a learner who prefers to work alone, use facts and data, is logical and spontaneous, is called an ISTP (the first letter of introverted, sensing, thinking, perception). For an online test based on Jung-Myers-Briggs typology, go to the Website http://humanmetrics.com/cgi-win/JTypes2.asp.

Kolb/McCarthy Learning Cycle

An underlying assumption of the Kolb/McCarthy model is that all learning includes a cycle of four learning modes, but each individual is apt to feel most comfortable in one mode along the dimensions of Perception and Processing. Kolb's four-stage theory is based on a model with two dimensions expressed in the form of a Learning Style Grid. The first dimension (s-axis) is based on the individual's preferred way of learning a task. The left end of this dimension identifies a preference for doing tasks, and the right end indicates a preference for observing a task. The second dimension (y-axis) is based on an individual's thought and emotional processes. The top end of the dimension indicates preference for learning through feelings, and the bottom indicates a preference for learning based on thinking (Montgomery & Groat, 1998; Kolb, 1984).

He placed educators in the Type 4 learning style, which he named Accomodators. He viewed faculty with this kind of learning style as evaluators/remediators. Sample activities for this learning style are using open ended problems, learner presentations, design projects, subjective exams, and simulations. Other learning styles included Divergers (Social Science and Humanities), Assimilators (Physical Science), and Convergers (e.g., Engineering).

Kolb suggests following a learning cycle that addresses each of the following questions in order (Kolb, 1984). By teaching through the cycle, all the various learning styles of nursing learners will be addressed. The questions include:

- "Why are we learning this?"
- "What are the key points of this issue?"
- "How do I use this knowledge?"
- "What are the implications of this information in other contexts?"

Kolb (1984) envisioned a four-stage learning process requiring the following abilities:

- Concrete experience,
- Reflective observation,
- Abstract conceptualization, and
- Active experimentation.

Felder-Silverman Learning Styles Model

The learning style model developed by Richard Felder and Linda Silverman (Felder, 1993; Felder and Silverman, 1988) incorporates two aspects of the Myers-Briggs and Kolb models. The Perception dimension (sensing/intuitive) is analogous to the Perception of both Myers-Briggs and Kolb. The Processing dimension (active/reflective) is also found in Kolb's model. Felder and Silverman also propose additional dimensions of input (visual/verbal), organization (inductive/deductive), and understanding (sequential/global). Felder (1993) advocated balancing the extremes of each learning dimension by:

- Providing a context for concepts by making connections to learners' everyday experiences (global),
- Balancing theory and models (intuitive),
- Using demonstrations and diagrams (visual),
- Using simulation (sensing, inductive) to illustrate abstract concepts (intuitive, deductive), and
- Providing time for learner reflection about information presented (reflective).

■ Nurse Educator Challenge

Which learning style model requires reflective observation?

Grasha-Reichmann Learning Styles
Anthony Grasha and Sheryl Hruska-Reichmann developed a learning styles model different from the other three models (Grasha, 1996). Their model was based on learner responses to classroom activities, not a general assessment of cognitive or personality traits, and included the following styles: competitive (prefers teacher-centered class activities), collaborative (prefers learner-led small groups), avoidant (prefers anonymous environment), participant (prefers lectures with discussion), dependent (prefers clear instructions and little ambiguity), and independent (prefers independent study and projects).

Grasha (1996) pointed out that matching teaching style to learning style is not a panacea that solves all classroom conflicts. He also underlined the importance of the following educator actions:

- Working out potential conflicts and misunderstandings with learners that can undermine learning
- Reflecting on pedagogical goals and strengths as an educator
- Gradually introducing class activities that expand learner style preferences

---

■ Nurse Educator Challenge

Which learning style model uses collaboration?

Learning Style Research

Several nursing researchers have examined learner preferences. Abu-Moghli, Khalaf, Halabi, and Wardam (2005) examined learning styles of Jordanian nursing learners. They found the majority of baccalaureate learners identified themselves as independent learners who were curious to learn and who could identify learner goals. A serendipitous finding of the study was that a low percentage of learners indicated having good study skills and ability to concentrate while studying, and they needed assistance using study time efficiently.

■ Nurse Educator Challenge

If you were the nurse educator in the class studied by Khalaf, Halabi, and Wardam, what action would you take? Base your answers on the research findings.

Wetzig (2004) focused on the differences in learning styles of a group of twenty RNs in Intensive Care. She used the Index of Learning Styles (ILS) devised by Soloman and Felder. Participants were asked to indicate their perceived accuracy of the assessment, and provide suggestions for improvement in educational support. Results showed the majority of learners identified a preference for visual learning while the learning program utilized mostly written learning strategies. Based on learner evaluation, educational support and teaching strategies changed.

■ Nurse Educator Challenge

If you were teaching the Intensive Care RNs, would you change your teaching strategies based on the findings of the study? Justify your answer.

Hauer (2005) assessed the learning style preferences of learners enrolled in various allied health programs, including nursing. He noted there have been many studies assessing the learning styles of learners in various health-related disciplines. These assessments include Three Representational Modes (Trim), VAK (Visual, Auditory, Kinesthetic), Kolb's Learning Style Inventory, and Howard Gardner's Multiple Intelligences (Clark, 2000).

Hauer used the Kolb Learning Style Inventory LSI-IIa, which is based on John Dewey's belief that learning must be grounded in experience, Kurt Lewin's belief in active learning, and Jean Piaget's theory of intelligence.

Eighty-nine learners from various allied health care programs enrolled at a small Midwestern university participated in the study. The nursing and speech-language pathology learners showed a slight preference for concrete experimentation, whereas the OT and physician assistant learners preferred abstract conceptualization.

Learning Style Implications for Teaching
The learning style implications for teaching include:

- Striving to provide a variety of learning experiences so all learning styles are addressed.
- Including some applications that will help the sensing learner understand the reason for learning abstract concepts.
- Grouping projects, case studies, and in-class presentations that engage sensing learners.
- Including both rote problems and open-ended questions to challenge both sensing and intuitive learners.
- Including both individual and group work to satisfy both introverts and extroverts.
- Making sure all of Kolb's four types are accommodated by using open-ended questions, learner presentations, projects, subjective exams, simulations to satisfy accommodators, homework, computer simulations, field trips, reports, demonstrations, motivational stories, group discussion, lectures, textbook reading, demonstrations by instructor, and independent research and objective (Montgomery & Groat, 1998).

■ Nurse Educator Challenge

Which of the suggested learning style implications for teaching have been introduced into your classroom? How could you help introduce at least one?

One assessment tool to use with learners is shown in Box 1–6. Environmental, emotional, social, and physical aspects of learning preferences are surveyed. Note that questions 39–49 begin to assess levels of cognitive complexity and moral development.

Box 1–6 Assessing Learner Preferences

Ask learners at the beginning of a semester to check whether they sometimes, always, or never need or like the following situations. Build your classroom accordingly.

	Always	Sometimes	Never
1. I need quiet in order to learn.	❏	❏	❏
2. I need to discuss things with others in order to learn effectively.	❏	❏	❏
3. I require bright light in order to learn.	❏	❏	❏
4. I require soft, low light in order to learn.	❏	❏	❏
5. I need a cool room to learn in.	❏	❏	❏
6. I need a warm environment to learn in.	❏	❏	❏
7. I like a table and chairs or a desk arrangement when learning.	❏	❏	❏
8. I like to sit on the floor and/or move my chair around when learning.	❏	❏	❏
9. I like to receive input from the educator about how I'm doing and what is important knowledge.	❏	❏	❏
10. I can learn as much, if not more, from fellow learners than I can from the educator.	❏	❏	❏
11. I have a short attention span.	❏	❏	❏
12. I can concentrate for long periods of time.	❏	❏	❏
13. I need positive comments from the instructor.	❏	❏	❏
14. I need support from fellow classmates.	❏	❏	❏
15. I like detailed instructions from the educator about how to proceed.	❏	❏	❏
16. I like to "take off" on an assignment and create my own learning experience.	❏	❏	❏
17. I like to pace my own learning.	❏	❏	❏
18. I like the educator to set deadlines for me.	❏	❏	❏
19. I give up easily on a learning task.	❏	❏	❏

Box 1–6   Assessing Learner Preferences (continued)

	Always	Sometimes	Never
20. I work harder when the task eludes me.	❑	❑	❑
21. I take responsibility for what I learn.	❑	❑	❑
22. I expect the educator to take responsibility for what I learn.	❑	❑	❑
23. I prefer to learn things on my own.	❑	❑	❑
24. I like to learn with one other classmate.	❑	❑	❑
25. I like to learn by working with a small group.	❑	❑	❑
26. I prefer to learn by working with the educator.	❑	❑	❑
27. I seem to learn best by listening to others speak.	❑	❑	❑
28. I seem to learn best when I can look at the material I'm supposed to learn.	❑	❑	❑
29. I seem to learn best when I can pick up and touch learning materials.	❑	❑	❑
30. I seem to learn best by acting, moving, or trying out a learning experience.	❑	❑	❑
31. I seem to learn best through a combination of seeing, hearing, touching, and/or acting (cross out those that don't apply).	❑	❑	❑
32. I like to take frequent breaks when learning.	❑	❑	❑
33. I like to finish a task or class and then take a break.	❑	❑	❑
34. I like to get up out of my chair occasionally and/or stretch and move around the room.	❑	❑	❑
35. I like to sit in my chair until I've finished the task.	❑	❑	❑
36. I learn best in the morning.	❑	❑	❑

(continues)

Box 1–6   Assessing Learner Preferences (continued)

	Always	Sometimes	Never
37. I learn best in the afternoon.	❏	❏	❏
38. I learn best in the evening.	❏	❏	❏
39. I like to learn things that are unambiguous and clear-cut where there is little conflict in the group.	❏	❏	❏
40. I like to weigh the effects of different ways of approaching a problem and to hear others' views even if they differ from mine.	❏	❏	❏
41. I like to learn about my classmates and clients more than about techniques or strategies.	❏	❏	❏
42. I like to negotiate rules and ways of proceeding and learning with my teacher and peers.	❏	❏	❏
43. I like to try to see how widely divergent theoretical frameworks might interrelate or be used at different times with different experiences.	❏	❏	❏
44. I believe that if the educator says something is right, it must be right.	❏	❏	❏
45. I'll give in to a fellow learner or educator only if they'll give in to me.	❏	❏	❏
46. I feel very loyal to the learner group.	❏	❏	❏
47. I tend to do things because they please others in the class or the educator.	❏	❏	❏
48. I tend to follow through on a contract or agreement once I've agreed to do so.	❏	❏	❏
49. I tend to agree on a contract or agreement only if it fits with my own internal set of ethical standards.	❏ ❏	❏ ❏	❏ ❏

Learner's name _____

Date _____

Cognitive Complexity

According to Joyce and Weil (1972), there are three or four levels of **cognitive complexity**.

Although the assessment tool in Box 1–6 taps only learner-reported levels of complexity, it is a beginning step toward individualizing cognitive learning needs.

> Cognitive complexity begins at the lowest level with black/white categorical thinking, and moves through various levels until it is possible to relate and compare different systems of interacting variables.

The **lowest level of cognitive complexity** is one characterized by black/white categorical thinking, a minimal tolerance of conflict, and a preference for a quick closure of discussion. The **moderate level of cognitive complexity** is one where people have several alternative ways of structuring the world and can weigh the effects of their own behavior from several vantage points simultaneously. **High cognitive complexity** is indicated by an ability to relate and compare different systems of interacting variables. Thinking is highly abstract and learners can adapt to complex, changing systems.

Although nurse educators might wish that all learners were able to think on the high cognitive complex level, many are not. Once cognitive complexity can be assessed, the learner can be assisted to the next higher level by matching the individual to an appropriate learning environment (Box 1–6).

Learners at a low level of cognitive complexity become even more rigid in thought without some structuring of the environment. Instruction must be supportive, directions must be given clearly, and information must not be too far removed from present belief systems; if information is too different, learners will reject it. Stress should be placed on self-delineation and on negotiation within the environment.

Jessie, a beginning BSN learner, asked for many rules for behavior. When the nurse educator asked the class to play a simulation game. the longer the game went on, the more questions Jessie asked.

■ Nurse Educator Challenge

What level of cognitive complexity is Jessie demonstrating?

Learners in a moderate level of cognitive complexity rebel against authority and resist external control. Learning experiences should emphasize negotiation in interpersonal relationships and divergence in the development of rules and concepts.

> David, a beginning master's level nursing education learner, questioned the instructor about the source of many of her comments, and refused to follow the class syllabus for assignments and their due dates.

Learners in a moderate-to-high level of cognitive complexity tend to overplay interpersonal relationships and neglect learning tasks. Learning experience should guide learners to keep working on the task. Overprotection will decrease conceptualization and ability to learn how to function in task-oriented situations.

■ **Nurse Educator Challenge**

What level of cognitive complexity is David demonstrating?

Learners at a high level of cognitive complexity can balance task functions with maintenance or interpersonal functions and can negotiate rules with others as well as ways of approaching abstract problems. Learners can operate at the highest level when placed in interdependent, information-oriented, complex environments, and take responsibility for his or her own learning and structure (Joyce and Weil, 2004). Another aspect of learning that is important to nurses is moral development.

Moral Development

Moral development is an important issue in nursing because nurses are increasingly being faced with ethical dilemmas. Nurses must be assisted to higher levels of moral development so they can deal effectively with ethical dilemmas.

Many developmental psychologists use stage theories to explain moral development. Kohlberg, probably the best known theorist, developed six stages of moral development (Barger 2000; Kohlberg, 1981).

Stage one and two of Kohlberg's moral development are preconventional stages. Stage one is characterized by avoidance of punishment and unquestioning deference to power; nurses who attain a moral level no higher than stage one are apt to do whatever anyone in power tells them to do, regardless of its effect on patient care. At stage two, right action consists of what is satisfying to self and (occasionally) to others.

Reciprocity in sharing is based on "you scratch my back and I'll scratch yours," not on loyalty, gratitude, or justice. Nurses at this development level may help clients or doctors only if they are helped in return.

The conventional level of moral reasoning includes stages three and four. At stage three, people choose to behave well so that others will approve of them; nurses at this level will be most likely to seek out approval and to try to be nice to others. At stage four, the keeping of rules, the completion of one's duty, and the maintenance of the status quo are important. Nurses at this stage are apt to give medications on the dot, not to question rules, and to live up to their job descriptions.

Stages five and six are postconventional or autonomous levels of moral reasoning. Since nursing seems to be moving toward independent practice, it would seem reasonable to expect nurses to function at the postconventional level; yet many do not. At stage five, right action is defined after critical examination and joint agreement.

Contracts and free agreement bind obligation. Nurses at this developmental level tend to contract with clients about health care issues.

At stage six, right action is defined by individual conscience in accordance with self-chosen ethical principles based on logical comprehensiveness, universality, and consistency. Universal principles of justice, equal rights, and respect for the dignity of individuals are used as measures.

> The preconventional stage of moral development is exemplified by the nurse who does whatever anyone in power tells them to do (stage one), and by the nurse who does what is satisfying or what is based on reciprocal sharing (stage two).

> The conventional stage of moral reasoning is exemplified by the nurse who seeks out approval and tries to be nice to everyone (stage three) and the nurse who maintains the status quo (stage four).

> The postconventional or autonomous level of moral reasoning is exemplified by the nurse who contracts with clients about health care issues (stage five), and the nurse who acts based on logical, consistent, comprehensive, and universal ethical principles (stage six).

> Edward, a master's degree learner, is always checking with the nurse educator to make sure he's doing all right and doing extra credit assignments, even though he's already assured an A.

■ **Nurse Educator Challenge**

What level of moral development does Edward exemplify?

Even though she was a learner of Kohlberg's, Gilligan disagreed with him and decided to develop her own moral development stages. She complained that Kohlberg's stages were male-centered, and indeed, Kohlberg did develop his theory based on a male population. Her complaint was that it is not good psychology to leave out half the human race.

Gilligan (1982) proposed a stage theory of moral development for women. She took umbrage at basing the theory on justice and guilt. From her careful interviews with women making momentous decisions in their lives, Gilligan concluded that these women were thinking more about the caring thing to do rather than the just thing to do.

Gilligan's five stages, which she called an "Ethic of Care," focused on connections among people and included:

1. The preconventional stage—the goal is survival.
2. The transitional stage—movement from selfishness to responsibility to others.
3. The conventional stage—self-sacrifices are good.
4. The transition stage—from goodness to truth that a woman is a person too.
5. The postconventional stage—may never be attained and includes the principle of nonviolence of not hurting others or self.

Nursing Research on Moral Development

Krawczyk (1997) conducted a study to determine the development of moral judgement in first-year and senior baccalaureate nursing learners. A sample of 180 learners enrolled in three separate nursing programs. The courses differed significantly in ethical content. Program A included an ethics course taught by a professor of ethics. Program B integrated ethical issues into all nursing theory courses. Program C included no ethical content in the theory courses. The independent variables were the amount of ethics taught in the nursing programs and the level of academic education. The dependent variable was the development of moral judgement as measured by Rest's Defining Issues Test. The senior nursing learners from Program A scored significantly higher than the other senior groups on the Defining Issues Test. Krawczyk concluded that an ethics course with group participation and a decision-making element significantly facilitated nursing learner development of moral judgment.

Kim and colleagues (2003) used a longitudinal study to examine moral judgement level and related factors. Thirty-seven nursing learners and twenty medical learners comprised the sample. She collected data using the Korean version of the Defining Issues Test. She found no significant change in score at each academic year in either group. The researcher suggested that ethics education be developed and evaluated.

Using Research and Theory to Enhance Learner Moral Development

Moral reasoning can be influenced in the direction of higher levels by exposing people to them (Barger, 2000). It is important to structure learning experiences so that learners will be exposed to the next higher stage of reasoning. It is important for them to be exposed to situations that pose problems, to contradictions in the current level of reasoning, and to an atmosphere of interchange and dialogue where values can be identified. Value clarification (see Chapter 5) is a beginning step toward identifying values.

This chapter has explored challenges nurse educators face and suggested some ways of dealing with these challenges in a positive manner. Chapter 2 provides information for designing effective learning systems.

EXERCISES FOR NURSE EDUCATORS

Directions: It's always wise to try out exercises yourself to make sure they work and determine how they work. Feel free to adapt them for your use after trying out each one. When using any of these exercises with learners in the classroom, allow a 10-15 minute period for debriefing the learning. Some questions to ask learners include:

- What was the exercise like for you?
- What did you learn from doing this exercise?
- What changes would you suggest in the exercise?
- How could you use this exercise when teaching learners?
- What questions do you have about this exercise?

1. Philosophy of nursing education

Study Figure 1–1. How might it help you to develop your own personal philosophy of nursing education? What other materials or experiences do you think you need to develop such a philosophy? What steps do you plan to take to consolidate your philosophy? Develop a written plan with deadlines for achieving each step.

2. Ideal classroom/dreaded classroom

Imagine a pleasant scene, where you are relaxed and away from the dreaded classroom. You are composed and about to enter your ideal classroom. Picture your ideal classroom in your mind:

- What are learners doing that you consider ideal?
- How are you acting, feeling, and thinking in your ideal classroom?
- To whom are learners talking?
- What actions do you observe?
- Where are people located in the room?
- What does the room look like?
- What are you feeling?

Imagine that you are about to face a classroom full of learners. Pretend that some dreaded situation occurs as you step into the classroom. Picture this classroom in your mind.

- What are learners doing that you dread?
- What are you doing?
- Who is talking to whom?
- What are the physical characteristics of the room?
- Where are people sitting?
- Who is moving?
- What is the movement?
- What are you feeling?

Consider steps you can take to make your dreaded classroom more ideal. Share your results with your classmates. This exercise can be used to prepare learners for clinical experiences by changing the term "dreaded classroom" to "dreaded clinical experience."

3. Risking success

Choose a teaching/1earning situation where you would feel comfortable taking a risk by demonstrating your lack of competence as a strategy to enhance learning. Plan how you will implement the strategy. Try it out, and evaluate the results in part by asking for feedback from at least three learners.

4. Finding uniqueness

A large classroom of learners can lead to a blurring of individual learner differences and unique qualities. Devise a way of finding out at least one personal or unique quality about each learner. You might consider using one of the following strategies:

- Asking learners to write down a unique thing about themselves,
- Asking learners to go around the class and report one thing about themselves they consider unique, or
- Greeting one new learner at the beginning (or end) of each class and finding out one thing about their wishes, aspirations, or unique qualities.

Write down your results and share it with at least three other learners.

5. Teaching/learning challenges
Identify one teaching/learning challenge you have. Devise a strategy for correcting it. Ask three learners for input and/or assistance with the problem. Share your results with at least three learners.

6. Facing your fears
Most educators have fears of losing control or not taking a positive direction in a classroom. Think about your fear(s). Devise a strategy for facing your classroom fear(s). Try out your strategy and share your results with at least three learners.

7. Empathy
Conduct an experiment to identify the empathy level(s) you use in your classroom. You may wish to use audiotape, videotape, written self-report, or learner feedback as part of your experiment. If you find you are functioning lower than at level three, devise a strategy for improving your empathic skill. Share your results with at least three learners.

8. Ethics/moral development
Compose a list of possible ethical/moral dilemmas nursing learners or graduate nurses might face. Poll other nursing instructors, learners, and nurse practitioners. Do some reading about ethics and moral development. Devise learning experiences for learners that will help them to function at a higher ethical or moral development level. Test it out with three other learners or collaborate with another learner to try out your experiences. Share your findings with the class or at least three other learners.

9. Managing the classroom
Make a list of the pros and cons of being a manager of classroom experiences. Be sure to include feelings, attitudes, or biases that motivate you to accept or reject the concept. What skills do you need to develop to adopt the position of classroom manager? What skills do you already have that would assist you? Make a written plan for enhancing your classroom management skills.

10. Journaling
Read at least one article on journaling and start your own journal detailing your process of becoming a nurse educator. Resist the urge to rewrite anything. If you have additional ideas, just add them as they occur to you. Every week, reread your entries and summarize what you've learned, what questions you wish to bring to class, and what goals remain for you.

ADVANCED LEARNING EXPERIENCES

11. Learning Challenges
Complete a small research project by comparing one nurse educator's learning challenges with three learners'; or compare 3-10 learner self-assessed learning challenges at the beginning and end of the course

12. Problem Statement
Devise a problem statement for a study of learning challenges for nurse educators or nursing learners.

13. Mastery through overfamiliarity
Interview three nurse educators using the questions in Nurse Educator Tips in the "Mastery through Overfamiliarity" section of this chapter.

14. Transfer
Chose one of the research questions regarding transfer from Box 1–1. Develop a problem statement and research design in collaboration with an advanced doctoral learner in a related discipline.

15. Developmental Helping Model
Choose one of the nurse educator actions for learners at level one, two, or three of the developmental helping model and develop a research design. Test your chosen action with three to ten nursing learners.

16. Feedback
Study the Nurse Educator Tip on feedback (page 54) and choose one of the principles to follow up on by taking a leadership role, a legislative/policy role, or a research role. Take action and write up the results.

17. Environment
Work in conjunction with a nurse educator to help create an environment for creative learning.

18. Learning Styles

Choose one of the reasons why nurse educators must understand learning styles and pair off with a fellow learner. Flip a coin to decide who will take the rationale as stated, and who will take the other side of the argument. Debate the issue.

19. Moral Development

Decide on a plan for enhancing the moral development of a group of learners. Put your plan into action.

References

Abu-Moghli, F. A., Khalaf, I. A., Halabi, J. O., & Wardam, L. A. (2005). Jordanian baccalaureate nursing learners' perception of their learning styles. *International Nursing Review, 52, 39-45.*

Akinsanyz, C., & Williams, M. (2004). Concept mapping for meaningful elearning. *Nurse Education Today, 24*(1), 41-46.

Allen, G., Rubenfeld, M. & Scheffer, B. (2004). Reliability of assessment of critical thinking. *Journal of Professional Nursing, 20,* 15–22.

American Association of Colleges of Nursing. (1998). *The essentials of baccalaureate education for professional nursing practice.* Washington, DC: AACN.

Anderson, E. T., & Mercer, Z. B. (2004). Impact of community health content on nurse practitioner practice: A comparison of classroom and web-based teaching. *Nursing Education Perspectives, 25,* 171–176.

Anderson, L., & Krathwohl, D. (Eds.). (2001). *A taxonomy for learning, teaching and assessing.* New York: Addison Wesley Longman.

Attewell, A. (1998). Florence Nightengale. *Prospects, The Quarterly Review of Comparative Education, 28*(1), 153-166.

Baumberger-Henry, M. (2005). Cooperative learning and case study: Does the combination improve learners' perception of problem-solving and decision making skills? *Nurse Education Today, 25,* 238-246.

Beckie, T., Lowry, L., & Barnett, S. (2001). Assessing critical thinking in baccalaureate nursing learners: A longitudinal study. *Holistic Nursing Practice, 15*(3), 18–26.

Billings, D. M., Connors, H. R., & Skiba, D. J. (2001). Benchmarking best practices in web-based nursing courses. *Advances in Nursing Science, 23*(3), 41–52.

Bloom's Taxonomy. (2003). Retrieved December 2, 2003 from http://www.olemiss.edu/depts/educ_school2/docs/stai_manual/manual10.htm

Bransford, J. D., Brown, A. L., & Cocking, R. R. (1999). *The design of learning environment: How people learn: Brain, mind, experience and school.* Washington, DC: National Academy of Sciences.

Callaghan, G. M. (2006). Functional analytic psychotherapy and supervision. *International Journal of Behavioral and Consultant Therapy, 2*(3), 416-431.

Candela, L., Dalley, K., & Benzel-Lindley, J. (2006). A case for learning-centered curricula. *Journal of Nursing Education, 45*(2)59–66.

Carkhuff, R. (1969). *Helping and Human Relationships* (Vol. 1). New York: Holt, Rhinehart & Winston.

Cashwell, C. (1994). *Interpersonal process recall.* Retrieved September 23, 2006 from http://www. eric.ed.go ED372342 1994-04-00

Clark, D. (2000). *Learning styles or, how we go from the unknown to the known.* Retrieved September 23, 2006 from http://www.nwlink.com/~donclark/hrd/vak.html

Cote-Arsenault, D. (2004). Planning for a new baby: A creative approach to learning. *Nurse Educator, 29*(1), 6-9.

Cottrell, S. (2002). Suspicion, resistance, tokenism and mutiny: Problematic dynamics relevant to the implementation of clinical supervision in nursing. *Journal of Psychiatric and Mental Health Nursing, 9,* 667–671.

Davies, P. (2000). Approaches to evidence-based teaching. *Medical Teacher, 22*(1), 142–159.

Davis, D., Stullenbarger, E., Dearman, C., & Kelley, J. A. (2005). Proposed nurse educator competencies: Development and validation of a model. *Nursing Outlook, 53*(4), 206–211.

DeVito, J. A. (2005). *The Interpersonal Communication Book.* Old Tappan, NJ: Pearson, Allyn & Bacon.

Diekelmann, N. (2002). "Pitching a lecture" and "reading the faces of learners": Learning lecturing and the embodied practices of teaching. *Journal of Nursing Education, 41,* 97–100.

Ekstein, R., & Wallerstein, R. (1971). *The Teaching and Learning of Psychotherapy* (2nd ed.). New York: International Universities Press.

Ellerman, C. R., Kataoka-Yahiro, M. R., & Wong, L. C. (2006). Logic models used to enhance critical thinking. *Journal of Nursing Education, 45*(6), 220–227.

Facione, P. A. (1992). *Test Manual: The California Critical Thinking Dispositions Inventory* (2nd ed.). Millbrae, CA: California Academic Press.

Felder, R. M., & Silverman, L. K. (1988). Learning styles and teaching styles in engineering education. *Engineering Education, 78*(7), 674-681.

Felder, R. M. (1993). Reaching the second tier: Learning and teaching styles in college science education. *Journal of College Science Teaching, 23*(5), 286-290.

Foley, B. J., Redman, R. W., Horn, E. V., Davis, G. T., Neal, E. M., & Van Ripper, J. (2001). Determining nursing faculty development needs. *Nursing Outlook, 51*(5), 227–232.

Forehand, M. (2005). *Bloom's taxonomy: Original and revised.* Retrieved November 5, 2006 from http://www.coe.uga.edu/epltt/bloom.htm.

Gilligan, C. (1982). *In a different voice: Psychological theory and women's development.* Cambridge, MA: Harvard University Press.

Ginsburg, S. (2004). The professionalism movement. *The American Journal of Bioethics, 4*(2), 14-15.

Grasha, A. F. (1996). *Teaching with style: A practical guide to enhancing learning by understanding teaching and learning styles.* Pittsburgh, PA: Alliance Publishers.

Hesook, K., & Kollak, I. (2005). *Nursing Theories* (2nd ed.). New York: Springer.

Hauer, P. (2005). Learning styles of allied health learners using Kolb's LSI-IIa. *Journal of Allied Health, 34,* 177-182.

Ibarreta, G. I., & McLeod, L. (2004). Educational innovations. Thinking aloud on paper: An experience in journal writing. *Journal of Nursing Education, 43,* 134-137.

Ironside, P. (2004). "Covering content" and teaching thinking: Deconstructing the additive curriculum. *Journal of Nursing Education, 43,* 5–14.

James, W. B., & Gardner, D. L. (1995). *Learning styles: Implications for distance learning.* East Lansing, MI: National Center for Research on Teacher Learning. Eric Document Reproduction Service No. ED514356.

Jeffries, P. (2005). A framework for designing, implementing, and evaluating: Simulations used as teaching strategies in nursing. *Nursing Education Perspectives, 26,* 96-103.

Joyce, B. R., & Weil, M. (1972). *Models of Teaching.* Englewood Cliffs, NJ: Prentice-Hall.

Kagan, N. (1975). Influencing human interaction—eleven years with IPR. *Canadian Counsellor, 9*(2), 74–97.

Kautz, D. D., Kuiper, R. A., Pesut, P. K. B., & Daneker, D. (2005). Promoting clinical reasoning in undergraduate nursing learners: Application and evaluation of the Outcome Present State Test (OPT) Model of Clinical Reasoning. *International Journal of Nursing Education Scholarship, 2*(1), 1–15.

Kearns, L., Shoaf, J., & Summey, M. (2004). Performance and satisfaction of second-degree BSN learners in web-based and traditional course delivery environments. *Journal of Nursing Education, 43,* 280–285.

Kim, Y. S., Park, J. W., & Son, Y. J. (2003). A longitudinal study on moral judgment development in nursing and medical learners. *Tachan Kanho Hakkoe Chi, 33*(6), 820-828.

Knowles, M. (1990). *The adult learner: A neglected species.* Houston, TX: Gulf Publishing.

Knowles, M. S., Holton, E. F., & Swanson, R. A. (1998). *The adult learner: The definitive classic in adult education and human resource development* (5th ed.). Houston, TX: Gulf Publishing.

Kohlberg, L. (1975). The cognitive-developmental approach to moral education. *Phi Delta Kappan, 56*(10), 670–677.

Kohlberg, L. (1981). *Essays on moral development, volume 1: The philogosophy of moral development.* New York: Harper & Row.

Kolb, D. A. (1984). *Experiential learning: Experience as the source of learning and development.* Englewood Cliffs, NJ: Prentice-Hall.

Krawczyk, R. M. (1997). Teaching ethics: Effect on moral development. *Nursing Ethics, 4*(1), 56-65.

Leasure, A. R., Davis, L., & Thievon, S. (2000). Evaluating reflective writing for appropriateness, fairness, and consistency. *Journal of Nursing Education, 39,* 149–155.

Leenerts, M. H. (2003). Teaching personal knowledge as a way of knowing self in therapeutic relationship. *Nursing Outlook, 51,* 158-164.

Luckowski, A. (2003). Concept mapping as a critical thinking tool for nurse educators. *Journal for Nurses in Staff Development, 19,* 225-230.

Marino, T. (2000). *Using technology to create a safe, humantistic classroom.* Retrieved January 26, 2007 from http://www.Tltgroup.org/resources/rmarinosafe2.html

McCarthy, P., Schuster, P., Zehr, P., & McDougal, D. (1999). Evaluation of critical thinking in a baccalaureate nursing program. *Journal of Nursing Education, 38,* 142–144.

Mester, J. (2003). *Transfer of learning: Issues and research agenda.* Report of a workshop on transfer of knowledge held at the National Science Foundation in Arlington, VA, March 21–22, 2002. Retrieved January 28, 2007 from http://www.nsf.gov/pubs/2003/nsf/03212/nsf03212_.pdf

Montgomery, S., & Groat, L. (1998). *Learner learning styles and their implications for teaching.* Center for Research on Learning and Teaching. Retrieved April 14, 2002 from http://www.crit.umich.edu/occ10.html

National Council of State Boards of Nursing. (2006). *Fast facts about alternate item formats and the NCLEX examination.* Retrieved September 14, 2006 from http://www.ncsbn.org/pdfs/01_08_04altitm.pdf

National League for Nursing Accrediting Commission. (1997). *Interpreting Guidelines for Standards and Criteria* (Rev ed.). (Publication No. 15-7681). New York: NLN Accrediting Commission.

Papes, K. A. (1998). *The relationships among nursing program attributes, nurse faculties' personal attributes and preferences for learn-centered instruction.* Unpublished doctoral dissertation, Florida Atlantic University. Retrieved January 25, 2007 from http://digitalcommons.fau.edu/dissertations/AA19913292

Phillips, J. M. (2005). Syllabus selections: Innovative learning activities. Chat role play as an online learning strategy. *Journal of Nursing Education, 9,* 43-44.

Profetto-McGrath, J. (2003). The relationship of critical thinking skills and critical thinking dispositions of baccalaureate nursing learners. *Journal of Advanced Nursing, 43,* 569–577.

Reising, D. L. (2004). Syllabus selections. The outcome-present state-testing model applied to classroom settings. *Journal of Nursing Education, 43,* 431-432.

Rosignol, M. (1997). Relationship between selected discourse strategies and learner critical thinking. *Journal of Nursing Education, 36,* 467–475.

Scriven, M., & Paul, R. (2004). *Defining critical thinking.* Retrieved September 14, 2006 from http://www.criticalthinking.org/aboutCT/definingCR.shtml

Sellappah, S., Hussey, T., Blackmore, A. M., & McMurray, A. (1998). The use of questioning strategies by clinical teachers. *Journal of Advanced Nursing, 28,* 142–144.

Sharif, F., & Masoumi, S. (2005). *A qualitative study of nursing learner experiences of clinical practice.* Retrieved September 7, 2006 from http://www.biomedcentral.com/1472-6955/4/6/

Shell, R. (2001). Perceived barriers to teaching critical thinking by BSN nursing faculty. *Nursing and Health Care Perspectives, 22,* 286-291.

Shin, K., Jung, D. Y., Shin, S., & Kim, M. S. (2006). Critical thinking dispositions and skills of senior nursing learners in associate, baccalaureate, and RN-to-BSN programs. *Journal of Nursing Education, 45*(6), 233–237.

Southern Regional Education Board Council on Collegiate Education in Nursing. (2002, February). *SREB study indicates serious shortage of nursing faculty. Faculty Shortage Committee 2001 Survey Report.* (Report 02N3). Atlanta, GA: Author.

Spelic, S., Parsons, M., Hercinger, M., Andrews, A., Parks, J., & Norris, J. (2001). Evaluation of critical thinking outcomes of a BSN program. *Holistic Nursing Practice, 15*(3), 27–34.

Staib, S. (2003). Teaching and measuring critical thinking. *Journal of Nursing Education, 42,* 498-508.

Stock-Ward, S. R., & Javorek, M. E. (2003). Applying theory to practice: Supervision in learner affairs. *NASPA Journal, 40*(3), 77-92.

Stone, C., Davidson, L., Evans, J., & Hansen, M. (2001). Validity evidence for using a general critical thinking test to measure nursing learners' critical thinking. *Holistic Nursing Process, 15*(3), 27–34.

Stuart, G. W., Hoge, M. A., & Tondora, J. (2004). *Theory and evidence-based teaching strategies: Implications for behavioral health.* Retrieved September 7, 2006 from http://www.annapolis-coalition.org/pdfs/Teaching_Strategies+2-02-04.pdf

Su, W., Osisec, P., & Starnes, B. (2004). Applying the revised Bloom's taxonomy to a medical-surgical nursing lesson. *Nurse Educator, 29,* 116-120.

Su, W., Osisec, P., & Starnes, B. (2005). Using the revised Bloom's taxonomy in the clinical laboratory: Thinking skills involved in diagnostic reasoning. *Nurse Educator, 30,*117-122.

Tomey, A. M. (2003). Learning with cases. *Journal of Continuing Education in Nursing, 34*(1), 34-38.

Torrance, E. P. (1962). *Guiding Creative Talent.* Englewood Cliffs, NJ: Prentice-Hall.

Valiathan, P. (2002). *Blended learning modes.* Retrieved April 6, 2007 from http://www.learning circuit.org/2002/aug2002/valiathan.html

Valiga, T. (2003). Teaching thinking: Is it worth the effort? *Journal of Nursing Education, 42,* 479-480.

Wagner, P. S., & Ash, K. L. (1998). Educational innovations. Creating the teachable moment. *Journal of Nursing Education, 27,* 278-280.

Walker, J. T., Martin, T., White, J., Elliot, R., Norwood, A., Mangum, C., & Haynie, L. (2004). Generation (Age) differences in nursing learners' preferences for teaching methodology. *Journal of Nursing Education, 45*(9), 371-374.

Walsh, C. M., & Seldomridge, L. A. (2006). Critical thinking: Back to square two. *Journal of Nursing Education, 45*(6), 212–218.

Watson, G. B., & Glaser, E. M. (1994). *Watson-Glaser Critical Thinking Appraisal Form S Manual.* San Antonio, TX: Harcourt Brace.

Wetzig, S. M. (2004). *Learning style preferences and learning strategies in intensive care nurse education.* Retrieved January 25, 2007 from http://eprint.uq.edu.au/archive/00001272

Yancey, N. R. (2004). Witnessing change with aspiring nurses: A human becoming teaching-learning process in nursing education. *Nursing Science Quarterly, 17*(1), 36-41.

TWO

Effective Learning Systems

■ **INSTRUCTIONAL GOALS**

Upon completion of this chapter and the nurse educator learning experiences, the learner will be able to:

- ■ Critique learning objectives using Bloom's taxonomy
- ■ Apply Mager's instructional objectives theory to written examples
- ■ Demonstrate Gagne's nine instructional events
- ■ Apply Bandura's cognitive learning theory
- ■ Write a definition of a learning system
- ■ Devise written evaluation procedures
- ■ Demonstrate sequencing of learning content
- ■ Choose active learning teaching methods from a list of strategies
- ■ Discuss learning system problems with a group of learners
- ■ List essential aspects of learning contracts
- ■ Verbalize the difference between a curriculum and a learning system

Upon completion of this chapter, the more advanced nurse educator will be able to:

- Model a procedure for classmates or nursing learners and use Bandura's social cognitive principles to evaluate her performance and identify teaching or research implications
- Devise a table comparing Gagne's conditions of instruction with Bloom's taxonomy and give examples of each that are pertinent to teaching nurse learners
- Teach three novice nurse educators how to construct behavioral objectives using Bloom's taxonomy and Mager's goal theory
- Build a curriculum for a nursing program starting with the course objectives and content by level and matching them to school, college, or program goals
- Design a research problem statement with motivation of learners as the theme

Key Terms

Affective learning domain	Learning systems
Bandura's social cognitive theory	Lesson plans
Behavioral objectives	Motivation
Cognitive domain	Post-test
Criterion-referenced grading	Pretests
Curriculum	Preview method
Deductive learning	Problem solving
Discovery method	Productive & reproductive learning
Disputation method	Prompts
Educator/learner contract	Psychomotor domain
Evidence-based learning	Purpose of instruction
Fidelity	Reliability
Generation X & Y learners	Taxonomy
Inductive learning	Validity

Introduction

Learning occurs when effective learning systems are in place. This chapter provides theory and specific ideas to help nurse educators design, implement, and evaluate effective learning systems and shows how learning systems relate to a nursing curriculum and learning objectives. Specific topics covered include: formulating learning objectives based on Bloom's taxonomy, using Gagne's conditions of learning theory to insure effective learning, examining examples of Bandura's cognitive learning and self-efficacy theory, considering Mager's goal theory, sequencing content, timing the presentation of material, dealing with environmental restraints, identifying and changing ineffective learning systems, developing learning contracts, evaluating learning, and aspects of evidence-based learning.

Designing Effective Learning Systems

Designing effective **learning systems** requires knowledge of learning, learning theory, learning systems, and the learner. It also includes skills in writing behavioral objectives and learning contracts, and building a curriculum. A beginning question for nurse educators who hope to develop effective learning systems is, "What kinds of learning are there?" There are four basic types of learning systems, which include:

1. trial and error
2. deductive and inductive approaches
3. discovery
4. social cognitive learning.

Trial and Error Learning

The least efficient way to learn is through trial and error learning, trying one approach and then another, with no guiding theory or principles. This is like reinventing the wheel every time the learner wants to progress.

Deductive Learning

Giving a definition and following it with examples is the **deductive** approach to learning. An example of deductive learning is giving a definition of anxiety and then following it up with examples of anxiety.

> Deductive learning includes giving a definition first and then providing examples.

Inductive Learning

The opposite process to deductive learning is **inductive learning**. Giving examples of a concept and then following it with a definition or assisting learners to formulate the definition is the inductive approach. When learners are asked to "discover" the definition, the **discovery method** of learning is used, a type of inductive learning. When using this approach, it is imperative that examples of a concept are clear and demonstrate only one characteristic difference. It is also useful to provide examples of situations that do not fit the concept (nonexamples). Examples and nonexamples must be plentiful, and the instructor must be vigilant so learners do not formulate the wrong definition. To monitor movements toward a wrong definition, provide counterexamples. For example, a learner might make the false discovery that crises are unexpected events if no examples of developmental crises are available.

> Inductive learning includes giving examples of a concept and then following it with a definition.

> The discovery method of learning includes asking learners to discover the definition by being presented with examples and nonexamples of a concept.

In addition to examples and nonexamples being presented to learners, preview and advanced practice can be used to assure concept learning. When using the **preview method,** learners are given time to inspect materials or equipment, to read related articles, to view films, or to participate in a mini-exercise or simulation that depicts the concept. All preview materials should underline the important aspects of the examples in order to focus the learners' attention on these. Once learners are able to discriminate between simple examples and nonexamples, more complex examples are used, with properties that are not easily identified and with many properties included in the definition. Examples may differ on more than one property, and there should be no prompts or cues to the learner to attend to aspects of the examples (Diamond, 1998; Davis, 1974).

> In the preview method, learners inspect materials or equipment, and participate in mini-exercises or simulations that depict the concept.

Social Cognitive Learning

Bandura (1977, 1986, 1997, 2001) developed a **social cognitive theory** that has been widely used and accepted (Graham & Weiner, 1996). Bandura wrote that individuals possess self-beliefs that can enable them to exercise control over their thoughts, feelings, and actions.

Self-efficacy, or the belief in one's ability to perform adequately, has proven to be a more consistent predictor of behavioral outcomes than other motivational constructs (Graham & Weiner, 1996). Learners with high self-efficacy expect higher grades and put forth the effort to get them. They approach difficult tasks as challenges rather than as situations to be avoided. Certain environmental characteristics can result in even highly self-efficacious and well-skilled learners choosing not to behave in concert with their beliefs and abilities if they:

- Lack the incentive
- Lack the necessary resources
- Perceive social constraints

Bandura wrote that learning would be laborious and hazardous if learners had to rely on only themselves (1977). Luckily, learners have educators to model appropriate behavior for them. This vicarious learning permits individuals to learn novel behaviors without going through the arduous task of trial and error learning.

Bandura emphasized the importance of modeling behaviors, attitudes, and emotional reactions (1977). He believed that it was the human capability to symbolize that allowed learners to:

- Extract meaning from the environment
- Construct guides for action
- Solve problems cognitively
- Support well thought-out courses of action
- Gain new knowledge by reflective thought
- Communicate with others at any distance in time and space
- Use self-reflection to make sense of their experiences, and
- Engage in self-evaluation and alter their thinking and behavior accordingly (Bandura, 1986).

■ Nurse Educator Challenge

Based on what you know about Bandura's theory, what is the role of the educator in relation to learners?

Social Cognitive Theory Principles

Principles of Bandura's theory include:

1. The highest level of observation learning is achieved by first organizing and rehearsing the modeled behavior symbolically and then enacting it overtly.
2. Coding modeled behavior into words, labels, or images results in better retention of information than does simply observing.
3. Individuals are more likely to adopt a modeled behavior if it results in outcomes they value, if the role model has admired status, and if the behavior has functional value.
4. Self-efficacy beliefs are paramount; level of motivation, affective states, and actions are based more on what learners believe than on what is objectively true.

Jason, a seasoned nurse educator, had been using Bandura's social learning theory for many years. Just recently, he'd been experimenting with several of the principles from Bandura's theory. Jason set up a role playing situation he wanted to use in class. He planned to ask participants to wear signs around their necks indicating the main concept they were portraying.

■ Nurse Educator Challenge

Which of Bandura's principles was Jason demonstrating?

Implications of Bandura's Social Cognitive Theory

The implications of Bandura's social cognitive theory are that nurse educators take care to role model positive behaviors, attitudes, and emotional reactions when teaching learners. Nurse educators must also provide a learning environment that allows learners to extract meaning from it and use social persuasion based on attainable success to help learners create and develop high self-efficacy beliefs. Other implications of Bandura's social cognitive theory are that nurse educators must remove real or imagined social or resource constraints to increase incentives to produce competent performances, help learners use self-reflection and self-evaluation to alter their thinking and behavior toward high self-efficacy, and provide learning incentives and adequate resources, as well as remove social constraints.

Devon, a seasoned nurse educator, planned to role model the most effective way to obtain an intake interview, allow learners to practice small segments of the interview process, and ask them to evaluate their learning experience in a journal.

■ **Nurse Educator Challenge**

Which of Bandura's principles did Devon overlook and how would you supply them?

Learning Systems

A **learning system** is an interdependent combination of people, media, and materials that interact to achieve a goal. In the systems approach to instruction, the teaching/learning process is planned to facilitate learning. A specific methodology is used to design, implement, and evaluate the teaching/learning process. This methodology is directed at achieving

> A learning system is an interdependent combination of people, media, and materials that work together to achieve a goal.

specified objectives and is based on research in human learning and communication (Diamond, 1998; Davis, 1993).

> Alexander, a new nurse educator, wasn't sure what kind of teaching/ learning activity to plan for his first classroom experience. After planning first a role playing situation and then a case study, he finally decided to keep it simple. He asked the learners to read an article and report back on their findings.

■ **Nurse Educator Challenge**

What evidence is there that Alexander provided a learning system? Give a rationale for your answer.

The minimum requirements for a learning system consist of:

■ A learner
■ A learning goal
■ A procedure for achieving the goal

By this definition, self-paced or individualized materials, programmed instructional materials, and small-group exercises used by learners according to specified instructions are learning systems. A learning system need not include an educator except in its design. Some learning systems do include visibly present educators or facilitators. A group of learners who have been given a learning goal and then receive a lecture compose one type of learning system. Many learning systems added together constitute a curriculum.

In the past, memorization of predigested amounts of information was sufficient. Now, process goals such as creativity, inquiry, and inductive thinking require that objectives be tied to the curriculum, teaching/learning strategies, and learner needs (Kizlik, 2006; Joyce and Weil, 2004).

Choosing Teaching/Learning Methods

The choice of teaching method is dependent on educator style and repertoire of skills, learner preferences and learning needs, and the qualities or teaching effectiveness of the available methods. The skill repertoire of the nurse educator can be increased by studying and using the methods that appear in the remaining chapters in this book. Learner preferences can be assessed using Box 1–3 in Chapter 1. Learning needs can be assessed by devising a written, verbal, or action pretest.

> **Fidelity is the quality associated with practicing in a realistic setting that is similar to the real-life situation.**

There are some guidelines based on learning method qualities that can help to select the teaching method of choice. The more realistic the practice component of the teaching method, the more likely the learner will be to apply learning in the referent situation. This quality is called **fidelity**.

Sonya, a nurse educator, selected two learning methods that were of equal fidelity. She knew she wouldn't have time to use both in one class and wasn't sure what to do.

■ Nurse Educator Challenge

What should Sonya do? Give a rationale for your answer.

When methods are equal in effect, the least expensive should be used. This is the *quality of cost*. If methods are equal in effect and cost, the safest one should be utilized. This is the *quality of safety*, and it can apply to safety for the client or the learner. Safety for the learner includes practice that will not unduly expose the learner to negative learning experiences.

When methods are equal on all qualities, use the one that provides practice experiences not readily available in the real world. This is the *quality of completeness* (Davis, 1993; Davis, 1974). Box 2–1 compares the methods presented in later chapters by their qualities.

It is possible to modify qualities of some methods. For example, by only using videotape with small, cohesive groups of learners, they can be protected from unnecessary exposure of their lack of skill or of their thoughts and feelings. Likewise, if nurse educators are skilled in developing their own inexpensive simulations, simulation games, self-paced materials, and programmed instructional materials and in operating their own audio- and videotape or videoconferencing equipment, cost may be decreased. Subsequent chapters assist nurse educators to develop their own teaching materials.

Box 2–1   Comparison of Learning Methods and Their Qualities

| Method | Quality | | | |
	Fidelity	Cost	Safety	Completeness
Simulations, simulation games	Excellent	Inexpensive to expensive	Safe	Incomplete
Peer supervision	Moderate to good	Inexpensive	Possibly unsafe	Quite complete
Self-paced materials	Moderate to good	Inexpensive to expensive	Safe	Complete
Video and audiotape	Moderate to good	Expensive	Possibly unsafe	Complete
Perceptual exercises, journal writing, value clarification	?	Inexpensive	Safe	Complete
Programmed instruction	Moderate	Inexpensive to expensive	Safe	Complete
Small groups	Moderate	Inexpensive	Possibly unsafe	Complete

Teaching/learning methods are chosen based on the purpose of instruction.

In addition to the qualities of fidelity, cost, safety, and completeness, the tips that follow can help in the selection of teaching/learning methods based on the **purpose of instruction**.

1. If objectives such as learning to learn and learner responsibility for learning are the focus, self-paced materials are appropriate.
2. If learning objectives include pre-practice in a safe environment and an integrated cognitive, affective, and perceptual-motor approach, simulations and simulation games are appropriate.
3. When immediate feedback and presentation of self to others are important, audio- and videotape and videoconferencing methods can be used.
4. When content can be broken down into small, sequential bits of knowledge and when learners learn individually, programmed materials are useful.
5. When learners are blocked from other learning, affective learning is important, and perceptual exercises, journal writing, and/or value clarification are effective when values, moral development, or ethics are the focus.
6. Peer supervision or small-group methods are helpful if input, collaboration with peers, and learning leadership qualities are essential learning objectives.

Learner-Centered Syllabus

According to Diamond (1998), a learner-centered syllabus can help:

- Define learner responsibilities and help manage time by providing a clearer idea of what is expected and a time frame for accomplishing it
- Improve learner note-taking and studying
- Reduce anxiety by providing sample test questions, readings that may be difficult to obtain, and important handouts
- Improve learner efficiency by including detailed descriptions of major assignments with sample expected responses

Possible content for a learner-centered syllabus includes:

1. Title and number of course
2. Letter of welcome to the learner describing the intent, purpose, and overall goal(s)
3. Table of contents
4. Purpose of the learner manual and how to use it

5. Introduction including how the course fits in the general program and for whom it was designed, general directions for learners, where notices, grades, and related items will be posted

6. Personnel involved in the course and how to contact them, office hours, and an e-mail address

7. Overview of the course, including course outline, module outline, options, and course objectives

8. Evaluation and grading procedures including credits, grading system, scales, or forms

9. Logistical forms including change option, notification form of faculty of problems with learning materials

10. Textbook(s) including where to get it, how to get it, and how to use it

11. Calendar that includes topics by class meeting, projects due, and deadlines

12. Facilities that will be used

13. Checklist for due date of assignments

14. Self-tests for learners to evaluate their ability to meet course objectives

15. Additional information on using the library and/or computing center

16. Online segments including description of how to log online to the course, how to contact the school or university's Help Desk, how to use the e-mail system, the nurse educator's email address, where to find online postings of the class syllabus and schedule, and any additional other information such as forums, online exams, etc.

Lesson Plans

In the traditional lecture approach, a **lesson plan** that contains sequential components is used. It contains the following phases:

> A lesson plan contains sequential learning components.

1. *Motivation*—a specified period of time is spent or materials are used to evoke learner interest in the topic.

2. *Aim*—a specified period of time is spent in activities to help learners focus on learning objectives and formulate a problem or question.

3. *Development*—a specified period of time is spent in lecture, demonstration, laboratory, audiovisual experiences, or discussions to permit learners to learn cognitive, affective, or perceptual-motor skills.

4. *Pivotal questions*—a specified period of time is spent or materials are used to draw out ideas, detect learning difficulties, and move the interaction forward. Questions are used to help learners recall material presented to date and to tie past learning to new material. Acquisition and coding are enhanced by this process.

5. *Summary and evaluation*—a specified period of time is spent (and materials may be used) to summarize and evaluate what has been presented.

6. *Assignment*—a specified period of time is spent (and materials may be used) to prepare learners for accompanying work or the next class period. Assignments that enhance transfer and provide for practice or review will promote retention of material.

7. *Additional items*—a specified period of time is spent in assisting learners to work through learning problems with the teacher, report on related events, or share learning experiences with peers. Effective learning can be enhanced and resistances to learning and sharing can be decreased in this period.

The amount of time spent on each of the seven categories will vary by nurse educator, content, and learner population.

Timing Presentation of Materials

Timing of learning materials is an important issue for the nurse educator. If the method chosen to present material is lecture (or a modified version), the issue of timing is often resolved through the use of a lesson plan. When self-paced materials are used, learners time their own work. Whenever classroom time is used for learning, the educator must consider how to use the time to best advantage. Lesson plans are one way to do this.

> Jim, a nurse educator, was planning a class period. He tried to make sure he divided the time between all seven categories. When he thought about class, it soon became clear he'd made a mistake in his planning. He decided to forget about his lesson plan and wing it. He dumped his learning plan into the waste receptacle.

■ **Nurse Educator Challenge**

Do you agree with Jim's action? Give a rationale for your answer.

Novice nurse educators tend to disregard classroom plans and even whole learning systems when there are indicants that the plans or systems are ineffective in some way. Prior to discarding any plan or learning system, an evaluation of each part of the system should be made, including use of learning theory, presentation of content, structure of materials, and evaluation and sequencing difficulties.

In addition to assessing what was wrong with a class period or learning system, it is important to identify what was right or useful and to make written comments on both aspects. This will assist in obtaining a more objective and balanced view of classroom work. It can also serve as a goal to work toward as well as a reward for having achieved some success. The Nurse Educator Tip that follows provides a way to evaluate lesson plans.

Nurse Educator Tips

Evaluate Your Lesson Plans

To evaluate your lesson plans, ask:

- Was motivation lacking or ineffective?
- Were learners effectively assisted in focusing on the chosen topic?
- Was the wrong method used to develop the topic?
- Were questions unclear, always directed to the same learners, or irrelevant?
- Was insufficient time allotted to accomplishing the objectives?
- Were activity directions unclear?
- Were learners observing, rather than being actively involved?
- Were there difficulties with equipment or materials?
- Was the summary omitted, too brief, or unprofitable?
- Was the assignment inadequately covered?
- Was insufficient time allotted for emerging teaching or learning problems or for feedback and sharing among learners?

Learning Contracts

The design of a learning system will be influenced by the quantity of educator and learner input. A major issue in instructional procedures is the **educator/ learner contract**.

> Educator/learner contracts can be educator or learner assigned or made.

There are a number of basic contracts including:

- *The educator-made and educator-assigned contract*—in this kind of contract, the teacher makes all the decisions concerning the content and sequence of learning activities. This contract is most commonly used in individualized instruction approaches.
- *The educator-made and learner-assigned contract*—learners are able to select a contract based on their own choices and preferences. The educator prepares a number of contracts, and learners choose those that appeal to them.
- *The learner-made and learner-assigned contract*—this contract is based on areas identified by learners as those where they have interest or are academically weak. Once learners begin to learn to assess their own instructional needs and special areas of interest or nursing specialty, such a contract has implied objectives and potential for learning to learn and lifelong learning.

The jointly written contract is developed between educator and learner during a series of meetings. The content of the contract and the procedures surrounding it are discussed and forged through discussion. This type of contract has potential for teaching cooperative and collaborative skills, for working through two-person teaching/learning difficulties, and for developing mentor or sponsor relationships where educators and learners are on a more equal basis than in traditional learning situations. A learning contract of this type includes:

- An initial description of the learner's work,
- The specific goals, purposes, and time frame for the work,
- A description of learning activities and resources, and
- The evaluation criteria to be used to evaluate attainment of learning goals.

Nurse educators who use this method have a special opportunity to assist learners in developing and maximizing their own unique abilities and their own learning styles. When learner input and independence is great, they cannot help but influence the ability to function as an independent practitioner in referent situations.

How can independent learners be educated in traditional classrooms when the educator makes all relevant decisions and learners are passive and dependent? Box 2–2 shows a sample written collaborative contract for a course in group dynamics.

Box 2–2   Sample Nurse Educator/Learner Collaborative Contract

---

Collaborative nurse educator/learner contract between:
Sylvia Tyrone and Carolyn Chambers Clark

Course: Group Dynamics

A. **My goals:** I hope to work in pediatrics and I would like to become skilled in group work with children.

B. **Group skills I have:** I have taught church school and Girl Scouts for three years. I participated in a sensitivity group for a weekend marathon.

C. **Group skills I need:** I need to develop ways of directing the movement of a group more effectively. I tend to sit back and let the group lead itself. I need to read on the subject of group theories and practice applying them with (simulated) groups.

D. **To help improve my group skills, I plan to do the following:**
   1. Survey the literature and (with assistance from the instructor) choose appropriate readings.
   2. Lead a group of hospitalized children for eight sessions.
   3. Participate in group simulations and videotape replay of my participation in these simulations as pre-practice for actual group leadership.
   4. Complete the programmed instructional unit on recording in groups.
   5. Complete three recordings of group sessions to criterion.
   6. Present excerpts of three process recordings to the instructor verbally, using the brief presentation form to evaluate my work.
   7. Present excerpts of three group process recordings to a peer verbally, using the brief presentation form to evaluate my work and obtain feedback from the student.

Building a Curriculum

Jessie, a PhD nursing education learner, plans to develop a nursing curriculum as one of her requirements to obtain her degree. She has no idea where to start and when she does an Internet search, she doesn't find much information. Because their school recently revised its curriculum, Jessie decides to interview several nursing educators and find out more about how to develop a curriculum. Here's what she discovered.

A **curriculum** is an educational program designed to meet specified goals. The nursing curriculum is an example. It consists of all the content and teaching approaches used to meet identified goals (learning systems).

> A curriculum includes all the content and teaching approaches used to meet program learning goals.

A nursing curriculum flows from a philosophy of nursing education. Major concepts are threaded throughout courses. Examples of major concepts are:

- Evidence-based practice
- Informatics/communication
- Interdisciplinary teams
- Client-centered care
- Mind-body-spirit (holism)
- Learner centered environments

Organizing frameworks for curricula include:

- NLN competencies, such as provider of care and manager of care.
- NCSBN Core Competencies, such as professional behaviors, communication, assessment, clinical decision making, caring interventions, teaching and learning, or collaboration.
- NCLEX Test Plan, including safe, effective care environment, health promotion and maintenance, psychosocial integrity, physiological integrity, functional health patterns, and systems.
- The American Holistic Nursing Association (AHNA) standards, theories, and concepts including nurses as models of wellness, promoting client self-responsibility and self-care, the nurse as a healing environment, meaning and wholeness, and the holistic nursing process.

■ Nurse Educator Challenge

What framework should Jessie choose? Give a rationale for your position.

Building a curriculum is an interactive process. Educational outcomes or terminal objectives (what the learner will be able to do upon graduation) specify the curriculum and relate back to major concepts identified in the philosophy. Level objectives or course objectives move the learner toward terminal objectives. Levels of a program demonstrate progression and provide the framework for clinical evaluation. The objectives for the final course are the same as the educational outcomes or terminal objectives.

■ **Nurse Educator Challenge**

Develop three terminal objectives for the framework you chose.

Course objectives determine the content for each course, with the organizing framework providing structure for the content. Objectives should be achievable and reflect the philosophy of nursing. Because it is impossible to cover every topic, the challenge in designing a curriculum is to identify critical concepts.

■ **Nurse Educator Challenge**

Study the curriculum and learning objectives for your school or college. Are there any concepts or objectives that could be deleted? Give a rationale for your decision.

When the curriculum is in harmony with teaching approaches, learning goals are met. A curriculum sketches the framework and broad design, while the teaching/learning process actualizes it (Joyce and Weil, 2004.)

Evidence-Based Learning

The most common method of teaching continues to be standing in front of the class and transmitting knowledge via lecture. This method often continues even though evidence shows that active, self-directed, problem-based learning (evidence-based learning) is more effective than traditional, lecture-based learning (Beers and Bowden, 2005; Hill et al., 1997; Jamrozik, 1996; Schwartz, Donnelly, Nash, and Young, 1992; Shin, Haynes, and Johnston, 1993; Schmidt, 1993; Patel, Groen, and Norman, 1991; Friedman, DeBliek, and Norman, 1990; Woodward, 1990), and better liked by learners.

> Evidence-based learning means learning that is based on research findings.

Problem-based approaches can also be more effective than lecture in the areas of communication and self-directed learning, level of independence, and satisfaction with the course (Rideout et al., 2002), effective performance (Smits et al., 2003), and in positive attitude toward course content (Pugsley and Clayton, 2003).

For learners to use new information, they need to structure, organize, and integrate the information with their previous knowledge. But there appears to be a disconnect between what faculty want to do—*cover content*—and what adult learners need and request—*active, problem-based learning* (Sharif and Masoumi, 2005; Candela, Dalley, and Benzel-Lindley, 2006).

Many nursing faculty believe they must cover content but what learners need to learn is usually covered in their textbooks or assigned readings. As Candela, Dalley and Benzel-Lindley (2006) remind nurse educators, teacher-centered education is no longer adequate to prepare today's learners to perform adequately in the complex health care system. Instead of asking, "What do I need to cover in class?" nurse educators need to ask, "What do learners need to and want to learn to feel equipped to function as a professional in clinical situations?"

Clinical Learning

One example of what learners need that may not be provided in many settings was made apparent in one study. The nursing learners in the study reported their dissatisfaction with the way they were prepared for their clinical experience. They described feeling incompetent and lacking professional nursing skills, and having a need to learn ways to handle their anxiety about performing while being evaluated (Candela et al., 2006).

■ **Nurse Educator Challenge**

If you were teaching the nurse learners in the Candela study, what would you do?

Age Differences in Learning

Learner needs may differ by age. For example, **Generation X learners** (born between 1965 and 1976) tend to:

- Be highly independent,
- Challenge authority frequently,
- Solve problems independently, and
- Multitask.

Generation Y learners (who began entering college in 2000) are:

- The most culturally diverse group of all time,
- Self-reliant,
- Questioning,
- Technologically advanced,
- Expecting others to earn respect, and
- Addicted to visual media.

Nurse educators must develop teaching methods that align with the expectations, values, and needs of these learners (Walker et al., 2006).

> Generation X learners are highly independent, challenging, problem solving, multitasking.

> Generation Y learners are culturally diverse, self-reliant, questioning, technologically advanced, expecting others to earn respect, and are addicted to visual media.

Health Care Shifts and Learning

In addition to learner needs, changes in the health care environment dictate a shift in nurse educator goals. With the shift from acute to chronic health care, and from curing to caring, lifestyle has become an essential component in health promotion (Stark, Manning-Walsh, and Vliem, 2005). Being a healing presence to clients requires that nurses learn to care for and nurture themselves (Burkhardt and Nagai-Jacobson, 2001).

Credentialing and Learning

One area of nursing that has not kept up with learning theory is credentialing and certifying examinations for practice. The questions on these exams are only weakly linked, if at all, to performance in clinical practice (Harden, Grant, Buckley and Hart, 1999). Teaching to exams and state boards in no way guarantees learners will be proficient in clinical care.

Active Learning Processes

What is a nurse educator to use to promote critical thinking and self-directed learning if lecturing is not the answer? Studies show that active learning procedures are more apt to promote critical thinking. Chapters 3-6 explore ways to design and use active learning systems that enhance critical thinking, including:

- Structured role play,
- Simulations and simulation games,

- Peer supervision,
- Self-paced learning materials,
- Programmed instructional materials,
- Audiovisual and computer methods of learning,
- Perceptual exercises,
- Journal writing, value clarification, small-group methods, and
- Other novel strategies that work well even with large classes.

No matter what type of learning system is being developed, behavioral objectives are crucial.

Behavioral Objectives

Behavioral objectives are statements of what learners are to be like when they have successfully attained the criterion. Behavioral objectives are tied to criteria, tests,

> Behavioral objectives are statements of what learners are to be like when they've attained the criterion.

and other measures of successful achievement in a course. Since it is impossible to look inside a learner's head and know if they understand a concept, nurse educators depend on objectives that detail observed behaviors. Without clear behaviorally-defined objectives that are shared by nurse educator and learner, measures of achievement can be misleading, irrelevant, unfair or useless.

Learning objectives spell out expected learning outcomes, but they are not a substitute for a philosophy of instruction or for expertise in teaching/learning methods. Learning objectives are not course descriptions or lists of what the teacher hopes to accomplish in the course, but precise ways of stating instructional goals (Kizlik, 2006).

Taxonomies of Learning Objectives

Just as nursing philosophy guides curriculum, learning objectives guide the development of a learning system. A Committee of Colleges led by Bloom, Englehart, Furst, Hill, and Krathwohl developed a taxonomy of cognitive or thinking objectives in 1956. These objectives were revised by Anderson and Krathwohl in 2001. Bloom's taxonomy continues to be one of the most universally applied models. Simpson (1972) developed the psychomotor taxonomy for manual skills. Later, Krathwohl, Bloom, and Bertram (1973) developed the education objectives for the affective (feeling, valuing) domain.

A **taxonomy** is an orderly classification. In this case, Bloom and associates classified thinking skills into learning objectives.

> A taxonomy is an orderly classification.

They appear in six levels, from the most basic (remembering, understanding, and applying) to the higher order levels of thinking (analyzing, evaluating, and creating). At the graduate level, most learning objectives are usually developed at the higher levels of thinking. The purpose of writing behavioral objectives is to define what is to be mastered by the end of a course. Using detailed objectives will help learners understand the purpose of each classroom activity by clarifying the learning outcome. It is best to avoid using verbs that do not define an explicit performance, such as know, appreciate, internalize, and value (Mager, 1997).

Websites Using or Explaining Bloom's Taxonomy

Stella, a new nurse educator, was planning a new community education course on family health. She went online to some of the Bloom Web sites including:

http://rite.edu.qut.edu.au/oz-teachernet/training/bloom.html
http://www.tedi.uq.edu.au/Assess/Assessment/bloomtax.html
http://www.officeport.com/edu/blooms.htm
http://www.utexas.edu/learner/utic/handouts/1414.html
http://www.coun.uvic.ca/learn/program/hndouts/bloom.html
http://www.kent/wednet.edu/KSD/MA/resources/blooms/teachers_blooms.html
http://eduscarpes.com/tap/topic69.htm
http://coe/sdsu.edu/eet/articles/bloomrev/index.htm

Once Stella had a basic understanding of Bloom's objectives, she created the cognitive objectives listed in the next section.

Cognitive Behavioral Learning Objectives

The **cognitive domain** involves knowledge and the development of intellectual skills. This includes the recall or recognition of specific facts, procedural patterns, and concepts that serve in the development of intellectual abilities and skills. There are six major categories that are listed in order below, starting from the simplest behavior to the most complex. The categories can be thought of as degrees of difficulties. The first level of the hierarchy must be mastered before the next level can take place (Clark, 2001). Sample learning objectives for each of Bloom's six categories of cognitive behavioral learning objectives follow.

> The cognitive domain focuses on knowledge, including recall or recognition of specific facts, procedures, and concepts.

Cognitive Domain: Remembering

Remembering is the most easily attained level of cognitive learning objectives. Some verbs to use when developing learning objectives include recalling information, recognizing, listing, describing, quoting, naming, and finding (Anderson and Krathwohl, 2001). Some examples of cognitive behavioral learning objectives Stella wrote at the lowest level of Bloom's taxonomy, remembering, are:

1. **List** three cardinal rules for teaching relaxation procedures.
2. **Describe** the anatomy and physiology of the heart.
3. **Name** four side-effects of SSRIs.

■ **Nurse Educator Challenge**

How well did Stella meet Bloom's criteria for remembering? Provide a rationale for your answer.

Cognitive Domain: Understanding

Understanding is the next category on Bloom's hierarchy. Understanding includes explaining ideas or concepts. Key words to use to develop objectives include interpreting, summarizing, paraphrasing, exemplifying, classifying, and comparing (Anderson & Krathwohl, 2001). Some examples of cognitive behavioral learning objectives Stella wrote for understanding are:

1. **Explain** the importance of stress theory to clients in three clinical situations.
2. **Paraphrase** Orem's theory of self-care using your own words.
3. **Compare** Gagne's Conditions of Instruction with Bloom's taxonomy

---

■ **Nurse Educator Challenge**

How well did Stella meet Bloom's criteria for understanding? Provide a rationale for your answer.

Cognitive Domain: Applying

Applying is the last of the simpler cognitive behavioral objective categories. Applying is the ability to use information gained in another familiar situation. Key words to use to develop objectives include implementing, carrying out, using, and executing (Anderson & Krathwohl, 2001). Some examples of cognitive behavioral learning objectives for applying Stella composed are:

1. **Apply** the steps of the diagnostic conclusions handout to draw diagnostic conclusions from a given case history.
2. **Implement** a plan of care for a specified client using assessment data from an intake interview, lab findings, and observations of the client.
3. **Use** information you gained from participating in the ICU simulation game in your clinical practice in the ICU tomorrow.

■ **Nurse Educator Challenge**

How well did Stella meet Bloom's criteria for applying? Provide a rationale for your answer.

Cognitive Domain: Analyzing

Analyzing is the first step up the ladder to more difficult cognitive tasks. Analyzing includes breaking information into parts. Key words to use to develop objectives include exploring relationships, organizing, deconstructing, questioning, and defending (Anderson & Krathwohl, 2001). Sample analyzing behavioral objectives Stella created are:

1. **Organize** a class presentation in a logical and understandable fashion.
2. **Analyze** the group dynamics that took place in class this semester.
3. **Defend** research findings.

■ **Nurse Educator Challenge**

How well did Stella meet the criteria for analyzing? Provide a rationale for your answer.

Cognitive Domain: Evaluating

Evaluating is the second to the most difficult cognitive task. Evaluating includes justifying a decision or a course of action. Key words to use to develop objectives include checking, hypothesizing, critiquing, experimenting, and judging (Anderson & Krathwohl, 2001). Some examples of evaluating objectives Stella wrote are:

1. **Hypothesize** about the meaning of class behavior during the role playing situation.
2. **Critique** your thinking strategies this semester by keeping a journal of events.
3. **Experiment** with assertiveness approaches with three people this week.

■ **Nurse Educator Challenge**

How well did Stella meet Bloom's criteria for evaluating? Provide a rationale for your answer.

Cognitive Domain: Creating

Creating includes generating new ideas, products, or ways of viewing things. Key words to use to develop objectives include designing, constructing, planning, producing, inventing (Anderson & Krathwohl, 2001). Sample learning objectives Stella devised were:

1. **Plan** a role playing situation demonstrating a communication problem you encountered.
2. **Invent** a way to teach a blind and mute person how to brush his teeth.
3. **Design** a way to reduce medication errors on one clinical unit.

■ **Nurse Educator Challenge**

How well did Stella meet Bloom's criteria for creating? Provide a rationale for your answer.

Major Cognitive Knowledge Dimensions

Bloom's revised taxonomy also provides information on types of knowledge, including:

■ *Factual knowledge*—professional terminology and specific details, such as the normal anatomy and physiology of body systems.

■ *Conceptual knowledge*—knowledge of classifications and categories such as medications, herbs, and diets. Standard care procedures are also part of conceptual knowledge, and so is knowledge of theories, models, and structures, such as Orem's self-care theory, Gagne's instructional theory, and so forth.

■ *Procedural knowledge*—includes information about how to do something, such as nursing procedures; criteria for using skills, such as nursing process; and criteria for using appropriate procedures, such as when to use a lab test, when to teach post-operative home care, and when to use relaxation procedures with clients.

■ *Metacognitive knowledge*—includes thinking about your thinking, such as self-critiquing your abilities, or defending how you planned or executed care.

■ **Nurse Educator Challenge**

Which, if any, of the three types of knowledge are missing from the behavioral objectives Stella composed? Provide a rationale for your answer.

Developing Affective Learning Objectives

Bloom's **affective learning domain** focuses on the manner in which learners deal with situations. This domain targets feelings, values, appreciation, enthusiasm, motivations, and attitudes (Krathwohl, Bloom, & Bertram, 1973; Clark, 2001)

> The affective learning domain targets feelings, values, appreciation, enthusiasm, motivations, and attitudes.

Jeff, a new nurse educator, was charged with developing affective learning objectives for a new course on self-care he planned to teach with two colleagues through the community outreach and adult education department at his university. One of his colleagues, a more seasoned nurse educator, pointed him toward the Internet for help in finding Krathwohl's, Bloom's, and Bertram's affective taxonomy handbook. Jeff found that affective objectives were classified in a hierarchy beginning with receiving phenomena, moving next to responding to phenomena, then to valuing, organizing values, and ending with internalizing values.

Affective Domain: Receiving Phenomena

Receiving phenomena includes awareness, willingness to hear, and selected attention. Key words to use to develop behavioral objectives include asks, chooses, describes, follows, gives, holds, identifies, locates, names, points to, selects, sits, erects, replies, and uses (Krathwohl, Bloom, and Bertram, 1973; Clark, 2001). Jeff wrote the following receiving phenomena affective behavioral objectives:

1. **Asks** questions that are focused on the topic.
2. **Listens** to others with respect and does not interrupt or look away.
3. **Sits** in a calm and open way, indicating receptiveness to others' comments.

■ **Nurse Educator Challenge**

Did Jeff meet Krathwohl's and Bloom's criteria? Provide a rationale for your answer.

Affective Domain: Responding to Phenomena

Responding to phenomena includes active participation in class and paying attention to particular phenomena. Key words to use to develop objectives include answers, assists, aids, cooperates, discusses, greets, helps, presents, reads, recites, reports, selects, tells, and writes (Krathwohl, Bloom, and Bertram, 1973; Clark, 2001). Learning outcomes emphasize active interest in responding, willingness to respond, or satisfaction in responding (motivation). Jeff wrote the following responding to phenomena affective behavioral objectives:

1. **Participates** in class discussions in a prepared manner.
2. **Questions** concepts, models, and procedures to understand them.
3. **Practices** ethical and empathic communication in class.

■ **Nurse Educator Challenge**

Did Jeff meet Krathwohl's, Bloom's, and Bertram's criteria? Provide a rationale for your answer.

Affective Domain: Valuing

Valuing is the worth or value attached to a particular object, phenomenon, or behavior. Valuing ranges from simple acceptance to the more complex state of commitment. Key words to use to develop objectives include completes, demonstrates, differentiates, explains, follows, forms, initiates, invites, joins, justifies, proposes, reads, reports, selects, shares, studies, and works. Valuing occurs when values are internalized, but clues to values are often expressed in learner overt behavior, and making them identifiable (Clark, 2001). Jeff created the following affective behavioral objectives:

1. **Proposes** a social plan to aid the community and follows through.
2. **Demonstrates** belief in ethical behavior.
3. **Informs** class about matters one feels strongly about.

■ **Nurse Educator Challenge**

How well did Jeff do with valuing objectives? Provide a rationale for your answer.

Affective Domain: Organizes Values

Organizes values into priorities by contrasting different values, resolving conflicts between them, and creating a unique value system. The emphasis at this level is on comparing, relating, and synthesizing values. Key words to use to develop objectives include adheres, alters, arranges, combines, compares, completes, explains, defends, formulates, generalizes, integrates, modifies, orders, organizes, relates, and synthesizes (Clark, 2001). Jeff created the following affective behavioral objectives:

1. **Generalizes** new ethical standards to clinical practice.
2. **Defends** professional ethical standards by speaking up in class.
3. **Organizes** values into priorities through participating in a simulation.

■ **Nurse Educator Challenge**

Did Jeff's objectives meet the criteria for this level? Provide a rationale for your answer.

Affective Domain: Internalizing Values

Internalizing values includes having a value system that controls behavior and is pervasive, consistent, predictable, and characteristic of the learner. Key words to use to develop objectives include acts, discriminates, displays, influences, performs, practices, qualifies, revises, serves, solves, and verifies. Jeff constructed the following learning objectives:

1. **Practices** self-reliance when working independently.
2. **Displays** teamwork in group activities.
3. **Revises** judgments and changes behavior in light of new evidence.

■ **Nurse Educator Challenge**

Did Jeff meet the criteria for this level? Provide a rationale for your answer.

Psychomotor Domain

The **psychomotor domain** includes physical movement, coordination, and use of motor skills. Development of these skills requires practice and is measured by precision, procedures, or execution of techniques. Sometimes speed of performance is a factor, especially in life-threatening situations. The following seven major categories appear from the simplest behavior to the most complex behavior (Clark, 2001; Simpson, 1972).

> The psychomotor domain includes physical movement, coordination, and use of motor skills.

Psychomotor Domain: Perception

Perception is the ability to use sensory cues to guide motor activity. Important processes include sensory stimulation, cue selection, and translation of messages. Key words to use to develop objectives include chooses, describes, detects, differentiates, distinguishes, identifies, isolates, relates, and selects.

> Daisy, a clinical lab instructor, was asked to revise the psychomotor behavioral objectives for learners who used the lab. She pulled out the notes she'd taken on the psychomotor domain in her master's program and went to work on the objectives.

The psychomotor objectives Daisy constructed appear below:

1. **Detects** nonverbal communication cues.
2. **Identifies** client anxiety.
3. **Estimates** correct body placement and force needed to complete an IM injection.

■ **Nurse Educator Challenge**

How did Daisy do? Do her behavioral objectives fit with perception criteria?

Psychomotor Domain: Readiness to Act

Readiness to act includes the mental, physical, and emotional sets necessary to perform. These three sets are dispositions that predetermine response to a situation. These dispositions are sometimes called "mindsets." Key words to use to develop behavioral objectives include begins, displays, explains, moves, proceeds, reacts, shows, states, and volunteers (Simpson, 1972; Clark, 2001). Daisy developed the following objectives for this category:

1. **Displays** correct equipment to perform a nursing procedure.
2. **States** correct side effects to medication before dispensing it.
3. **Explains** steps in a procedure prior to beginning.

■ **Nurse Educator Challenge**

Did Daisy meet the criteria for this level? Provide a rationale for your answer.

Psychomotor Domain: Guided Response

Guided response occurs in the early stage of learning a complex skills. Imitation and trial and error learning are prevalent. Adequacy of performance is achieved through practice. Key words to use to construct objectives for this domain include copies, traces, follows, reacts, reproduces, and responds (Simpson, 1972; Clark, 2001). Daisy developed the following psychomotor objectives:

1. **Performs** accurate treatment setups.
2. **Responds** to instructor hand-signals while learning to work with simulated client.
3. **Follows** simulation directions.

■ **Nurse Educator Challenge**

How well did Daisy meet the criteria for this level? Provide a rationale for your answer.

Psychomotor Domain: Mechanism

Mechanism is the intermediate stage in learning a complex skill. Learned responses have become habitual and the movements can be performed with some confidence and proficiency. Key terms to use to construct objectives for this domain include assembles, calibrates, constructs, dismantles, displays, fastens, fixes, grinds, heats, manipulates, measures, mends, mixes, organizes, and sketches (Simpson, 1972; Clark, 2001). Daisy constructed the following objectives for this domain:

1. **Organizes** Web site information
2. **Displays** statistical information
3. **Measures** liquid pediatric medication

■ **Nurse Educator Challenge**

How well did Daisy meet the criteria for mechanism? Provide a rationale for your answer.

Psychomotor Domain: Complex Overt Response

Complex overt response indicates the skilled performance of motor acts that involve complex movement patterns. Proficiency at this level is indicated by adjectives such as quick, accurate, and highly coordinated performance requiring a minimum of energy. This category includes performing without hesitation in an automatic manner.

Key words are the same as for mechanism, but adverbs or adjectives indicate a better, quicker, or more accurate performance (Simpson, 1972; Clark, 2001). Daisy constructed the following objectives for this level:

1. **Pours** medications quickly and accurately.
2. **Organizes** equipment for a procedure quickly and accurately.
3. **Displays** competence while communicating with a client.

■ **Nurse Educator Challenge**

How well did Daisy meet the criteria for this level? Provide a rationale for your answer.

Psychomotor Domain: Adaptation
Adaptation means skills are well developed and the individual can modify movement patterns to meet special requirements. Key words to use to formulate objectives are adapts, alters, changes, rearranges, reorganizes, revises, and varies (Simpson, 1972; Clark, 2001). Daisy developed the following objectives for the adaptation domain:

1. **Responds** effectively to ED crises.
2. **Modifies** nursing procedure to meet client needs.
3. **Revises** instruction to meet learner needs.

■ **Nurse Educator Challenge**

Did Daisy meet the criteria for adaptation objectives? Provide a rationale for your answer.

Psychomotor Domain: Origination
Origination involves creating new movement patterns to fit a specific situation or particular problem. When skills are highly developed, creativity is possible. Key words include arranges, builds, combines, composes, constructs, creates, designs, initiates, makes, and originates (Simpson, 1972; Clark, 2001). Daisy composed the following objectives for the origination level:

1. **Constructs** a theory.
2. **Develops** a teaching module.
3. **Creates** a new imagery protocol.

■ **Nurse Educator Challenge**

Did Daisy meet the criteria for the origination level?

Articles Citing the Use of Bloom's Taxonomy

A number of articles cite Bloom's taxonomy. Goldman and Torrisi-Steele (2004) used the taxonomy to design educational multimedia for an undergraduate learning system about child sexual abuse. Holcomb (2004) used Bloom's taxonomy to develop an online master's degree program in rehabilitation.

Xu, Carne, and Ryan (2002) applied Bloom's taxonomy when evaluating learning outcomes in an educational program for an underserved population. Shuldham (1993) used the taxonomy to guide the curriculum design of a masters program in cardio-respiratory nursing. Mikol (2005) reported using behavior, cognitive, and psychomotor objectives that coincide with simulated and clinical laboratories and class discussions in a nursing course taught without lecturing. Duan (2006) examined how to select and apply taxonomies for learning outcomes, using a nursing example.

Mager's Goal Theory

Mager (1997) took learning objectives a step farther. What Mager called instructional goals, Bloom and colleagues called a taxonomy for classifying learning outcomes. Mager specified objectives. Using his theory, useful learning objectives contain:

- An audience (the learner),
- A terminal behavior or performance (what the learner is expected to do),
- Test conditions under which the performance is to occur, and
- A criterion for success (how well the learner must perform to be acceptable).

■ **Nurse Educator Challenge**

Compare and contrast Bloom's taxonomy with Mager's theory of learning objectives.

Box 2–3 lists some terminal behaviors, test conditions, and performance standards.

Box 2–3   Learning Objective Components and Examples

Terminal behaviors	Test conditions	Performance standards
Label the circulatory system	Given a diagram of the circulatory system	Labeling nine of the numbers drawn on the diagram
Present a teaching session on the emotional aspects of diabetes	Given one hour of class time	Covering six of the seven aspects covered in class
Identify by underlining the side effects of tranquilizers	Given a written test and a time period of 20 minutes	Answering nine of ten questions correctly
List in writing the major theories of the etiology of depression	After viewing a film on depression	Completing quiz in 15 minutes after viewing film
Give a bedbath	Given a simulated client	Completing bedbath in 20 minutes, following all steps listed in procedure manual
State the feelings of a client	Given a simulated client	Completing a 15-minute interview using the Communication Skills Checklist
Conduct a group session with peers	Given a topic to cover	Ensuring all students speak at least once

Examples of Instructional Goals and Their Learning Objectives

Some examples of instructional goals and their learning objectives follow:

Instructional goal: For the learner to demonstrate empathy in a nurse/client interaction.

Learning objective: With a simulated client, the nursing learner will conduct an intake interview for 15 minutes, using level three empathy as defined by Carkhuff (1969).

Instructional goal: For the learner to teach pertinent skills to a client with diabetes.

Learning objective: With a simulated client, the nursing learner will conduct three 20-minute teaching sessions that include an assessment of what is known by the client about diabetes and its treatment and interventions to fill cognitive, affective, and/or perceptual-motor learning deficits as defined in class.

■ **Nurse Educator Challenge**

Delineate two instructional goals and their learning objectives.

Common Pitfalls to Writing Instructional Objectives

Novice nurse educators sometimes put two verbs in an instructional objective. This leads to a false performance, false givens, objectives focused on teaching strategies, gibberish, educator performance, and false criteria.

False Performances

Below are examples with a false performance in each one.

1. Have a thorough understanding of the anatomy of the hand.
2. Demonstrate a comprehension of the main arteries of the heart.
3. Be able to relate to clients with empathy.
4. Be able to understand special diets.

■ **Nurse Educator Challenge**

Revise the four false performances above to make them into objectives with an audience, performance, condition, and criterion.

False Givens

False givens describe the instructional process itself, not the specific conditions the learner must have or be denied when demonstrating achievement of an objective. Some examples of false givens are:

1. Given adequate practice, the nursing learner will be able to calculate dosage for three medications.

2. Given that the learner has completed Module 10, the learner will be able to interview three clients.
3. Given that the learner received an A for the previous course, the learner will be able to complete three IM injections.

■ **Nurse Educator Challenge**

Turn the false givens into specific objectives with an audience, performance, condition, and criterion.

Objectives Focused on Teaching Strategies

When objectives focus on teaching strategies, they can't be focused on the learner. Although this pitfall is similar to false givens, this statement describes a practice exercise, teaching point, or some other aspect of classroom activity. Describing a classroom activity is not constructing an objective. Some examples of focusing on teaching strategies include:

1. Be able to choose the right instruments for surgery.
2. Be able to choose a nursing procedure that illustrates a related point.
3. Be able to explain the case histories handed out in class.

■ **Nurse Educator Challenge**

Turn the three objectives focused on teaching points into useful objectives with an audience, behavior, condition and criterion.

Gibberish

Gibberish is the use of unclear and incomplete statements. Gibberish loses the reader in flowery terms and nonspecific phrases. Sometimes two verbs are used in an effort to be more thorough. Unfortunately, the result is an unclear objective that leads to unclear communication with learners. Examples of gibberish include:

1. Have a deep and increasing awareness and thorough professional grasp of nursing.
2. Demonstrate a thorough comprehension of bed baths.
3. Relate and encourage with multiple approaches the necessity of an immune system.

> **■ Nurse Educator Challenge**
>
> Turn the three gibberish statements into instructional objectives that would make Mager proud.

Educator Performance

An instructional objective describes learner, not educator performance. Avoid saying anything about educator behavior. Examples of objectives focused on educator performance and not learner behavior include:

1. The nurse educator will encourage an atmosphere promoting the development of security, confidence, and self-esteem in learners.
2. Show learners the proper procedures for designing a learning system.
3. Demonstrate the ability to role play with a learner.

> **■ Nurse Educator Challenge**
>
> Turn the three educator-centered statements into learner-centered objectives.

False Criteria

False criteria are unclear, insignificant, and incomplete. Often these statements are missing one or more of Mager's critical components. Three examples of false criteria include:

1. Must make 80% on a multiple choice exam.
2. Must pass a final exam.
3. Must complete a procedure to the satisfaction of the instructor.

> **■ Nurse Educator Challenge**
>
> Put on your thinking caps and revise these false criteria to describe the conditions under which the performance is to occur.

Overcoming Barriers to Writing Instructional Objectives

Writing instructional objectives is not always easy because some performances may not be visible and no single behavior (or type of behavior) may indicate the presence of the experience.

Ramona, a new nurse educator, was having difficulty writing instructional objectives for a course she planned to teach. She had tried Bloom's taxonomy, but wasn't satisfied with it. She felt something was missing. When a more experienced nurse educator told her another theory might work for her, she was glad to try it.

Mager's goal analysis theory (1997) can be used to objectify experiences that refer to attitudes and values. Mager suggests using the following four strategies to describe the goal to be attained.

1. Answer the question, "What will I take as evidence the goal has been achieved?"
2. Given all learners, what is the basis to be used to separate them into two groups: those who have achieved the goal and those who have not?
3. Imagine you are telling someone else how to judge whether learners have met the goal; what instructions would you give?
4. Think of people who have attained the goal; tell why you think they have attained it.

An example of a goal in the nursing classroom might be to participate effectively in group discussions. Some indicators that this goal has been met might be that learners:

■ Allow speakers to finish presenting their views,
■ Act to prevent others from interrupting speakers,
■ Acknowledge information presented by others,
■ Return discussion to the assigned topic or task, and
■ State their own feelings without blaming others for their motivation or intent.

Covert Versus Overt Performances

Some verbs, such as identify or consider, refer to performances that cannot be observed. In this case, add an indicator behavior, such as write solutions, or circle, or point to, or another behavior you can observe the learner doing. Read the three objectives that follow and think of ways to make covert actions overt:

1. **Identify** the correct solution to a medication dosage.
2. **Identify** the correct answer to a client's question about overnight guests.
3. **Consider** the best way to assess a client's diabetes condition.

After mastering the writing of instructional objectives, the next step is applying a systematic approach to instructional design.

Implementing Learning Systems

Implementing learning systems includes teaching/learning principles, content sequencing, learning contracts, teaching methods, and giving feedback to learners,

Teaching/Learning Principles

Cognitive learning usually begins with the teaching of concepts that are generalized from particular instances. Examples of concepts include anxiety, conflict, frustration, empathy, responsibility, relationships, communication, roles, and competition. To teach concepts, give a definition or allow learners to develop an operational definition (all processes in order of their occurrence).

Concepts are combined to form principles. These principles specify relationships between events, leading to an ability to predict consequences, explain events, infer causes, control situations, and solve problems (Breslow, 2001; Davis, 1974).

Three phases must be experienced to learn a principle:

- Curiosity
- Identification of the principle, and
- Its application.

Curiosity

Some learners may ask questions that imply they are curious:

"Why did the client . . . ?"

"Why doesn't . . .?"

"How come . . . ?"

These questions can be used as a lever to introduce nursing principles such as family systems or death and dying principles. If no questions are forthcoming, the nurse educator can promote curiosity by making a provocative statement. Some examples are:

"Nurses cannot decrease client pain."

"Families cannot be changed by nursing intervention."

"There's nothing a nurse can do to help a dying client."

An alternate method is to ask a thought-provoking question. Some examples are:

"How can you apply what you learned about the teaching/learning process to your relationship with clients?"

"Can nursing care affect client anxiety?"

■ **Nurse Educator Challenge**

Think of two other provocative statements to use to promote learner curiosity.

Another method of enhancing curiosity is to demonstrate a relationship or event that reveals a new idea; for example, asking learners to predict what will happen to the use of other senses if a client becomes blind, then blindfolding them and asking for their observations.

Identify the principle

Once curiosity is aroused, learners are usually ready to identify the principle(s) involved. Four approaches can be used.

1. **Ask learners questions until the principle is fully stated.**

    Nurse Educator: What sensations did you notice while blindfolded?

    Learner 1: I was scared to walk around.

    Learner 2: I was much more aware of how I felt.

    Learner 3: I didn't know where anyone else was at first.

    Learner 4: I looked for other cues to where things were.

    Nurse educator: Those are all good points. What skills did you begin to depend on?

    Learner 5: I used my sense of hearing and touch to orient myself.

    Nurse educator: Good. What does this experience tell you about how newly blind people might be expected to act?

    Learner 6: That they will be scared at first, but then they will try to use their other senses.

    Nurse educator: How can we state your findings so they will be useful to you when assisting newly blind clients?

    Learner 7: Expect newly blind people to show fear, followed by a search of ways to use their other senses.

    In this approach, the nurse educator reinforces and encourages further learner comment with statements that summarize, reward, or lead to the principle.

2. **An approach to learning principles that is related to the discovery approach is the disputation method.** In this approach, the curiosity of the learner is aroused via a provocative statement such as:

"Primary nursing entails more independent practice than does team nursing."
"Families should be encouraged to allow a dying family member to die at home."
"Nurses who counsel for abortions are acting unethically."
"Clients who are recovering from a heart condition should be cautioned against having sex."

Learners are then directed to obtain data from books, journals, consultants, and other sources to support or refute the statement during classroom debate. Learners can choose which disputes and which side of the dispute they wish to participate in. Some learners may choose to be moderators; their role is to summarize the discussion and state the solution agreed upon through debate. The role of the teacher is to serve as resource person, guide and stimulator.

> The disputation method arouses curiosity by presenting a provocative statement that leads to debate.

3. **The third approach to teaching principles is to tell learners the principle.** This approach can be used when there is insufficient time or when there is no need to have learners empathize with the client.

4. **The fourth approach is to demonstrate applications of the principle.** For example, a film depicting the reactions of newly blind people could be shown to illustrate how they cope with blindness.

Principles and Problem Solving

Principles are used to solve problems. A problem occurs whenever a goal cannot be reached. **Problem solving** involves five steps including problem sensing, problem formulation, searching for solutions, evaluating the solutions and selecting the best one, and trying out and evaluating the solutions.

Problem Sensing

The first step in the problem solving process is problem sensing. The educator's role in this step is to teach learners to recognize a problem when they see one. Questions to use to alert learners to a problem include:

"What did the client say about his functioning?"
"What do you make of his response?"
"Does this indicate a problem?"

Problem Formulation

The second step in problem solving is problem formulation. In this step, the educator helps learners to formulate the nature of the problem and its elements in question form; for example:

"How can the nurse assist clients to comply with nursing orders?"

"What is the most effective way to conduct a nursing interview?"

"How can the nurse assess client readiness to learn?"

> Problem solving includes problem sensing, problem formulation, searching for solutions, evaluating solutions and selecting the best one, and trying out and evaluating solutions.

Searching for Solutions

The third step in problem solving is searching for solutions. Information from many sources is collected to find a solution. The educator's role in this step is to assist learners to develop hypothetical solutions to be tried out. Some questions to ask learners are:

"What hunches do you have about what's happening with the client?"

"Who has an idea of what to do?"

"Don't be shy. Give your idea a try. Nobody knows all the answers—not even me."

Evaluating Solutions and Selecting the Best One

The fourth step is evaluating potential solutions and selecting the one most likely to be effective. The nurse educator's role is to assist learners in weighing the pros and cons of each possible solution to the problem.

Trying Out and Evaluating Solutions

The fifth step of problem solving is trying out and evaluating the most feasible solution. To assist learners through the problem-solving process, educators specify learning objectives focused on action verbs such as sense, formulate, search, select, and evaluate.

Learners must be given the opportunity to sense the problem, formulate it, search for solutions, select one, try it out, and evaluate it. Practice conditions should simulate

Nurse Educator Tip

Questions to ask to help learners weigh pros and cons:

"Which one of the solutions is the best and why?"

"If you had to weigh each of the ideas, what are the pros and cons of each one?"

encounters outside the classroom. Although maximum uncertainty is desirable, learners who are at a low level of cognitive complexity may become more rigid and less able to problem solve if faced with too much ambiguity. To prevent rigidity, learners should be presented with simple problem-solving practice conditions until those are solved. Only then should learners be placed in more ambiguous practice situations.

Developing Problem-Solving Learning Experiences

When developing problem-solving learning experiences for learners, it is important to exclude prompts or cues that alert them to the problem. Situations where potential problems exist but are unidentified and unformulated are necessary to teach and evaluate problem-solving skills.

Problem solving cannot be taught via the lecture method, but there are other methods that can be used in the classroom to encourage problem solving in learners, including:

- *Providing classroom experiences that include specific strategies and techniques for solving problems in the referent situation.*
- *Sharing clinical experiences and past experiences in nurse/client situations to assist learners to problem-solve and transfer classroom learning to other situations.* To use this option, nurse educators need to be excellent practitioners in order to have a backlog of clinical situations from which to choose when developing strategies and sharing experiences with learners.
- *Using the "think aloud" process* developed by Jack Lochhead and Arthur Wimbey (Breslow, 2001). Two learners work together to solve a series of problems. One learner is the problem solver who reports out loud everything going on in her head while attacking the problem. The other learner is the

Nurse Educator Tip

Modeling Problem-Solving

Nurse educators can increase the effectiveness of modeling effective problem-solving by:

- Labeling each step as it is performed, and
- Pointing out antecedent conditions, relationships, and consequences of any principles that were used.

listener who listens carefully, takes notes, and stops the problem solver whenever necessary by saying, "I don't understand; say it in other words," or "I'm not sure that's correct. I think you need to check that."

- *Modeling ways to solve problems.* When the nurse educator models the ways of solving a problem, learners are provided with the rare experience of observing an expert successfully performing the problem-solving process. Going down a blind alley to see if learners are listening can also be beneficial (Breslow, 2001).

Programmed materials, group methods, journal writing, simulations, and simulation games can also be used to teach problem-solving skills (see Chapters 3–6).

There are a number of rules and strategies to be used when implementing problem-solving practice situations.

1. **Describe a problem and then encourage learners to scan all the elements of a situation.** Ask learners to list as many factors affecting the system or problem as possible. Becoming bogged down in habitual ways of solving problems is antithetical to creative problem solving.

2. **Provide experiences viewing problems from different physical or symbolic positions.** Learners need experience in asking:

   How else can this object be used?
   How else can the elements of the situation be related?
   How can the behavior of the nurse or client be varied to change the problem?
   How is the nurse like a client?
   What would happen if the nurse were to take the client's place for a day?

3. **Encourage learners to list basic questions to use in solving a problem, such as:**

   Who can help solve the problem?
   Where can information about the problem be found?
   Which limits can be controlled or changed and which are fixed?
   What is allowed in solving the problem and what is ruled out?
   What rules could be changed or modified to solve the problem?
   Where can we go to be closer to the problem?
   How many solutions to the problem are there?
   Who can we discuss the problem with to clarify thoughts, feelings, or solutions?

4. **Suggest learners stop working on the problem when progress is impeded and return to it later.**

5. **Provide practice for learners in listening empathically to others' ideas and in being critical of their own.** For example, assign a paraphrasing exercise where one learner is to listen to another learner for five minutes and then paraphrase what the other said without judging, persuading, or reacting to what the other said.

6. **Encourage learners to continue to generate solutions to a problem past the point of previous solutions.** For example, post a large sheet of paper on the bulletin board or chalkboard so that all learners can see the formulated problem. Ask learners to use a felt-tip pen to write solutions to the problem on it, whenever one occurs to them. When the paper is filled, categorize the solutions using every solution suggested, decide on one, and try out and evaluate the agreed-upon solution.

7. **Ask learners to go to a new place or person each day for ideas, such as a new laboratory, a different school of nursing, a consultant, and so on.** Encourage them to bring back something that attracts them while visiting. Suggest that they should not be concerned initially with categorizing their acquisitions or whether the object is related to the problem. After a specified number of days, ask learners to try to relate their collection to the problem.

8. **Ask learners to devise a list of all the nursing theorists, practitioners, researchers, and educators they consider important.** Then ask them to pretend they are those people and explain how they might solve the problem.

9. **Ask learners to expand the problem by asking, "What is the problem?" and following it with, "And what is that about?" to each learner response that is given, until no one can go any further with the problem.** This allows learners to see the interrelationships among problems, principles, and situations.

10. **Ask learners to contract the problem to its essential base.** First, state the problem; then ask, "Why is that a problem?" Continue responding, "Why is that a problem?" to each learner response until no one can go any further with the problem.

Problem Solving and Perceptual-Motor Skill

Learning problem-solving skills often requires a great deal of thought and discussion; the development of perceptual-motor skills requires a different approach. As with any learning experience, learners should be provided with precise, clear objectives. Providing a picture, demonstration, description, film, or tape recording of the criterion performance is helpful. This model performance provides the learners with an overview of the task. The overview should be brief and move the learner to direct practice in the task.

Educators need to keep in mind:

- Early in the training period, the learner needs maximum verbal guidance about how to proceed as well as demonstrations by the educator or others who have mastered the task, including peers.
- In complex tasks, such as learning to give an injection, learners can be given practice to criterion level in each of the subtasks of calculating medication, drawing up/mixing medication, and giving the injection. Once each of the subtasks has been mastered, a dry run through the entire task can be scheduled prior to actually giving the injection to a client.

■ Nurse Educator Challenge

Besides showing learners the subtasks in tasks, what would you do to enhance learning? Give a rationale for your answer.

Giving Feedback to Learners

Instructor feedback that can assist learning is the kind that helps to point out critical cues or prompts. Constructive comments are helpful, such as,

- "That's the way, wipe the vial off with the alcohol swab."
- "Pull back a few c.c.'s on the plunger and notice that there may be a bit of resistance to your pull."
- "Use the mnemonic device we discussed in class to help you remember."
- "Don't forget to remind the client why you're there."
- "Remember not to censor anything you say during this brainstorming phase."

By analyzing and describing subtasks, cues and prompts important to learning the complete task can be isolated. In addition to supplying cues or prompts, it is useful to provide the struggling learner with motivation to learn the task.

Motivation may be enhanced by making a positive comment after a subtask has been performed correctly (Bandura, 1997) such as,

- "Good; you drew that up without contaminating the needle."
- "Good job, you remembered the mnemonic."

According to Bandura (1997), any verbal or nonverbal communication after a learner action can reinforce it and increase the chance it will recur. It is important not to make negative comments when a subtask is not performed correctly. Negative comments such as, "Not that way," or "That's wrong," not only discourage the learner, they increase learner anxiety, and do not give information on ways of correcting the fault.

Time intervals between attempts to master a task or subtask should be brief. This is critical if the learner has made many errors and the learner or the educator is upset about this. When repeating the task practice, it is suggested that the nurse educator reestablish the learner's progress toward learning by making a comment before repeating the task such as "Remember to begin by . . . then . . . next . . . ."

If time does not intervene between practice sessions, the educator briefly brings the learner to a salient point with a comment such as, "Remember the last time you tried this, you _____; this time, remember to _____."

This kind of learning is best done in a simulated situation, where clients are not kept waiting for medication or treatment, and when no other health personnel are nearby to distract learners from the task. Once the task has been performed to criterion, learners are ready to try it out in a real-life nurse/client situation.

At the end of a practice session, learner and educator should review and summarize the practice session, or a learning aid such as a videotape or audiotape can be replayed as an evaluative tool and a way of comparing learner performance with the expert performance demonstrated on the tape.

Nurse Educator Tips

Criterion Performance

- Avoid setting the criterion of satisfactory performance too high at first when learners are beginning a task.
- Set criteria for satisfactory performance appropriately. This will lead to a higher rate of success and more highly motivated learners.
- Shape the learner's behavior by commenting positively on all approximations to the criterion performance.

The object of a postsession after practice is also to make factual and positively reinforcing comments, such as, "You were able to do _____ well, next time focus on _____."

Learners who find it difficult to master tasks may be given the assignment to rehearse the task mentally or to practice the movements of a task without actually handling the equipment or materials. This kind of practice between actual practice sessions helps the learner to focus on essential skills.

Regardless of the method chosen, the nurse educator needs to be concerned with how learning theory is applied. The following questions can be of help in assessing this aspect:

- Do I make sure that learners review behavioral objectives prior to beginning a learning system?
- Do I use cues or prompts to direct learners to important aspects of the matter to be learned?
- Do I present material in a way that is meaningful to learners?
- Do I provide remedial learning experiences, extra credit offerings, and between-class practice for learners who do not have prerequisite skills?
- Do I use my assessment of individual learning styles and preferences to point learners toward appropriate learning experiences?
- Do I underscore and positively comment on approximations to the goal?
- Do I set learning tasks that are neither too high nor too low?
- Do I actively involve learners in the teaching/learning process?
- Do I allow sufficient time for leadership, critical thinking, or psychomotor skill practice?
- Do I use modeling to increase the probability of learner performance to criterion?

Summary of Learning System Design

As this chapter has indicated, the process of analyzing the current status of the learning environment (analysis), formulating learning objectives, developing content and sequencing learning experiences (design), and evaluation are interactive and ongoing processes that are part of learning system design. See Figure 2–1 for a summary of the interactive quality of learning system design.

Figure 2–1 Flow chart for learning system design

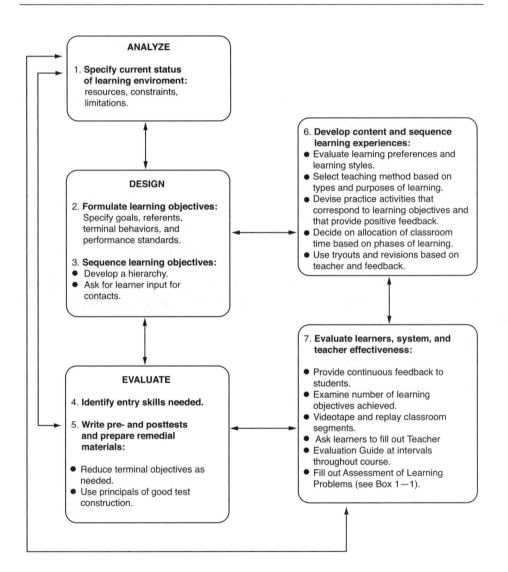

Gagne's Learning Theory

Psychologist Robert Gagne was the foremost researcher and contributor to the systematic approach to instructional design and training. He believed instruction should be designed to include a variety of instructional methods to meet the needs of different learners. Gagne is often called a behaviorist because his focus was on the outcomes or behaviors that result from training. His four outcomes or objects of learning included:

- Verbal information
- Intellectual skills
- Cognitive strategies
- Motor skills

In his book, *The Conditions of Learning* (1995), Gagne identified the mental conditions for learning. He based his theory on an information processing model and created a nine-step process he called the Events of Instruction.

What makes Gagne's nine steps or events of instruction superior to Bloom's taxonomy is that learning conditions for each learning outcome are clearly recommended. These recommendations can help nurse educators develop instructions. The nine steps Gagne identified are:

1. Gaining attention
2. Informing the learner of objectives
3. Stimulating recall of prerequisite learning
4. Presenting the stimulus (learning content)
5. Providing learning guidance
6. Eliciting performance
7. Providing feedback about performance
8. Assessing performance
9. Enhancing retention and transfer

Step 1: Gaining Attention

Donna, a new nurse educator, complained to one of the more seasoned nurse educators that learners in her nursing theory class nodded off and looked bored. The learners never asked questions and rarely answered hers. The more seasoned nurse educator shared information about Gagne's theory. The next class,

Donna dressed like Florence Nightengale, carried a lamp and shared details in first person of her days nursing during the Crimean War.

Learners will be more ready to learn if they are physically and emotionally comfortable in the learning environment. After identifying learner learning styles and preferences (see Box 1–5 in Chapter 1) the educator uses this information to create a comfortable learning environment.

Once learners are comfortable, the nurse educator strives to gain learner attention. One way is to distribute a course or class period outline. Another way is to focus the learners' attention through the use of unusual materials or presentation of self, or use a thought-provoking question or interesting fact to begin the class. Curiosity motivates learning and attracts learner attention. Music or a multimedia program can also capture learner attention. Learners are more apt to be motivated if the material is not too technical or complex, and if it is meaningful to them. Another method is to add differential cues or prompts such as signs, written directions, or media that alert learners to new information to be focused upon. Stating objectives to learners, pointing out relationships, using reinforcing pictures or props to get a point across, and asking questions that will evaluate whether learners understood the objectives and how to attain them are all ways of facilitating the attention process.

■ Nurse Educator Challenge

What advantage to learning is there to stepping up the podium in front of a class of learners? Give a rationale for your answer.

Educators can count on prior learning to gain learner attention. For example, the educator stepping up to the lecture podium is often a cue to the audience that information is forthcoming (Gagne, Briggs and Wagner, 1992).

Step 2: Informing Learners of the Objectives

Early in each class, it is important to discuss learner-centered objectives to be achieved that day, e.g., "Upon completing today's class, you will be able to..." This not only activates interest in learning, but it gives learners a goal to strive toward. Handing out written objectives will provide a more permanent reminder of what was achieved.

Step 3: Stimulating Recall of Prerequisite Learning

A topic takes on added meaning when it can be related to the learner's everyday experience (Gagne & Medsker, 1995; Gagne, Wager, Golas, and Keller, 2004). Learners will be highly **motivated** to learn if they have the prerequisite skills.

The nurse educator directs efforts toward specifying the prerequisite skills needed to accomplish the learning goal, identifying learners who do not have those skills, and directing those learners to learning experiences that will provide them.

Learners will be less motivated when learning tasks are set too low. For this reason, it is important to identify the current state of learner knowledge. Some ways of achieving this are by asking the learner to tell or demonstrate what is known or by giving a written pretest. An online pretest or hard copy can be completed prior to class. Another option is to ask for a show of hands to 5-10 questions that exemplify content for that class. The way to create links to long-term memory is by tapping into personal experience and knowledge. A simple way to stimulate recall is to ask questions about previous related experiences, an understanding of previous concepts, or a body of knowledge.

Step 4: Presenting the Stimulus (New Content)

To obtain the best response, learners can complete a Web tutorial of the material or read chapters in their textbook. By presenting material in small, achievable steps, and organizing it in a meaningful way, learning is more apt to occur because moti-

Nurse Educator Tip

Modeling or Demonstration

When using the modeling (or demonstration) approach:

- Label the important aspects of the behavior being modeled,
- Be sure the modeling is done in an atmosphere where rewards for performing the behavior are forthcoming,
- Be careful not to punish learners for their behavior with words, facial expressions, or actions, and
- Use modeling when teaching technical and/or interpersonal skills.

vation is increased when success is more reachable. After each small step is achieved, it is important to provide praise (Gagne et al., 2004).

> Motivation is enhanced by positive expectations, success in learning situations, meaningful material, and knowledge of goals to be achieved.

During the class, skills are explained first, then demonstrated. To appeal to different learner styles and preferences, nurse educators use a variety of strategies (see Chapters 3-6 for more information).

Corrine, a RN-BSN learner, was scheduled to make a class presentation the next week. She told her instructor, a nurse practitioner with stress management skills, that she got so stressed when she had to speak in front of a group that she nearly passed out. Her instructor gave her a schedule with small steps, including picturing herself making the presentation and getting up the morning of the presentation while remaining calm. Corrine worked through the schedule before her presentation, stopping to relax herself when a step made her feel anxious. She completed the hierarchy before class started and felt confident entering the classroom because she'd mastered each step.

Step 5: Providing Learning Guidance

To help learners encode information for long term storage, use the following guidance strategies: examples, non-examples, case studies, role playing, simulations, graphical representations, mnemonics, and analogies (Gagne et al., 2004).

Nurse Educator Tip

Motivating Learners

Make a classroom with pleasant learning conditions by:

- Setting learning tasks that guarantee success by breaking large tasks into a series of small ones,
- Giving learners frequent reports on their performance, with suggestions for improvement; for example, "That was good; now try it and make eye contact", and
- Rewarding learner performance immediately after attaining the goal and consistently after the attainment of each goal.

Step 6: Eliciting the Performance (Practice)

This step includes the learner practicing the new skill or behavior. Eliciting performance provides an opportunity for learners to confirm their understanding, and repetition increases the likelihood of retention and transfer to clinical practice (Gagne et al., 2004). Role playing, simulation, simulation gaming, lived case studies (such as the previous Nightengale example), simulated clients, and practicing procedures in the nursing laboratory can be helpful in this stage.

Step 7: Providing Feedback

Dr. Jefferson, a new nurse educator, tried her first simulation in class. She'd handed out written instructions for peers to provide feedback and stood around watching learners take over their own learning. She wasn't sure what to do until a learner raised her hand, indicating a need for help. That's when Dr. Jefferson hurried to the pair of learners and began to coach them and provide hints of what to do next in the procedure.

Prompts are another way to increase learning. At the beginning of practice, learners need many prompts, hints, and directions. Prompts could be anything from a word, a hand signal, a list of steps, a symbol, a flag or sign, or anything that provides information to learners about how to proceed. As learning progresses, these should gradually be withdrawn (Gagne et al., 2004). For example, when first being taught physical assessments skills, learners require step-by-step directions or clues about what comes next. As learning accrues, learners may need only beginning, middle, and end assessment directions. If prompts are withdrawn too quickly, learners can begin to make errors (Gagne, Briggs, and Wagner, 1992). Nurse educators must think through how to fade out learning prompts gradually to reduce errors.

> Prompts are anything nurse educators use to remind learners of appropriate procedures.

While learners practice new behaviors, the nurse educator or a peer provides specific and immediate feedback of their performance. (If peers provide feedback, the nurse educator provides simple written instructions for them, including words to say.) Before pairing off learners, the nurse educator demonstrates the procedure in front of the class with at least one learner to solidify peer feedback skills, and answer any questions. Once all questions have been answered, learners pair off and begin practice.

> ### ■ Nurse Educator Challenge
>
> Once learners are paired off, the best thing for the nurse educator to do is go sit in the back of the room and observe, true or false? Give a rationale for your answer.

The nurse educator's role isn't over. At this point, it is important to circulate around the class, coaching, giving hints about what to do next, and praising approximations to the goal. This role modeling behavior can help peer learners move along in competence, and provide feedback that might be missing from a peer. This kind of formative feedback can help learners correct their performance and achieve success as they repeat the task until the criterion is met. A commonly accepted level of mastery is 80% to 90% correct (Mager, 1997).

Step 8: Assessing Performance

After mastering the instructional module or class procedures, learners complete a verbal or written post-test, demonstrate their skill, or both. This assessment is not used for formal scoring. It is a method of enhancing comprehensive and encoding purposes. Learners are encouraged to ask questions and the nurse educator shares information and tips about how to improve performance. Or, if a written test is anticipated, the nurse educator discusses the questions and their answers, giving tips and additional information as needed.

Step 9: Enhancing Retention and Transfer

The final step in the learning process is retention and transfer (Gagne, Briggs, and Wagner, 1992). It is not yet completely clear how the retention phase can be influenced, yet some learning principles may be applicable. For instance, learning is more likely when the learner takes an active part in practice that is structured to achieve the learning objective (Gagne, Briggs, and Wagner, 1992).

Requiring learners to answer questions (verbally or in writing), asking them to reorganize or pass on to other learners the information they have learned, or using games and simulations as teaching strategies are ways of involving learners in active, whole learning situations. Games and simulation are especially likely to assist in the retention of learning, since affect associations are attached to concrete actions in

Nurse Educator Tip

Need for Repetition

Some questions to ask when assessing the need for repetition are:

- How new or complex is this material?
- How long is the attention span of the learner?
- How anxious or uncomfortable is the learner?
- What questions does the learner ask that imply need for repetition?
- What nonverbal clues does the learner give that imply need for repetition?

game playing and not merely to abstract symbols, as in information-processing or memorization (Digital Media Center, 2004).

Retention of material may be facilitated through repetition. When learners are physically, psychologically, or socially uncomfortable in their learning environment, material that is presented may not be retained. To counteract this, repetition of learning materials can be used to enhance learning. Factors such as newness and complexity of material, short attention span of learners, and learner anxiety indicate the need for more than one type of learning material or increased frequency of presentation (Gagne et al., 2004).

Jacqueline, a new nurse educator, prepared a test using all of Gronlund's ideas for test preparation. When half the class failed, she had no idea what to do. She had to do something fast or fail twenty learners. She made an appointment with a more seasoned nurse educator and asked him what to do.

Whenever learners fail to learn, the nurse educator needs to locate the difficulty by examining a number of instructional areas including unclear learning objectives, direction, evaluation, content and sequencing method, and constraints. This begins the evaluation phase of the learning system process.

Evaluation and Learning Systems

Evaluation procedures are used to assess learning and to detect problems with learning systems. When learners fail to learn, a good place to start is to examine the behavioral objectives for clarity.

Unclear Learning Objectives

The first area to be examined when learners fail is initial structure or direction. When a problem exists here, learning goals or objectives are unclear or not understood by learners. The result is that learners try to outguess educators.

Grading and Evaluation Difficulties

Once the nurse educator has determined that the learning system problem is not caused by unclear objectives, evaluation procedures should be examined. When there is a problem with evaluation, unfair, unreliable, or invalid testing and grading procedures are used.

When learners are graded on the basis of having obtained a criterion level (Popham, 2001) rather than on their scores in relation to other learners', there are fewer difficulties in explaining a grade. Using Mager's theory (1997), the highest level of achievement of learning objectives would then be equivalent to an A or the highest grade.

Some comments made by nurse educators that provide evidence of difficulties in test development are:

- How do I grade fairly?
- How do I know learners are learning what I think is important?
- What parts of the course should be changed?

Nurse Educator Tip

Indicants that learners do not understand course objectives are evident in comments such as:

- What is the purpose of learning this?
- What should we take notes on?
- What should we focus on when we study?

Possible solutions:

- Check to make sure learning objectives are clear and specific.
- Ask learners to read the learning objectives for the course.
- _____ (your idea)

Learner comments that reveal evaluation difficulties are:

- The test questions are ambiguous.
- Have I really learned anything in this course?
- What's the difference between an A or a B (or pass or fail) in this course?

■ **Nurse Educator Challenge**

What is the advantage of using criterion-referenced grading? Give a rationale for your answer.

Nurse Educator Tip

Grading

- Grade only on learning; avoid grading on class participation, attitude, and other nontangibles unless they are directly related to a learning objective and can be tested.
- Give learners feedback on their learning throughout the semester.
- Clearly state grading policies in writing on the course syllabus, including weight of various assignments, any allowances for extra credit, redone papers, or late assignments.
- Short tests or writing assignments every week or two are preferable to a midterm and final.
- Allow learners to choose learning methods to support what they know: for example, journaling critical issues and solutions, researching projects and reporting findings, developing a study guide or audiovisual materials for the course, or reviewing literature for a specific disease.
- Allow learners to drop their lowest grade or do extra credit.
- Ask disgruntled learners to wait a day after receiving a low grade and write down their complaint and justification for a grade change; resist pressures to change a grade due to personal reasons such as the need to do well in grad school, and focus on the exam and what was missing (Davis, 1993).
- When scoring a test, use a computer-programmed item analysis to find out how well your items discriminate among learners; throw out the worst, keep the best, and build a bank of test items (Oermann and Gaberson, 1998).

Criterion-Referenced Grading

Criterion-referenced grading is the kind of testing nurse educators need to learn about and use more often, if not exclusively (Mager, 1997). Criterion-referenced grading is consistent with the State Board Examination system, where it is assumed that the applicant is eligible for licensure when a score at or above a cutoff point has been attained, not when scores are curved and then assigned grades.

Criterion-referenced measurement is also consistent with a cooperative (rather than a competitive) learning environment, where learners are taught how to teach one another. Peer teaching and peer supervision not only give learners the idea that they are competent and responsible learners, but help to prepare them for

> Criterion-referenced grading means a learner is graded on the basis of having obtained a criterion level, not on their score in relation to other learners.

their own professional life, of which peer review and supervision of others is a part.

Content Sequencing Problems

> Oscar, a nurse educator who'd mastered test construction, was surprised to overhear two learners discussing his class. "I can't follow where he's going. And the syllabus isn't any help. It doesn't go in order and I'm having a hard time with this course. I like the teacher, but I'm going to fail if I don't get some help." Oscar took their words to heart and decided to fix whatever was wrong with the course.

If there are no indicants that evaluation is a problem, the next area to examine for difficulties is content sequencing. If important skills are not taught or are overtaught, or if they are taught out of sequence, learners may perceive the course as trivial, irrelevant, disorganized, or incomprehensible. Learner comments that indicate problems of content omission or sequencing are:

- I don't understand this course.
- The teacher talks over our heads.
- The teacher repeats things we already know.
- We aren't taught what we're tested on.

Educator Method Issues

Another area to examine is teaching method. When learning theory is not used to motivate learners and promote learning, learners may not learn, and they often complain of being bored, or they try to avoid class. Another indicant that a teaching method is inappropriate is low learner performance in clinical areas.

No one method is appropriate for all learning objectives. Teachers who have limited repertoires of classroom skills and methods are apt to have teaching/learning problems in this area.

Lack of Resources

Another area to examine is the constraints imposed by deficits in educator skills, learner abilities, and school resources. Some of these constraints result from educators not being oriented to essential institutional knowledge, being expected to teach in overcrowded classrooms, or being given too many administrative tasks. Educator expectations of learner abilities may be above or below what exists, and there may be a failure to use available instructional resources, or a lack of these resources. No instructional environment is completely conducive to learning; when the nurse educator is faced with overwhelming institutional constraints, learning will be difficult, if not impossible, despite the effectiveness of direction, evaluation, content, and method.

Evaluating Learning

Evaluation is an ongoing process. It is goal directed and requires the use of appropriate measures and tools for collecting information. To evaluate effectively, an educator can collect information that answers the following questions:

"Did the learning system succeed?"

"What should be changed in the learning system?"

There are three sets of evaluation questions to be concerned about—entry skill questions, instructional procedure questions, and terminal objective questions.

Entry skill questions include the following:

1. Which learners have the entry skills needed to proceed?
2. Which skills does each learner lack?
3. What modifications or extra practice is needed to bring skills of all learners up to entry level?
4. What feedback will be helpful to learners about their skill level?

Grades in previous courses usually do not give a good measure of entry skills. The nurse educator prepares tests for measuring entry skills. If courses have been established using the method espoused in this chapter, the final examination of a previous course or unit may provide an entry skill test or pretest if terminal objectives have been specified. If this is not the case, the educator develops a pretest to determine the entry skills of learners.

Uses for Pretests

When the major criterion of teaching effectiveness is learner achievement, effective instruction occurs when most (if not all) learners achieve the objectives. A good way to test the clarity and specificity of an objective is to write a test item to assess learner achievement (Kizlik, 2006).

Pretests can be used to evaluate what level of learning a learner has reached at that moment. Using differences in score from pretest to posttest (after instruction), they can also be used to measure the process of learning. Pretests can also be used to move learners to the next learning system if they attain a score of 90 or higher. In the latter case, there is no need to bore learners by requiring that they redo learning experiences they have already mastered.

A pretest could be a written examination, a verbal examination, or a demonstration of a skill. A final use of pretests is for research on the effectiveness of

> Use pretests to evaluate where the learner is now and to chart the process of learning to the posttest.

learning systems. For example, the educator may compare the attainment of terminal objectives achieved by learners at the end of instruction for each system. To use pretests in this fashion, the educator obtains two equivalent groups of learners and pairs them according to score on a pretest. Since research has demonstrated that the most critical self-reports are distorted by the person's desire to appear competent to others, observations can be biased by observers' "blind spots" (Gronlund, 2000).

Before developing test items, it is important to understand the concepts of reliability and validity.

Test Reliability

Jenna, a nurse educator, asked several graduate nursing learners to help administer her test to various sections of class. When she examined the results and found that the three sections tested by the graduate learners scored much lower on the written exam, she went back to her nursing research text to find an answer. In her rush to test her group of learners, she remembered she hadn't prepared the graduate nursing learners properly to administer the exam.

An important question to ask about a test is: How can I be sure I'm consistently measuring what I'm measuring over time and between different raters? This is the question of **reliability.** Unclear questions and inadequate scoring materials can lead to unreliable testing. Essay questions can be particularly open to unreliable results, unless a very specific scoring system is in place. It is important to develop a detailed scoring system prior to administering the test (Gronlund, 2000).

■ **Nurse Educator Challenge**

What would you do about the learners who scored so much lower?

Increasing Reliability of Evaluation Tools

Reliability is important because without it, tests cannot be valid, although the reverse is not true. Reliability provides the basis of consistency, which makes it possible for a test to be valid. Reliability is a statistical concept that can be estimated by

> Reliability is a measure of consistency over time and/or between raters.

- Giving the same test twice to the same group (test-retest method),
- Giving two forms of the test to the same group (equivalent forms method),
- Giving the test once and scoring two equivalent halves of the test (split-half method), or
- Applying the Kuder-Richardson formula (Gronlund, 2000).

Steps to take to increase the reliability of tests include:

- Providing a long test to lessen the possibility of chance guessing,
- Developing tests that are neither too easy nor too difficult by basing them on the level of ability of learners,
- Providing a sample unit on taking tests to reduce learner anxiety about failing,
- Deleting jargon words,
- Ensuring that test conditions fulfill stated behavioral objectives.

Tests should differentiate between learners who have fulfilled the terminal objectives and those who have not. One way to ensure differentiation is to give the test to learners who have already completed the learning system (or course). Test items that cannot be answered by these learners should be redone or eliminated (Gronlund, 2000).

A concept that is as important as reliability is validity.

Test Validity

A well-designed evaluation tool is both valid and reli-able. **Validity** is concerned with whether a test is measuring what is hoped to be measured. Content validity determines whether the tool measures the

> Validity is concerned with whether a test is measuring what is hoped.

behaviors under consideration (Gronlund, 2000) or something else.

Criterion-referenced measures are validated primarily in terms of how well they represent the criterion (Popham, 2001). Some questions to ask are:

- What is the criterion behavior I want to measure?
- What is the best way to measure this criterion behavior?
- How well does the test represent criterion behavior?

Developing Valid Test Materials

Essay questions must test more than recall of facts to be valid. Essay questions must make sure learners

- Compare and/or contrast important interventions,
- Outline steps or protocols,
- Explain and summarize effects or data,
- Apply concepts and theories to a situation, or
- Analyze multiple nursing interventions for a client and provide supporting rationales (Oermann and Gaberson, 1998).

Some test factors that influence validity are:

- Unclear directions on appropriate responses to items,
- Overly complex sentence structure or vocabulary,
- Use of obscure factual information,
- Inappropriate level of difficulty of test items,
- Poorly constructed test items,
- Ambiguity,
- Test items that are inappropriate to the (hierarchy) level meant to be measured,
- Too few test items used,
- Test items arranged improperly, or
- An identifiable pattern of answers (Gronlund, 2000).

Box 2–4 compares suitable compatibility among learning objectives, tests of the objectives, and practice conditions that can lead to valid tests.

Box 2–4   Planning Valid Reproductive and Productive Learning Tests

Reproductive Learning

Objective	Test practice	Condition
1. Given syringe, needle, and medication vial, the learner will draw up and administer precalculated IM medication.	1. The learner administers an IM injection to a manikin.	1. Give learners practice doing the procedure with syringe, needle, vial, and IM medication card.
2. Using the Diabetic Teaching Guide, the learner will conduct a 20-minute teaching session with a client who has diabetes.	2. The learner conducts a 20-minute teaching session with a simulated client who has diabetes, using the Diabetic Teaching Guide.	2. Give learners the Diabetic Teaching Guide to study and practice in presenting the information, listening to the client, eliciting questions or reactions, and ending the teaching session. Use prompts when necessary.

Productive Learning

Objective	Test practice	Condition
1. The learner will solve nine of ten medication dosage problems correctly.	1. The learner gives ten dosage calculations not encountered in practice.	1. Give information on calculation and practice in solving problems using corrective feedback. Give tests until the learner attains 90% correct on the test. Give remedial instruction if necessary.

Box 2–4   Planning Valid Reproductive and Productive Learning tests (continued)

Objective	Test practice	Condition
2. The learner will identify the group concept of conflict and identify examples of it in novel situations.	2. The learner identifies examples of group conflict in an unfamiliar videotaped scene.	2. Teach the concept. Demonstrate how to assess group conflict. Give the learner practice with feedback on identifying examples of group conflict.

When designing test questions, the educator must decide whether reproductive or productive learning is important. For **reproductive learning**, the learner knows the exact content of the test and has practice on that content. In this case, the pretest and posttest could be the same. For **productive learning**, the learner is taught principles and is given practice in solving problems, but the content or problem examples in the test differ from the practice content or problems (Briggs, 1991). In this case, the posttest would differ from the pretest in the specific problems given, but would cover the same concepts or principles. When learning objectives are closely tied to outcome measures, there is a greater likelihood that the evaluation tool is valid, whether productive or reproductive learning is focused upon.

> Reproductive learning is when the learner knows the exact content of the test and has practice on that content.

> Productive learning is when the content or problem examples in the test differ from the practice content or problems.

Box 2–5 illustrates some of these test construction difficulties and their correction.

Developing Items that Test for Critical Thinking

To promote and measure critical thinking, multiple choice questions should:

- Be up-to-date with current clinical practice in the area,
- Be at application or above cognitive level,
- Require multi-logical thinking, and
- Require a high level of discrimination among plausible alternatives (Morrison and Free, 2001).

Box 2–5   Poorly Constructed and Reworked Test Items

Poorly constructed item	Reworked item
Essay:	
Discuss the implication of learning theory to teaching. (unclear and simplistic question)	Describe how you would use learning theory when teaching (a) clients or (b) other learners. Include specific applications by identifying teaching strategies discussed in class and by giving a rationale for each strategy.
Completion:	
Observations are biased by _____ (Critique: more than one answer could apply)	What quality of the observer could bias observations? _____ (Suggestion: phrasing a question helps to qualify what precisely is being asked)
Multiple choice:	
Reliability is a A. Introductory measure B. Measure of consistency C. Useful adjunct to tests D. Enabling objective	Reliability is the A. Measure of consistency B. Primary measurement C. Enabling objective D. Best adjunct to teaching
1. A and B 2. A and C 3. A, C, D 4. A only (Critique: use of article, "a," provides a clue that the answer begins with a consonant; multiple-multiple choice is an overly complicated method that may confuse students)	

Box 2–5   Poorly Constructed and Reworked Test Items (continued)

Poorly constructed item	Reworked item
Matching:	
__ Validity A. Unclear directions	Directions: On the line to the left
__ Reliability B. Length of test	of each factor that influences test
__ Measurement C. Validity	characteristics, place the letter
__ Sampling error D. Nonrepresentative	from the test characteristic
(Critique: no directions on how to match)	column that is influenced. Each
	character may be used once, more
	than once, or not at all.
	Factors that influence test
	characteristics:
	__ Learning objectives A. Validity
	__ Validity B. Reliability
	__ Length of test C. Reproducibility
	__ Unclear directions
	__ Use of obscure
	information
	__ Reliability
	(Suggestions: clear directions on
	how to match responses decrease
	measurement error. Placing shorter
	responses on the right increases the
	efficiency of test taking. An unequal
	number of responses decreases
	chance guessing. Ensure there is
	homogeneity in test characteristics.)

To evoke critical thinking, questions assist learners to:

- Identify problems and issues to solve and their rationale for choosing them,
- Zero in on different points of view and the reasoning behind their answers,
- Describe how they plan to solve problems and give a rationale,
- Examine how key concepts and principles are used to analyze situations,

- Identify their assumptions and tell how they affect their thought process,
- Evaluate the evidence used to support a specific position, and
- Compare varied solutions and outcomes for a specific situation (Oermann and Gaberson, 1998).

Some techniques for writing multiple-choice questions that measure critical thinking ability include asking learners to identify the correct outcome of a given circumstance, map the relationship between two items in different contexts, understand a case study and tie it to theory, provide what is missing or needs to be changed within a provided scenario, and evaluate solutions based upon criteria provided.

Some examples of multiple-choice items that test for critical thinking ability follow:

1. You see Christa, a young married woman, in the clinic for a broken humerus, and her x-rays reveal past fractures. Circle the best option for the nurse:
   a. Ask her if her husband abused her.
   b. Call the police and report her husband.
   c. Show her the x-ray and ask her if she'd like to talk.
   d. Hand her information about a local shelter.
   e. Tell her calcium would help strengthen her bones.

To reveal the thought process of the learner, space is left to provide a rationale for the answer chosen.

2. A follow-up study of graduates of a nursing program revealed that 75% of the learners who received an A in psychiatric nursing worked as graduates in psychiatric nursing. Which of the following interpretations of this findings is most valid? Circle your response and provide a rationale for your choice.
   a. Receiving an A in psychiatric nursing may be related to future practice in that specialty. Rationale:
   b. Graduates of that nursing program are more likely to practice in psychiatric nursing than in other specialties. Rationale:
   c. If you get an A in psychiatric nursing as a learner, you will be prepared to work as a psychiatric nurse. Rationale:
   d. The more knowledge you have of psychiatric nursing, the better prepared your are to practice in that area. Rationale:

3. Mrs. Sears, a forty-five-year-old pregnant Catholic woman, is expecting her fifth child. She came to the wellness clinic today looked disheveled and crying. She tells you she doesn't want this child.

■ **Nurse Educator Challenge**

Choose an answer from those that appear below and give a rationale for your choice.

---

   a. Tell her she's too far along for an abortion. Rationale:

   b. Ask her if something's changed. Rationale:

   c. Refer her to a psychiatrist. Rationale:

   d. Refer her to a mental health nurse. Rationale:

   e. Refer her to her priest. Rationale:

4. You are in a new position working in a clinic that provides pain relief. You notice that the nurse uses relaxation measures and self-hypnosis to help clients reduce pain, while the nurse practitioner uses medication. Circle the best solution to this issue and provide a rationale.

   a. Ask the nurse and nurse practitioner separately for their results. Rationale:

   b. Take care of your own clients; this doesn't concern you. Rationale:

   c. Design a research study to compare the two approaches. Rationale:

   d. Mention it to the nursing supervisor and let her handle this. Rationale:

Another issue to considered when developing test questions is ensuring that course content is covered.

Ensuring Course Content Is Covered

Bess, a new nurse educator, tried to lecture on every point mentioned in the textbook until she found out there was another way to make sure important course content was covered.

To ensure that course content is adequately covered, a chart showing terminal objectives for each learning system should be prepared. Box 2–6 shows a table constructed for a learning system on families. Each objective is weighted according to its contribution to successful performance in the referent situation. Increased weight is given by assigning a greater number of points to questions that correspond to an objective or by assigning more test questions to them.

Box 2–6 The Number of Questions for a Test on a Learning System on Families by Behavioral Objectives

	Objectives						
	Knows		Understands	Demonstrates skill in			
Course content	terms	concepts	Influence of parts of the system	assessment	intervention	recording	total
The family unit	2	4	3				9
Problematic family interactions	3	2	3	2		2	12
Effective family interactions	2	2	3	2		3	12
Family roles	2	3	2	2		2	11
Communication skills with families	1	1	4	3	6	3	18
Total # of items	10	11	16	9	6	10	62
% of items	16	17	26	15	10	16	100

Weighting Course Objectives

When terminal behavior is complex and short-answer questions are not applicable, the nurse educator can make a subjective judgment about the importance of each objective and assign a weight of between one and three. A number of ways can be used to assign grades by this method:

1. Translating the total test score into a letter grade of A, B, C and so on.
2. Setting a fixed percentage of objectives as passing (often 80 or 90 percent).
3. Setting a fixed number of objectives as a criterion level; for example, if there are five objectives, learners who attain all five receive an A.
4. Ranking objectives by level of difficulty. Learners who attain the lowest level receive a C; learners who attain the highest level receive an A.

In each of these methods, the criterion for judging learning is the attainment of learning objectives, not how learners performed in relation to one another. Grading on the curve provides no information about attainment of learning objectives, gives ambiguous information about learner preparation for future learning systems or courses, and may be unfair to learners who have achieved many objectives but still receive a low grade. Assessing achievement of learning objectives may be the best method of measuring instructional effectiveness (Taylor and Runte, 1995).

Learners can also be queried about their judgments of instructional effectiveness. Some topics that could be evaluated by learners in a written or verbal survey are:

- Instructor involvement,
- Learner interest in the course,
- Nurse educator/learner interaction,
- Learning system demands,
- Learning system organization and structure,
- Grading and examinations,
- Relevance of the course or learning system to clinical work with clients.

Nurse Educator Tip

Meeting Learning Objectives: Determining Why Objectives Are Not Being Met

To find out why objectives are not being met by learners, ask yourself the following questions:

- Were objectives clear to the learners?
- Was subject matter organized so that objectives could be met?
- Was there adequate balance between structure and freedom in the objectives (to encourage learning)?
- Were sufficient examinations and demonstrations given?
- Was there sufficient opportunity for learners to practice skills?
- Did learners receive adequate feedback about what they were learning?
- Did learners lack prerequisite skills or knowledge?
- Were learning styles or preferences overlooked?

In addition to evaluating learners on the basis of end-of-system or end-of-course grades and questionnaires, it is helpful to have ongoing evaluation procedures in progress for both learners and educators. This method can provide valuable feedback and enhance learning. It also alerts learners to their progress or lack thereof.

Obtaining Feedback on Educator Practices

Thom, a seasoned nurse educator, was acting as a mentor for Tess, a new nurse educator. She asked him whether he used the school educator evaluation tool or whether he had his own. Thom told her that periodic post-class questionnaires or small group discussions can be used to obtain learner feedback regarding that day's classroom activities.

Some areas Thom suggested she cover in her daily class evaluation were:

- What was worst and best about the class period?
- What was accomplished, what prevented more from being accomplished?
- What questions and suggestions do learners have?

It is wise to ask for anonymous feedback about grading clarity and fairness after an assignment has been returned. Learners are more apt to be honest if they do not have to write their names on an evaluation.

Disgruntled learners who identify themselves and are obviously upset about their grade can be asked to wait a day, write down their complaint, and justify a grade change. Davis (1993) suggests resisting pressures to change a grade due to personal needs (Dean's List or grad school) and focus on having the learner explain the fault of a test question or justify the correctness of a paper.

■ Nurse Educator Challenge

What would you tell a disgruntled learner who wants a grade elevated because her parents would be very upset if she doesn't do well? Give a rationale for your answer.

Long-term feedback can be planned by involving learners as members of curriculum committees.

Nurse educators can devise evaluation guides to help learners develop skills needed to evaluate their teachers. Information gleaned from completed guides can provide useful feedback as well as teach learners to assess others' skills systematically. This is the kind of experience that may be readily transferable to clinical situations, where nurses use assessment skills to evaluate the performance of peers and clients.

Many educator evaluation forms are nonspecific and tend to reflect learner attitudes and opinions. Such evaluations may add to teaching/learning difficulties. To change to more constructive behavior, evaluations should provide specific, objective information on educator performance. Box 2–7 illustrates the kind of evaluation that can give specific feedback about teaching effectiveness. Such an evaluation can also provide useful information about learner ability to evaluate classroom instruction and their learning styles and preferences.

Box 2–7   Nurse Educator Evaluation Guide

Directions:

For me to be an effective nurse educator, I need your feedback on my performance. Please answer the following questions for the designated class period.

1. Which words did I use today that you did not understand?
2. Describe any situations where I punished or put down students in the class today.
3. Which of the questions that were asked today were not answered satisfactorily?
4. What led you to conclude that the question was not adequately answered?
5. Give specific examples of teacher indifference to student needs.
6. Give specific examples of how class discussions or individual student ideas were discouraged.
7. What other feedback would you like to give me? (Be sure to be specific.)

Feedback as Evaluation

Learners require continuous feedback. Tests should be frequent and educator reaction to learner progress should be given regularly. When the mastery learning method is used, learners know exactly what has been learned and what needs to be focused upon, since no learner can progress to the next learning system without satisfactorily meeting the objectives for the current unit.

Media can also be used to provide feedback to learners. Programmed instructional materials, simulation games, flash cards, value clarification exercises, and quizzes given and corrected by the learners themselves can provide feedback regarding knowledge of facts, concepts, and principles as well as their ability to work collaboratively with peers and to be self-directed in their learning. Videotape playback and educator demonstration with learner redemonstration can provide feedback concerning complex motor skills. Audio- or videotape playback, role playing with subsequent discussions, peer supervision, perceptual exercises, journal writing, and small-group exercises (see Chapters 3–6) can provide feedback about complex interpersonal or cognitive skills.

Giving Post-tests

When learners have mastered more complex discriminations, a **post-test** is given. Make sure that learners can discriminate examples that lay people would find difficult to distinguish. For example, lay people might be able to recognize that a client

> A post-test is administered at the end of a learning segment or learning system.

is upset, whereas a competent professional nurse would be able to identify indicants of levels of anxiety. It is important to include new examples on the post-test; otherwise, learners will be being tested for memory rather than for concept attainment. For anxiety, learners may be presented with a simulated anxious client, a film that depicts anxiety, or a written test that presents new examples as a post-test.

This chapter has provided information for planning, implementing, and evaluating learning systems. This chapter and all other chapters that follow provide beginning and more advanced exercises for nurses educators to help assist in active learning and critical thinking.

EXERCISES FOR NURSE EDUCATORS

1. Learn from other educators
Talk with, sit in on a class with, or examine course materials created by another nursing educator. Use the information presented in this chapter to evaluate the effectiveness of the learning system(s). Ask yourself: What did you learn from the other educator's mistakes and competencies?

2. Design a learning system

Using the information in this chapter, devise a learning system for one aspect of nursing. Pick a small, workable topic for initial practice. Ask yourself the following questions when designing the system:

- Did I specify institutional goals and constraints?
- Did I specify resources available for planning, evaluating, and trying out the learning system? (Include people, materials, and equipment.)
- Did I specify procedures for overcoming (or living with) constraints?
- Did I specify skills I need to develop in order to design a learning system?
- Did I formulate learning objectives, using learning theory, referent situations, terminal behaviors, and performance standards?
- Were learning objectives sequenced according to a hierarchy of difficulty or importance?
- Was learner input collected? For example, was a learning contract written or a guide for one developed?
- Were plans included to evaluate learner learning preferences and styles?
- Were learning experiences selected based on type and purpose of learning to be achieved?
- Were there sufficient directions and aids to assist learners to identify and reach learning objectives?

3. Transfer

List ways classroom experiences affect how learners interact with clients and other learners.

4. Application of learning principles

Devise ways to use the following in the classroom:

- Motivation
- Prompts and cues
- Active learning
- Repetition
- Recall
- Modeling
- Feedback

5. Process records

Begin a record or journal of your disappointments, triumphs, learning, frustration, inventions, and so on as you develop learning systems. They will be of use to you in future planning and can be used to guide others. Consider writing an article about your experiences in learning system design.

ADVANCED LEARNING EXPERIENCES

6. Gagne and Taxonomy
Devise a table comparing Gagne's conditions of instruction with Bloom's taxonomy and gives examples of each that are pertinent to teaching learners.

7. Communication Problem
Plan and execute a role-playing situation demonstrating a communication problem and its solution.

8. Motivating
Using the Nurse Educator Tip on Motivating Learners, try out the suggestions, and evaluate the results.

9. Research Problem Statement
Design a research problem statement regarding motivating nurse learners.

10. Bandura
Model a procedure for nursing learners or classmates using Bandura's social cognitive principles to evaluate your performance and derive implications of your findings.

11. Behavioral Objectives
Teach three novice nurse educators how to construct behavioral objectives using first Bloom's taxonomy and then Mager's goal theory. Seek feedback from your learners and redo your performance with another group, using their suggestions.

12. Curriculum
Build a curriculum for a nursing program, ensuring course objectives and content correspond to program and school or college objectives.

References

Anderson, L. W,. & Krathwohl, D. R. (Eds.). (2001). *A taxonomy for learning, teaching, and assessing: A revision of Bloom's taxonomy of educational objectives.* New York: Longman.

Bandura, A. (1977). *Social learning theory.* New York: General Learning Press.

Bandura, A. (1986). *Social foundation of thought and action: A social cognitive theory.* Englewood Cliffs, NJ: Prentice Hall.

Bandura, A. (1997). *Self-efficacy: The exercise of control.* New York: W.H. Freeman.

Bandura, A. (2001). Social cognitive theory: An agentic perspective. *Annual Review of Psychology, 52,* 1-26.

Beers, G. W., & Bowden, S. (2005). The effect of teaching method on long-term knowledge retention. *Journal of Nursing Education, 44*(11), 511–514.

Bloom, B. S., Englehart, M. D., Furst, E. J., Hill, W. H., & Krathwohl, D. R. (1956). *Taxonomy of educational objectives: The classification of educational goals. Handbook I: The cognitive domain.* New York: David McKay Company, Inc.

Breslow, L. (2001). Transforming novice problem solvers into experts. *Teaching and Learning, 13*(3). Retrieved September 24, 2006 from http://web.mit.edu/tll/tll-library/teach-talk/transforming-novice.html

Briggs, L. (1991). *Instructional design principles and applications* (2nd ed.). Englewood Cliffs, NJ: Educational Technology Publications.

Burkhardt, M., & Nagai-Jacobson, M. (2001). Nurturing and caring for self. *Nursing Clinics of North America, 16,* 23–31.

Candela, L., Dalley, K., & Benzel-Lindley, J. (2006). A case for learning-centered curricula. *Journal of Nursing Education, 45*(2), 59–66.

Carkhuff, R. R. (1969). *Helping and human relationships.* New York: Holt, Rinehart & Winston.

Clark, D. (2001). *Learning domains, or Bloom's taxonomies.* Retrieved January 30, 2007 from http://www.nwlink.com/~donclark/hrd/bloom.html

Davis, B. G. (1993). *Tools for teaching.* San Francisco: Jossey-Bass.

Davis, R. H. (1974). *Learning system design: An approach to the improvement of instruction.* New York: McGraw-Hill.

Diamond, R. M. (1998). *Designing and assessing courses and curricula: A practical guide.* San Francisco: Jossey-Bass.

Digital Media Center. (2004). *Games and simulations.* Minneapolis, MN: University of Minnesota.

Duan, Y. (2006). Selecting and applying taxonomies for learning outcomes: A nursing example. *International Journal of Nursing Education Scholarship, 3*(1), 1-12.

Friedman, C. P., De Bliek, R., & Norman, G. R. (1990). Charting the winds of change: Evaluating innovative medical curricula. *Academic Medicine, 32*(2), 8–14.

Goldman, J., & Torrisi-Steele, G. (2004). Education about child sexual abuse on interactive multimedia CD-ROM for undergraduate teachers. *Health Education Journal, 63*(2), 127-144.

Green, S. (2002). *Criterion referenced assessment as a guide to learning—The importance of progression and reliability.* Paper presented at the Association for the Study of Evaluation in Southern Africa International Conference, Johannesberg, South Africa.

Gagne, R., Briggs, I., Wagner, W. (1992). *Principles of instructional design.* (4th ed.). Fort Worth, TX: HBJ College Publishers.

Gagne, R., & Medsker, K. L., (1995). *The conditions of learning: Training applications.* Belmont, CA: Wadsworth Publishing.

Gagne, R., Wager, W., Golas, K., & Keller, J. M. (2004). *The principles of instructional design.* Belmont, CA: Wadsworth Publishing.

Graham, S., & Weiner, B. (1996). Theories and principles of motivation. In D. C. Berliner, & R. C. Calfee (Eds.). *Handbook of educational psychology.* New York: Simon & Schuster/Macmillan.

Gronlund, N. E. (2000). *How to write and use instructional objectives* (6th ed.). Upper Saddle River, NJ: Merrill.

Harden, R. M., Grant, J., Buckley, G., & Hart, L. R. (1999). BEME Guide No. 1: Best evidence medical education. *Medical Teacher, 21,* 533–561.

Hill, D., Stalley, P., Pennington, D., Besser, M., & McCarthy, W. (1997). Competency-based learning in traumatology. *American Journal of Surgery, 173*(2), 136–140.

Jamrozik, K. (1996). Clinical epidemiology: An experiment in learner-directed learning in Western Australia. *Medical Education, 30*(4), 266–271.

Holcomb, L. L. (2004). Leveling the playing field: The development of a distance education program in rehabilitation counseling. *Assistive Technology, 16,* 135-143.

Joyce, B. R., & Weil, M. (2004). *Models of teaching* (6th ed.). Upper Saddle River, NJ: Allyn & Bacon.

Kizlik, R. (2006). *Common mistakes in writing lesson plans (and what to do about them).* Retrieved January 30, 2007 from http://www.adprima.com/mistakes.htm

Krathwohl, D. R., Bloom, B. S., & Bertran, B. M. (1973). *Taxonomy of education objectives, the classification of education goals, handbook II. Affective domain.* New York: David McKay Co., Inc.

Mager, R. F. (1997). *Preparing instructional objectives* (3rd ed.). Atlanta, GA: Center for Effective Performance.

Mikol, C. (2005). Teaching nursing without lecturing. Critical pedagogy as communicative dialogue. *Nursing Education Perspectives, 26*(2), 86–89.

Morrison, S., & Free, K. W. (2001). Writing multiple-choice test items that promote and measure critical thinking. *Journal of Nursing Education, 40*(1), 17–24.

Oermann, M. H., & Gaberson, K. B. (1998). *Evaluation and testing in nursing education.* New York: Springer.

Patel, V. L., Groen, G. J., & Norman, G. R. (1991). Effects of conventional and problem based medical curricula on problem solving. *Academic Medicine, 66*(7), 38–39.

Popham, W. J. (2001). *The truth about testing—An educator's call to action.* Alexandria, VA: ACSD.

Pugsley, K. E., & Clayton, L. H. (2003). Traditional lecture or experiential learning: Changing learner attitudes. *Journal of Nursing Education, 42*(11), 520–523.

Rideout, E., England-Oxford, V., Brown, B., Fothergill-Bourbonnais, F., Ingram, C., Benson, G., Rosee, M., & Coates, A. (2002). A comparison of problem-based and conventional curricula in nursing education. *Advanced Health Science Education Theory Practice, 7*(1), 3–17.

Schmidt, H. G. (1993). Foundations of problem-based learning: Some explanatory notes. *Medical Education, 27*(5), 422–432.

Schwartz, R. W., Donnelly, M. B., Nash, P. P., & Young, B. (1992). Developing learners' cognitive skills in a problem-based surgery clerkship. *Academic Medicine, 67*(10), 694–696.

Sharif, F., & Masoumi, S. (2005). A qualitative study of nursing learner experiences of clinical practice. *BMC Nursing,* 4(6), 1-7.

Shin, J., Haynes, R. B., & Johnston, M. E. (1993). Effect of problem-based, self-directed undergraduate education on lifelong learning. *Canadian Medical Association Journal, 148*(6), 969–976.

Shuldham, C. (1993). Nurse education in a specialist environment. *Nurse Education Today, 13,* 435-440.

Simpson, E. J. (1972). *The classification of educational objectives in the psychomotor domain.* Washington, DC: Gryphon House.

Smits, P. B., deBuisonje, C. D., Verbeek, J. H., van Dijk, F. J., Metz, J. C., & ten Cate, O.J. (2003). Problem-based learning versus lecture-based learning in postgraduate medical education. *Scandinavian Journal of Work and Environmental Health, 29*(4), 280–287.

Stark, M. A., Manning-Walsh, J., & Vliem, S. (2005). Caring for self while learning to care for others. *Journal of Nursing Education, 44*(6), 266–270.

Taylor, G., & Runte. (1995). *Thinking about teaching.* Toronto, Canada: Harcourt Brace.

Walker, J. T., Martin, T., White, J., Elliot, R., Norwood, A., Mangum, C., & Haynie, L. (2006). Generational (age) differences in nursing learners' preferences for teaching methods. *Journal of Nursing Education, 45*(9), 371–374.

Woodward, C. (1990). Comparison of the practice patterns of general practitioners and family physicians graduating from McMaster and other Ontario medical schools. *Teaching and Learning, 2*(2), 70–88.

Xu, Y., Carne, P., & Ryan, R. (2002). School of nursing in an underserved multiethnic Asian community: Experiences and outcomes. *Journal of Community Health Nursing, 19,* 187-198.

Part II
Specific
Classroom Skills

THREE

Role Playing, Simulations and Simulation Gaming

■ **INSTRUCTIONAL GOALS**

Upon completion of this chapter and the nurse educator learning experiences, the learner will be able to:

- ■ Devise ways to use role playing in the classroom
- ■ Compare and contrast role playing, simulations, and simulation gaming
- ■ Find ways to utilize simulations in the classroom
- ■ Identify ways to use simulation games in the classroom

Upon completion of this chapter, the more advanced nurse educator will be able to:

- ■ Devise three ways to use process simulation theory
- ■ Plan and execute a role playing situation demonstrating a frequent communication problem and its solution.
- ■ Use the theory of mental simulation or chaos theory to plan, implement, and evaluate one or more educator/learner situations.
- ■ Design a problem statement for research related to using role playing, simulation, or simulation gaming issues.

Key Terms

Accommodative learning	Parallel simulation presentation
Active case-study simulation	Post-simulation discussions
Assimilative learning	Process simulation theory
Behavior rehearsal	Role playing
Chance	Role reversal
Chaos theory	Serial simulation presentation
Common simulation presentation	Simulation
Debriefing	Simulation game constraints
Experiential learning	Simulation game payoffs
External validity	Simulation game rules
Information processing	Simulation games
Internal validity	Symbolic replication of reality

Introduction

This chapter presents a rationale for the teaching/learning procedures explored; introduces the process simulation theory; examines differences and similarities among role playing, simulation, and simulation games; and delves into the evidence for their use. Methods of using each learning strategy and ways of designing and using learning systems for each approach are also presented. Process simulation theory is discussed first because it provides the underpinnings for the three teaching/learning strategies that appear in this chapter.

Process Simulation Theory

Process simulation theory provides a framework for understanding role playing, simulation, and simulation gaming, and stands at the center of self-directed action by examining rehearsals of likely future events and replays of past events.

Process simulation theory can provide a framework for understanding role playing, simulation, and simulation gaming. Process simulation stands at the center of self-directed action. Process simulation serves a problem-solving and emotional regulation function for turning imagined experience into action. It includes rehearsals of likely future events and replays of past events. Mental simulations make courses of action seem real or true. When individuals actively envision future events, they later express greater confidence the events will occur. This effect of simulation on enhanced likelihood may create a state of readiness. Because imagining how events are going to take place, simulation provides information essential to planning and checking on their viability in the real world. The information derived provides a plan of action (Pham and Taylor, 1999). For more information, see page 179 "Theories that Explain Simulation Processes."

Rationale for Active Learning Skills

The three procedures—role playing, simulation, and simulation gaming—all necessitate active learning and process simulation. Alternatively, rote memorization tends to emphasize **assimilative learning** that is very easy to forget. Thinking at a level of cognitive complexity requires an exercise of three interdependent categories of skills: problem-solving, communication, and self-awareness. Self-awareness need not be thought of as a psychological process. Self-awareness includes exploring cultural, group, and interpersonal dynamics, and reflecting on how one's own motives may interfere with thinking clearly about a problem (Blatner, 2002).

> Assimilative learning is rote memorization and is easily forgotten.

> Accomodative learning is learned by practicing skills that are learned in interaction with others and that provide feedback and encouragement.

Accomodative skills cannot be learned by reading a number of books. The kinds of skills nurse educators need are flexible, creative, rational, practiced, and learned in interaction, including risk-taking, self-expression, providing feedback, and encouragement. This kind of learning is called **accommodative learning** (Blatner, 2002).

Role Playing

The first active learning technique to be explored is **role playing**. What is role playing? How is role playing used with learners? What possible effects can participating in role playing have on learners? Role playing is a way of projecting oneself into the future in a "what if" scenario. Although the outcome cannot be controlled, if role playing is accomplished in a safe environment such as a respectful classroom, this teaching/learning strategy can be a flexible and an effective tool.

> Role playing is rehearsal for the future that focuses on an given situation that contains two or more different viewpoints or perspectives that are played out according to a brief description of their character.

In most role-playing situations, the learner practices taking the role of someone else. Spontaneity in role playing is a major goal, and too much briefing of characters is discouraged. Role playing is also called sociodrama. Sociodramatic situations always involve more than one person and are focused on problems that are relevant to the classroom group.

■ **Nurse Educator Challenge**

Name three times it would be beneficial to use role playing.

When to Use Role Playing

Role playing can be used to:

- *Learn helpful ways to relate to clients or learners*—learning to be a nurse educator consists of more than learning facts or procedures. It involves the process of learning a helpful way of relating to clients or learners. One of the most common sources of non-helpfulness is the misinterpretation of the other's behavior. Role playing provides practice in situations for which learners have little experience.

- *Change attitudes*—when nursing learners are able to play the client or learner role, they become sensitized to aspects of behaviors, thoughts, and feelings they may never have been conscious of before. This new awareness can be used to effect changes in the nurse educator's attitudes and behavior, and can lead to improvement in the quality of relationships, and to feelings of increased self-esteem and mastery (Miaskowski and Maxwell, 2002).

- *Involve the class in active learning*—although the role players are the most involved in the role playing situation, the whole class is involved in active listening, posing questions and comments about what they observed, sharing their observations with the rest of the class, and thinking of ways to use what was learned with clients or other learners. A sense of involvement and identification can develop even in those who are less verbally active.

- *Devise new teaching/learning perspectives*—when novice nurse educators are able to play the learner's role, they become more aware of what a class or individual learner may be going through. Insights come to light and new perspectives abound that can be used to enhance the teaching/learning partnership.

- *Enhance critical thinking*—role playing is a teaching/learning method that is particularly helpful when interpersonal relationships and/or critical thinking are the focus of learning objectives. Role plays dramatize an event or situation that can bring forth the process of critical thinking (University of New Mexico College of Nursing, 2006).

- *Meet related learning objectives*—role playing should be selected as a learning experience when learning objectives dovetail with potential benefits.

- *Forecast decisions*—role playing is the preferred method for predicting decisions in situations in which a small number of people are involved, they are in conflicts that involve large changes in the situation, and for which little information exists about similar events. Five case studies showed that role playing is more accurate (56%) than expert opinion (16%) for predicting decision-making outcomes, and provide better information than traditional methods to predict the success of novice doctors (Armstrong, 2000).

- *Resolve conflict*—role playing can be used when conflict occurs in the classroom or clinical setting (University of New Mexico College of Nursing, 2006). If a situation such as an argument between two learners arises spontaneously during class, the nurse educator can take the opportunity to have the two learners reverse roles and begin to understand the other's viewpoint.

- *Encourage synthesis and evaluation of information*—role playing takes learners out of their chairs and helps them "learn by doing" (Lovecraft, Chapin, Parker, and Sadler, 2006).

The next section provides some uses for role playing that have appeared in recent literature.

Uses of Role Playing Found in Literature

Role playing has been used to:

- Shed light on the impact of cultural context, assist with negotiation and dispute resolution, and bring realism and experience into the classroom (Frank, 2006; Meligrana and Andrew, 2003).
- Enhance learners' cultural competency (Cooper, 2004)
- Help counsel adolescents with substance abuse issues (Fagan, 2006)
- Help prevent substance abuse (Hecht and Kreiger, 2006)
- Teach families how to talk to their children about death (Gebara and Tashijan, 2006)

- Transport prevention interventions from research to real-world settings (Rohrbach, Grana, Sussman, and Valente, 2006)
- Teach parents how to control their anxiety (Fisak, Oliveros, and Ehrenreich, 2006)
- Show clients how to reduce anxiety and depression (Abramovich, 2006)
- Provide an approach with community mental health clients (Kirsh and Tate, 2006)
- Teach couples how to reduce their stress (Pinet, Bodenman, Shantinath, Cina, and Widmer, 2006)
- Teach nurses how to discuss smoking in a nonjudgmental way (Lee, Hajek, McRobbie, and Owen, 2006)
- Develop managers (Raelin and Coghlan, 2006)
- Practice effective job interview procedures (Marks and O'Connor, 2006)
- Teach staff how to help clients with developmental or cognitive disabilities (Arco and du Toit, 2006)
- Teach African American and Latina girls how to practice applying condoms as a way to reduce STDs (Mennick, 2005)
- Recruit nursing students to play a standardized patient with pharmacy students and then write a self-reflection paper (Haddad, 2006)
- Teach nurses skills for learning pain management ((Miaskowski and Maxwell, 2002)
- Teach nurses to enact end of life scenarios such as helping children deal with the death of a parent or loved one (Mayo Clinic, 2006)
- Teach ethics (Schwartz & Weber, 2006).
- Teach critical thinking (Staib, 2003)

■ **Nurse Educator Challenge**

Name three benefits that can be derived from role playing.

Benefits Derived from Role Playing

Some benefits that can be derived from role playing are:

1. Increased empathy that can be used in relationships with clients, peers, and nurse educators and can be acquired while learning to identify thoughts and feelings of others.
2. The opportunity to experience the results of hostility, threats, and suspicion.

3. The opportunity to experience the constructive results of tolerance and empathy.
4. The opportunity to fuse cognitive, affective, and perceptual-motor learning—learners not only hear about a problem, but live through it.
5. The opportunity to practice playing a role can help learners reach a criterion level of behavior for related learning objectives.
6. The opportunity to present information to others. For example, a subgroup can show the larger group what has occurred, rather than tell them or write about it.
7. The opportunity to discuss sensitive issues in a relatively safe environment, the classroom.
8. A stimulation of critical thinking through decision making and problem solving as verbal exchanges occur.
9. Immediate feedback about their communication skills and other behavior for role-playing learners (University of New Mexico College of Nursing, 2006).
10. The opportunity for collaborative application of what has been learned.
11. The opportunity to synthesize aspects of the topic in the creative process of formulating the role play itself.
12. The opportunity to reach a better understanding of the topic as the learner analyzes the role play after its presentation.
13. The opportunity to practice in relating education with experience that is the optimal path to true learning (Dewey, 1963).
14. The opportunity to lead to sustained knowledge, which is vastly different from facts that are superficially memorized.
15. It allows learners to evaluate each other further advancing knowledge and understanding, which corresponds to the highest level of Bloom's taxonomy (Bender, 2005).
16. It allows learners to remain anonymous and thus free to be more creative (Nelson and Blenkin, 2007).

Why Some Nurse Educators May Not Use Role Playing

Dr. Epstein had been using lecture for many years, but now her school was moving toward active learning. She had no idea how to help learners be more active, nor did she want to learn. When the Dean asked faculty to summarize their attempts toward active learning in their classroom, Dr. Epstein remained silent. A young nurse educator who was familiar with role playing tapped her senior colleague on the arm. "Why don't you sit in on my class on Tuesday. You can see how much students can learn from role playing."

Nurse educators may shy away from using role playing for two basic reasons: lack of awareness of its benefits and fear of its consequences. The nurse educator's fear of the consequences of role playing may be due in part to lack of exposure to the method and to lack of skill of the role-playing process. Learners, too, may feel anxious or fearful about role playing if they have had past negative experiences with the method or if they feel inadequate or unprepared. Written, verbal, or programmed instructional materials can be used prior to class to introduce learners to role playing.

Disadvantages of Role Playing

> Stuart, a new nurse educator, had read several articles on the benefits of role playing and was anxious to try it out with learners. He didn't have much time to prepare for class, but he figured he could talk learners through the process, even though he wasn't quite sure what to do or how to prepare learners.

Possible disadvantages, especially for inexperienced nurse educators, are that time is needed to develop and set up a role playing situation and some learners may be shy or anxious when asked to role play in front of the class (University of New Mexico College of Nursing, 2006). These disadvantages can be minimized through practice with the technique; like any skill, role playing requires practice. The nurse educator can ask members of the class to help set up the role-playing situation, suggest how to handle shy learners, and so on. This not only enhances their critical thinking and assertiveness skills, but helps the nurse educator, who acts as classroom manager throughout all three phases.

Using Role Playing Situations in Class

Role-playing exercises can take time to prepare and execute, but student motivation and accomplishment can be high. Novice nurse educators might take this set of behaviors one step at a time while more seasoned nurse educators may be ready to jump right in and start role playing with the next class (Teed, 2006).

■ **Nurse Educator Challenge**

What is the first step a nurse educator must take after deciding to use role playing in a classroom? Give a rationale for your answer.

Preparation for and Planning Role Plays

It is wise for novice nurse educators to participate in role playing practice prior to attempting the method with learners. Seasoned faculty members, friends, or even

Nurse Educator Tip

Considerations for Role-Playing Situations

There are three major phases in the development of a role-playing situation:

* Preparation.
* Action and discussion, and
* Evaluation and replay.

family members can be asked to assist in role-playing practice. Once nurse educators have gained some experience with the method themselves, it will be easier to direct learners.

Steps in using role playing situations include (Teed, 2006):

Step 1: Define objectives and ask questions

What topics or concepts should the exercise cover?

How much time is available to work on the exercise?

What will be expected of learners? (research, reports, presentations, or only in-class feedback?)

Will learners role-play in pairs or in front of the class?

Should a challenge or conflict element be introduced?

Step 2: Choose context and roles

Decide on a problem related to the chosen topic(s) of study.

Choose a setting—make it realistic, but not necessarily real.

Consider using or adapting material other educators have prepared.

Define each role player's goals, characteristics, and what happens if the goals aren't achieved.

Alternate approaches:

Assign learners to collect characters' background information via research.

For more advanced learners, provide the class with a role play demonstration, written steps to follow, and assign them to develop and implement the role play situation.

Generally, two learners are chosen to role play a situation, although more than two people may be required. To begin, it might be wise to limit role playing situations to two people. Choose role players randomly or because of their assertive characteristics, ask the class to draw a role playing card out of a hat or bowl, or ask for volunteers. It might be best to obtain volunteers from the population of learners who have had experience with role playing. This will make the educator's job easier and is more likely to lead to a better outcome. The role-playing situation should be chosen to depict problem situations that are relevant to all class members. It is useful to pretest the written description to make sure it is comprehensive and understandable (Armstrong, 2000). Otherwise, critical classroom time may need to be spent explaining the situation.

> Jenna, a new nurse educator, chose a role playing situation set in the middle of the emergency department. She instructed members of the audience to make some of the typical machine and voice sounds. With all the noise and confusion, no one was able to focus on the role playing situation.

It is helpful at first to choose problem situations that are not too complex or threatening; this allows the nurse educator and learners to gain confidence and achieve success with the method. Jenkins and Turick-Gibson (1999) found that using diabetes mellitus as the focus of a role-playing situation allowed learners to solve life-like problems, develop sensitivity and awareness of the client's life experience with illness, and generate empathy toward individuals diagnosed with diabetes. Use of double-entry journals also led to an increase in critical thinking behaviors as well.

The nurse educator may choose to present a particular problem situation, it may grow out of classroom or clinical difficulties, or a group of learners or the entire classroom group may volunteer to formulate a problem situation. Which of these is used depends on time constraints, the level of sophistication of the learners, and the learning objectives to be met. For example, if independent learning and peer collaboration are part of the learning objectives, the nurse educator would not choose the problem situation. Learners would be encouraged to become actively involved in choosing and detailing the problem situation.

> Roberta, a new nurse educator, decided to try out role playing after she learned about its many uses. Since the learner group was so small, she decided to use verbally agreed upon role playing situations. Many learners looked confused

and unsure of how to proceed. Roberta promised herself to provide handouts of the problem situation and how to develop a role playing situation prior to using the technique with learners again.

Step 3. Role Instructions

Instruct learners in their roles before they read the situation descriptions. Players are not to be over-briefed on their roles, as this may lead to restricted or overplayed roles. No attempt is made to tell players what to say or do in the role-playing situation; this is where spontaneity and creativity take over. Role players can be asked to talk among themselves about their parts and suggest any props and their placement in the setting. If learners look confused, it may be helpful to talk to them individually about the role, interview them "in role," and draw out their thoughts about playing the role, gently involving them in the situation (Blatner, 2002).

While the role players are reading their role descriptions, the nurse educator briefs the audience about their roles. Depending on the learning objectives, the audience may be asked to observe the general interaction of players or to watch for specific events. The nurse educator attempts to relax both players and observers to enable them to derive benefit from the exercise.

■ Nurse Educator Challenge

What information should instructions to role players include?

Role instructions should include:

- Telling learners which roles they will be playing before they read the written situation description.
- Asking role players to act as they themselves would act given the role and situation, or asking them to act as they believe the persons they represent would act.
- Instructing players to improvise but to remain in their roles (Armstrong, 2000).

Problem situations may be written out or verbally agreed upon. Written problem situations are probably best because role players can refer back to the facts, and copies can be distributed to the entire class for their edification. Role descriptions are only viewed by the role player the description pertains to. If it isn't possible to find seasoned role players, 5×8 role cards with specific role descriptions can be provided, and learners allowed 10–15 minutes to look over their character descriptions and get into their roles for the exercise. If learners voice reservations about their character, the nurse educator asks what their reservations are prior to the actual role-play. Learners may be unable at first to research an issue from a perspective very different from theirs because they may reinterpret objective data as support for their pre-existing world view (Teed, 2006).

Alternate approaches:
Assign roles prior to the role playing situation so learners can study their roles, obtain background information, etc.

Divide students into several small groups (groups of five are ideal) and present each group with a problem to role play.

As with any other educational tool, the role-playing situation is not considered an isolated item, but as part of a larger instructional plan. The nurse educator must decide whether skill training is desired or needed. The plan can include opportunities for testing out new insights by actual pre-practice prior to playing the role in class.

■ Nurse Educator Challenge

Dora wrote out a role play description, but everyone in the class looked confused. What might be the problem? Give a rationale for your answer.

The written role-playing situation and character descriptions must provide enough detail to make it seem real and to give sufficient direction for players and observers to understand the scene. Irrelevant situational facts or past history are omitted to minimize opportunities for the group to become sidetracked. Once the situation and role are set, both should be written out and provided to the role players.

Decisions regarding the description and casting of characters may be decided by a committee, the class group, or the nurse educator. If little is known about the class, it may be better to ask for volunteers than to assign parts in advance. If learners are known by the nurse educator, they can be chosen on the basis of their ability to play the role without becoming threatened. If learners are asked to play certain roles they are not comfortable with, they usually give a constricted performance that detracts from the usefulness of the exercise. If a role has unfavorable characteristics, it can be assigned to someone who has sufficient status and self-confidence to carry it out.

In some cases, the nurse educator might play this type of role to move the class more easily into the instructional method. The nurse educator might take on a role even if there is no role with unfavorable characteristics in order to decrease learner anxiety about performing and to demonstrate how to be spontaneous when playing it out. Beginners in the role-playing method are assigned to roles with which they are familiar or comfortable, or the nurse educator can ask for volunteers.

■ Nurse Educator Challenge

When should role players be allowed to take more difficult roles? Give a rationale for your answer.

Once learners have had some practice in role playing, they can be encouraged to take on more difficult roles during which greater insight and cognitive and affective learning can be gained. With experience, learners can also be trained in these aspects and take on peer-supervised roles. This can build leadership skills in learners. Once all these decisions have been made, the nurse educator moves on to Step 4.

Step 4. Introduce the exercise to the class
Engage learners by describing the setting and the problem. Determine how many learners have participated in role playing activity before by asking for a show of hands. If roles have been cast, this information is helpful in case one or more role players requires a coach or encouragement. The names of learners who have been involved in role playing situations should be collected for upcoming role playing situations.

Only the situation need be provided to the rest of the class. It is important to explain the relevance of the role-playing situation to the whole class. Information about the relevance of the situation and a brief summary can be written down and passed out to class members, or a short introduction that includes this information can be given by the nurse educator.

The nurse educator tells the class that role playing is the next activity, that it is not meant to focus on personal or private feelings, and that the task of the group is to watch carefully and analyze the role, not the person playing the role.

The members of the class are informed they are to serve as observers, clarifiers, analyzers, and sources of feedback to the role players once the exercise has

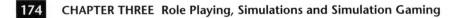

ended. Thus all learners are involved in this method, some more actively than others. The nurse educator encourages the rest of the class to remain quiet during the role playing, but to be observant, to take notes for later discussion, and to actively listen.

Step 5. Begin the role play
The nurse educator says something like, "Okay, let's start the role play." If the role playing is floundering or class members whisper, the nurse educator should ask everyone to remain quiet if they get caught up in the role play and speak. Remind them to "Please remain quiet." If any viewers make disparaging comments about one or more role players, the educator must cut off or rechannel remarks that attack or expose feelings or thoughts learners would prefer to keep private. The nurse educator sets the tone by reminding viewers to comment on the roles as enacted, not on the person playing the role.

> Dwayne was conducting his first role play and was perplexed. The role playing learners reached an impasse and looked to Dwayne to get them back on track. He couldn't come up with a solution so he decided to end the role play.

■ Nurse Educator Challenge

What would you suggest Dwayne do instead of ending the role play?

When learners reach an impasse because of miscasting, the nurse educator can step in and play the role or ask the class for a volunteer to help out. If players have been under-briefed, inadequately briefed, or are novice role players, the nurse educator can coach the players with comments such as, "You're being too easy on her; give her a hard time, the way it would happen in real life," or "Remember to stay in your role." Class members can also be chosen by the nurse educator and coached on how to give feedback and/or to serve as alter egos or coaches by standing behind the role players and whispering encouragement or suggesting what to say or do next.

Step 6. Timing and Ending a Role Playing Situation
> Timothy, a new nurse educator, kept looking at the clock once the role playing situation began. He hadn't given the group any direction on how long to stay

Nurse Educator Tip

A Sample Role Playing Situation

Situation: There is a physician on a medical unit who has angered many nurses by his rude, hostile, and verbally aggressive behavior. Tension on the unit has escalated and something has to be done.

Nurse educator role description: You just completed an assertiveness course and you believe it's up to you to discuss the situation with the physician and try to work out a more cooperative relationship with the man. Use assertiveness approaches such as Broken Record, Negative Assertion and Negative Inquiry, Assertive Probing, Content-to-Process Shift, Momentary Delay, Time Out, and Joining the Attacker.

Physician's role description: You don't understand the problem, don't have time to discuss the situation, and continue to be annoyed with the nurse. You use unfair criticism, procrastination, guilt induction, passive resistance, and intimidation to keep control in the situation.

in role and he wasn't sure how long to let it go on, especially since one of the role players kept getting out of role.

Sufficient time must be allowed for adequate coverage of the situation. The nurse educator sees to it that everyone moves into their roles at the same time; learners who talk as themselves, rather than in their assigned roles, can destroy the mood of the action. The nurse educator also encourages role players to stay in their roles and suggests an approximate time to play out the scene, for example, 10–15 minutes. The nurse educator will step in and stop interaction if the pertinent concepts have been demonstrated.

The role-play situation should not go on overly long. A role-play situation should be cut when:

1. Enough behavior has been exhibited to provide for appropriate discussion and class analysis.
2. The class can speculate about what would happen if the action were continued.

3. There is a natural closing, such as the end of an interview.

4. The learners reach an impasse because they have been miscast or not adequately briefed.

Step 7: Debriefing

Once action is cut by the nurse educator, the entire group is brought together to discuss and analyze the action. A large circle, or a circle within a circle, can be used to facilitate discussion. If the class is very large, small-group discussions can be formed by dividing the classroom into sections. Movable chairs are useful but not necessary. In large lecture sections where desks are not movable, learners can turn around or face sideways to join in a group discussion.

Each group is given a number of specific questions to discuss. These can be written on paper or on the chalkboard, or shown on an overhead projector. Following small-group discussion, the entire group can be reconvened, and the nurse educator can ask each group to present its findings. Points that were omitted or need underlining can then be discussed by the nurse educator or learners.

Sometimes the nurse educator may ask the players to comment critically on their performance, prior to others doing so. This allows the role players to set the tone for constructive class criticism. The nurse educator monitors criticism to ensure that comments about acting ability or personality traits are not the focus of discussion. Rather, the discussion is directed toward role-playing content and how it might illuminate the problem the group is attempting to solve. In addition, observers are directed to bring observations, not opinions, to the discussion.

If the class does not have the prerequisite skills to provide constructive feedback, the nurse educator might teach the group to make "I" statements when commenting by role modeling them, or hand out a list of rules for constructive feedback with examples:

- "I think the doctor was trying to make the nurse feel guilty,"
- "I noticed the doctor wasn't looking at the nurse."
- Comments that imply blame or inadequacy, such as "You should have been more convincing," or "Why didn't you . . . ," are to be avoided.

It might be best to provide a handout of rules prior to the role-playing situation and ask learners to be familiar with them when they come to class. That way, learners will know what kind of comments are helpful and start making them.

The nurse educator encourages classroom participation after the role play, including asking questions, evaluating, and suggesting ways to use what has been learned.

Step 8. Summary

At the end of the discussion, the nurse educator helps the group to summarize what was learned from the role-playing situation and to reach that can be applied to similar interactions. Examples of this type of statement are:

- "I think we have discussed several ways of dealing with the problem including . . . ,"
- "It seems important to try to understand the verbal and nonverbal behavior of others."

■ Nurse Educator Challenge

Once the role playing discussion is over, what options does the nurse educator have? Which is the best choice from the options? Give a rationale for your answer.

Step 9. Replay (optional)

At this point, the entire class may be given the opportunity to recast players and replay the scene to allow for further practice and to implement suggestions made by the class, or the players can be asked to reverse roles in order to gain insight into the others' behavior. **Role reversal** may be particularly useful if anger or conflict occurred in the role play; taking the other's role can provide information about why the other might be defensive or attacking. Another alternative measure is to develop a new role-playing situation and test out whether summary statements and generalizations hold in the new situation.

> Role reversal is taking the role of the other person for the purpose of understanding his or her viewpoint.

Step 10: Assessment

If grades will be given for a written project associated with the role play, presentations, questions asked of role players, and even involvement in interactive exercises can be graded. Special considerations for grading in-class role-playing exercises include (Teed, 2006):

- Playing in-character
- Working to further the character's goals
- Making statements that reflect the character's perspectives
- Stepping back and analyzing the characters' situations and making statements that indicate understanding or that relate to theory

Other Role Playing Possibilities

At least two other possibilities are available for role playing situations: assign an out-of-class role play and role play online (Gibbs, Doggett, and Frost, 2005).

Out-of-Class Role Play

The nurse educator can assign learners in pairs to role play a situation. They then report back in writing including:

- What was learned,
- The difficulties they encountered, and
- Any questions that remain.

Online Role Playing

Jade, a new nurse educator, was invited to learn about a new virtual learning environment used for role playing. On one online project she participated in an online role playing session with the computer. Jade entered the environment in the disguise of a character she chose, and participated by anticipating the way in which her given character would interact.

Gibbs, Doggett, and Frost (2005), Bender (2005) and Ip, Linser, and Jasinski (2002) extolled the virtues of the virtual world for role playing. Online role playing offers additional possibilities:

- Asynchronous learning can be used, giving the learner time to think about their responses and not be put on the spot to answer or role play.
- The nurse educator can monitor learner communication in their small groups as they discuss plans for their virtual role play; this not only provides information about their small group skills, but also about their ability to use critical thinking skills.
- Once a small group is ready to go live, the rest of the class become the audience and negotiate for future role playing roles.
- Learners compensate well for the lack of visual and auditory cues by writing in "Ring Ring Ring" for a telephone, adding information about facial expressions, mentioning when a role player is having an internal dialogue, and detailing actions through notes such as "They hug each other and sit down at a table."
- Members of the "cast" serve as discussion leaders, identifying the main themes, issues, and conflicts within their topics, and respond to questions and comments from the rest of the class.

- Immersion in the topic helps learners develop insight into real issues they have faced and helps them work through the issues in a meaningful way.
- Completing a role playing situation forces learners to incorporate all they have learned in class along with bringing in personal experiences.
- Online role playing can lead to feelings of enjoyment at the "fun" role playing was.
- Role playing can become more and more valuable when learners assume more and more responsibility over the process, when they are challenged to think and reflect, and when they can deploy significant facts rather than just memorize them.
- Assessment by both the role players and the audience occurs in which the value of the performance is assessed in terms of its organization as well as its relevance to the topic in general.

Simulation

In role playing, learners frequently adopt roles they will not play in real life. They often spontaneously create a role, and are given little or no instruction on what to say or do. In simulations, the roles played are controlled and structured to a greater degree by information and feedback. **Simulations** are focused on the adoption of the role that the learner will perform in real life, such as pretending to be a nurse educator prior to actually being a nurse educator.

> Simulations are controlled, structured, and focus on adoption of a future role.

A simulation is an operating model that displays processes over time. A model simplifies and introduces clarity through substitution. It is dynamic, because it shows how a system changes over time. A simulation extracts important aspects of a future performance. When using simulation, time can be compressed or expanded, feedback and emergency situations can be introduced to limit errors in transfer to real life, and variety in practice conditions can be planned. For example, learners may be asked to simulate what goes on in a classroom, at a bedside, or any other kind of situation they may be part of in the future.

Theories that Explain Simulation Processes

When many learners and factors are involved, simulations can become as hectic as any real-life situation. Leigh and Spindler (2004) introduced **chaos theory** as one framework for identifying the skills and knowledge nurse educators might need to anticipate

Chaos theory helps find the underlying order in apparently random data.

and respond to during the uncertainties generated during a large-scale simulation. Systems such as groups or classrooms units may appear disordered, but chaos theory is really about finding the underlying order in apparently random data. Use of this theory can allow nurse educators to quickly and accurately select and apply appropriate learning-centered interventions.

Knowing when to intervene and when to observe and stay quiet are skills nurse educators must develop to facilitate effective simulations. Many of these skills come with experience. As with role playing, it is suggested nurse educators try out their simulations and also be part of other faculty simulations prior to using them with learners.

Process simulation is another theory that explains how simulations harness the imagination using mental processes, and explores how they relate to self-regulation and coping skills (Taylor, Pham, Rivkin, and Armor, 1998). Humans can envision the future and then regulate their behavior and emotions to bring it about.

Social cognition researchers have studied how problem-solving activities can move learners toward an envisioned future. Taylor et al. (1998) reviewed the evidence for imagining hypothetical events and found at least nine empirical investigations demonstrating that people are more apt to believe events will actually occur following mental simulation as opposed to following other cognitive activities. This could be because when one envisions completing a procedure with a client or doing well on an exam, mental pictures are created that may lead to uncovering opportunities and problem solving in ways previously not considered. Rehearsing a process—either in the mind or with real objects—forces the learner to identify and organize the steps involved in the activities needed to get there and yields a plan for how to do it. According to Taylor et al. (1998), such behaviors also help regulate emotional states, such as performance anxiety.

Taylor et al. (1998) compared process simulations (imagining the steps in the process to get a good grade on an exam), and outcome simulations (imagining getting an A on an exam and feeling confident and proud). Learners who used process simulations for five to seven days before their midterms reduced their test anxiety and did better on their exams than those who just pictured themselves doing well. The same process also worked for learners assigned to complete a project. The researchers concluded that the process simulation enabled the learners to use planning and problem-solving skills to aid them in a timely completion of their projects. Simulation process skills can also be taught to clients to assist them to complete learning tasks, follow nursing advice, and be successful attaining their own goals.

> ■ **Nurse Educator Challenge**
>
> Explain one way to use mental simulation with learners. Demonstrate it to the class or to a small group of colleagues and obtain feedback.

Other Forms of Simulations

A simulation is designed to achieve learning objectives. It can be a group or individual activity. Roles could be written for a whole hospital staff or community group, thus allowing an active role for every member in a large classroom. Learners may interact with one another or with media such as written nursing notes and nursing care plans, computer printouts, film loops, or even simulated clients (manikins) and laboratories (Earle, 2006; Inglis et al., 2004; Barach, Satish, and Strenfert, 2001; Kendall and Harrington, 2003). Whatever the method, learners are always actively involved, because they must constantly interact with people or with materials.

By extracting a slice of life (the referent situation), highly complex situations can be simplified to increase skill practice. For example, by not including any information on the medical, nutrition, or other hospital departments, nursing behaviors can be focused on, thus simplifying the simulation.

Nurse Educator Tip

Helping Learners Do Well on Exams

Use a mental simulation exercise to help learners do well on exams. Read the following statement aloud, provide a handout with the words on it, and ask learners to complete this exercise for five minutes every day for a week prior to their exam:

See yourself studying and hold this picture in your mind. Eliminate all distractions by seeing yourself turning off the TV, radio, and any other sounds and declining any offers from friends to go out. See yourself sitting at your desk or at the library studying chapters and going over your notes. See yourself covering the material easily and calmly and learning a lot.

Learners are presented with cues and consequences similar to those that occur in real life and are asked to react to conditions as they would in the actual nursing situation. Simulations can provide an opportunity for learners to draw fragmented bits of information into a meaningful whole. Reading about a situation or even observing one never provides the feeling of what it is really like to be in the situation; simulation can.

Feedback in Simulations

Feedback in simulations is provided in ways that replicate natural channels. Educator/ learner personality clashes are avoided because materials and/or peers provide feedback. Potential danger for participants can be reduced by building in interpersonal and physical protection. High costs can be avoided by using inexpensive materials.

Potential Uses and Benefits of Simulation

Some types of learning objectives that lend themselves especially well to simulation are those that emphasize:

1. Affective behavior
2. Combined affective and cognitive and/or perceptual-motor learning
3. The learner's interaction with a complex and reactive environment
4. Incorporation of the behavior with the learner's self-image
5. Application of behavior in a variety of contexts
6. Problem-solving skill
7. The assimilation of the relationship between behavior and its consequences
8. Creativity and experimentation
9. Memory or practice drill

Whereas written multiple-choice or essay questions reveal how learners think they ought to behave, simulations place them in situations that elicit how they do behave. Examples of nurse/client or client/client situations that have been or could be simulated as learning experiences are:

- The dying process
- Aging
- The nurse/client relationship
- The nursing home experience
- Individual, group, or family nursing interviews

- Sessions of teaching, supportive, or task groups
- Physical assessment
- Nursing diagnosis with appropriate intervention
- Leadership and assertive behavior
- Community dynamics and emerging problems

Types of Simulations

Some simulations require that the learner(s) complete a series of assessments or carry out problem-solving procedures.

Active Case-Study Simulation

Jeffrey, a seasoned nurse educator, decided to use active case-study simulation with his graduate students. He gave them information about a case that matched the topic of the text he'd assigned for the week. Jeffrey gradually disclosed more and more information by having a colleague enter class halfway through, pretending to be a family member of the client under study, and disclosing genetic information to which the learners were not initially privy.

In the **active case-study simulation,** information is presented to participants in a preset pattern; additional material is gradually disclosed via the kind of source that would provide it in the real-life environment. For example, if new information is provided in real life via lab tests, lab information could be available on a unit computer at crucial times during the simulation.

> In an active case-study simulation, information is gradually disclosed to learners.

Simulation situations are designed to become progressively more complex. There are often critical decision points where several choices are presented; once a choice has been made, the learner is directed to a preset conclusion. This kind of simulation can be structured so that of the three choices, one is the most efficient and helpful, one is not harmful but is inefficient, and the other either impedes helpful actions or is harmful. The following example illustrates opening directions for a simulation portraying nursing leadership behaviors:

It is three o'clock, and you are the head nurse on a surgical floor. You are about to report off duty. Three unexpected admissions arrive, you find the unit manager drunk in the treatment room, and Dr. Jones, the senior resident, wants to make rounds with you. What happens in this situation depends on your leadership behavior. You may use any of the materials or people available to you to solve the problem. This simulation will end when you have solved each of the subproblems.

Some materials available for this simulation might be admission and history notes for the three new admissions, information about the past work record of the ward clerk, and data about the head nurse's previous relationship with the senior resident.

Available people might include role players such as a unit manager and/or senior resident. The complexity and completeness of the simulation would be dependent on learning objectives, the nurse educator's creativity, time constraints, and learner entry skill.

The simulation could call for learners to write down the simulations preselected points once they have consulted specific answers. Cues and prompts could be used or deleted according complexity level deemed to be important.

Symbolic Model Simulation (Manikins)

Another type of simulation uses symbolic models in the nursing laboratory. For example, various types of manikins have been developed to simulate cardiac arrest, colostomy irrigation, urinary catheterization, hip fracture care, and more (Currie, Hoy, Tierney, Bryan-Jones, and Lapsley, 2003; Lotz, 2007). Some manikins allow practice with many nursing skills. One targets key skills for in-hospital care including women's health, obstetrics, post-partum care, wound assessment and care, and general patient care. Pre-programmed scenarios provide standardized training while customizable scenarios and real time educator control allows adaptation to meet individual learner needs.

Flexible manikin platforms allow multiple accessory modules to be added, including trauma, NBC, and bleeding control for use in multiple clinical settings. Some features of manikins include anatomical landmarks, trachea and esophagus, along with simulated lungs and stomach that allow the practice of many procedures, including NG, OG, tracheal care, and suctioning. Normal and abnormal heart sounds, breath, and bowel sounds, and fetal heart tones provide skills in auscultation. Rhythm variants allow practice in interpreting ECGs using standard clinical monitors. A nurse educator-controlled blood pressure arm allows for realistic palpation and auscultation. Systolic and diastolic pressures, ausculatory gap, and volume are variable. An articulating IV arm allows for practice of IV cannulation, medication administration, and site care and maintenance

A manikin can allow for practice in medication dose calculations and administration through intramuscular injections at the deltoid, gluteal, ventrogluteal, and thigh sites. Optional modules can be added for breast examination, post-surgical mastectomy care, fundus massage skills, and assessment and care of wounds and surgical incisions.

> Cindy, a new educator, was assigned to the nursing lab. She received an orientation to SimWoman, a computerized manikin, that can be programmed by the nurse educator to interact with learners using a variety of phases. When three learners in hospital uniform arrived at the lab, Cindy watched while they practiced making life and death decisions, working with the manikin. The patient simulator had been programmed by faculty to react to the care given. The learners started by draping and screening the manikin, showing how to maintain privacy. The manikin spoke and told the learners how she felt. This gave them a chance to practice communication skills, and talk to the manikin, who responded. The learners explained each procedure they planned to undertake and asked appropriate questions. The learners identified an irregularity in the heartbeat, and although they performed the necessary treatment, the simulated client "crashed."

■ Nurse Educator Challenge

You are the nurse educator about to work with a group of learners and a manikin. What would be your first act? Give a rationale for your answer.

Working with Learners and Manikins

Manikins can be used to provide guided practice, more self-directed practice, and to evaluate learning. The learner may be presented with a specific manikin and directed to deal with the specific physical problem being demonstrated. At first the learner would be taught how to deal with the problem. Later, the learner might be asked to work with the manikin without cues or prompts; this time the physical situation could be used as an evaluation of what has been learned.

Advantages of working with a manikin are that they allow learners to experience situations they may never encounter during their regular rotations in hospitals, while providing a safe environment that can be regulated. At first, nurse educators write the scenarios. Advanced students may be given an opportunity to create a scenario as a class project.

Symbolic Replication of Reality Simulations

Symbolic replication of reality simulations or materials are used to evoke responses similar to those that would occur in the real-life situation. For example, although no alarm clocks go off at the change of shift, nurses are frequently working under the pressure of too little time to accomplish tasks.

> During symbolic replication of reality, time constraints and hierarchical relationships are portrayed symbolically.

By building in written time constraints or setting off an alarm clock or buzzer, the nurse educator can dramatize the constraints of time through the use of symbolic events. To represent hierarchical relationships symbolically, learners who are enacting doctor or nursing administrator roles sit in chairs, while learners who are playing staff nurse roles sit on the floor.

Behavior Rehearsal

Another type of simulation is the **behavior rehearsal**. In this simulation situation, nursing learners play themselves and say and do exactly what they would with an

> In behavior rehearsal, learners play themselves and obtain practice for upcoming situations.

actual client or learner. This can be a dry run for actual nurse/client interviews or teaching sessions. The nurse educator, a learner who has mastered the skill to criterion, or printed programmed instructional materials could serve as the client and as feedback

for the practicing learner. The example below illustrates the kind of dialogue that might occur when teaching a handicapped client how to deal with social situations by using the behavior rehearsal technique.

Learner nurse:	Let's pretend you're going to the party you mentioned. What's the first thing you think will happen?
Nurse Educator/Client:	I won't go in a wheelchair.
Learner:	Sure you can.
Nurse Educator/Client:	I don't think it would help to reassure me. Find out why I can't go in a wheelchair.
Learner:	Why can't you go in a wheelchair?
Nurse Educator/Client:	Everyone looks at me. They think I'm a freak.
Learner:	Perhaps you need to find a way to put them at ease. What about telling them or showing them how you want to be treated?
Nurse Educator/Client:	I can't.
Learner:	Try it.

Nurse Educator/Client:	Okay. Would you push my chair over to that tree?
Learner:	Then what would happen?
Nurse Educator/Client:	They would push me, I guess.
Learner:	Okay, then you know how to handle that; now let's go through that conversation.
Nurse Educator/Client:	Which one?
Learner:	Where you see me looking and you ask me to push you over near the tree.
Nurse Educator/Client:	Okay.
Learner:	(stares at wheelchair)
Nurse Educator/Client:	Would you mind pushing me over to that tree?
Learner:	Not at all.

In this illustration, cues and prompts were used, and cognitive, affective, and psychomotor practice were made available.

Debriefing a Simulation

George, a seasoned nurse educator, had facilitated a simulation of the emergency department after a fire had destroyed most of an elementary school. The class had dived into their roles and actively evaluated, treated, and/or referred the survivors to a physician. Even after George called "time," participants continued to play their roles.

Large simulations can exhilarate the classroom and start all kinds of learning processes. Even small simulations provide fodder for analysis of behavior that can enhance transfer to real-life nursing situations.

Debriefing or **post-simulation discussions** can enhance learning. The purpose of a debriefing or discussion after the simulation ends is to cool down and analyze what happened (Peters and Vissers, 2004). During the simulation, action is occurring and there may be little time for analysis.

In the case of an exploratory or first-time use of a simulation, the debriefing facilitator (usually the nurse educator) cannot claim to know exactly how to

> Debriefing or post-simulation discussions allow learners a chance to analyze what happened, ask questions, and process information.

proceed, but the basic focus is for participants to learn about perceptions of all other participants so they understand their effect on others. For this reason, a joint debriefing is suggested (Peters and Vissers, 2004).

Not only participants, but all learners in the classroom can also contribute to and learn from the simulation. Debriefing sessions can serve as a source of information about the naturalness and usefulness of the behaviors or role cards in the simulation, and participant views can also be used to validate observations or impressions observed by the nurse educator.

■ Nurse Educator Challenge

What is the purpose of debriefing after a simulation? Give a rationale for your answer.

Purposes of Debriefing

Debriefing can:

- Allow participants to exchange experiences without interference from the nurse educator
- Provide feedback to the nurse educator about the design and correctness of the simulation
- Enhance transfer of learning to real-life nursing situations
- Serve as a vehicle for retention of knowledge and skills
- Discuss ways learners can support each other in applying the acquired knowledge and skills in the real-life situation
- Provide simulated examples of mutual understanding, interpersonal conflict, communication skills (or lack thereof), creating a shared vision, team building, joint problem solving and decision making, assessment, and testing of procedures.

Debriefing Questions

After allowing learners to volunteer their reactions to the simulation, the nurse educator can ask one or more of the following questions to enhance transfer of learning:

1. What events and processes did you observe or experience?
2. How much do these events and processes resemble real-life processes?
3. What did you learn from participating in or observing this simulation that offers clues for action in real life?

4. How doable, desirable, and practical are these actions in the real-life situation and what obstacles or barriers would have to be overcome?
5. How could you overcome these barriers to provide high-level care?

Although these questions are provided in a linear fashion, a more cyclical process often occurs. Analysis of a given simulation situation can give rise to a revision of the facts presented, amended observations, and even refuted earlier explanations (Peters and Vissers, 2004). The more open to discussion the nurse educator is, the more likely analysis will rise to a higher level of critical thinking.

■ **Nurse Educator Challenge**

How could you extend the simulation learning experience for learners? Give a rationale for your answer.

Simulation-Related Assignments

The nurse educator can also give a homework assignment to use journal writing (see Chapter 5) to extend the analytical learning process. This requires each learner to organize the material and debrief on an individual basis. The richness of responses can be increased in this activity as learners weave their own personal thread of observations and reactions through others' statements and behaviors, and link them to theoretical concepts. Another benefit of adding this step to the learning process is that writing provides a permanent record of each learner's experience (Petranek, Corey, and Black, 1992).

All of the comments in this section are applicable to debriefing simulation games. The only differences are that if a simulation game is played in rounds, the nurse educator may wish to debrief after each round.

Simulation Use and Design

Prior to attempting to design a simulation, the nurse educator needs to try out and use already developed simulations. Participation in a simulation is a first step. Next, the nurse educator might try running or facilitating a simulation. A walk-through, either alone or with friends or peers, or a practice session is necessary prior to using the simulation with learners. The nurse educator needs to be familiar with all materials and directions; it is suggested that a checklist of activities, procedures, and materials be used to help to guide the educator and learners through the simulation. The checklist can also be used to plan follow-up discussions and introductory comments.

If learners have never used simulations, a short lecture or description of the method or programmed instructional materials can be used to introduce them to the concept of a simulation. Then the learners might first be exposed to relatively simple simulations and be directed in a summary or evaluation session. Learners who have had experience with simulations can be exposed to more complex ones, and in this case the nurse educator would take a less directive role, playing the role of facilitator in a post-discussion (debriefing) to consolidate learning, or even allowing a learner to take that role.

A simulation is one kind of learning system; as such, its design should follow all the principles discussed in Chapter 2. A simulation would be designed or used only when called for by the learning objectives. System constraints must be examined to ensure that there is sufficient freedom to innovate and enough time allotted for designing the simulation. Task or goal analysis would reveal appropriate content and its sequencing.

Once simulation is chosen as the method, an essential question to ask when designing one is, "How much reality information is needed to achieve learning objectives and involve the learner?" To answer this question, a situation is whittled down to its basic core elements and then choose those that fit with learning objectives and can be demonstrated relatively easily and inexpensively.

There are certain basic frameworks that can be adapted to changing content. For example, in the active case method, materials and directions are changed depending on objectives, but the basic process of design remains the same. Likewise in a practice or symbolic model simulation, materials, directions and/or problem-solving situations change, but the format remains. Simulations are based on learning objectives that lead to a specific model of reality to be enacted. In the following objective, a specific model is presented:

> Using the family interview guide, learners will conduct a forty minute initial interview with a simulated family.

Forty minutes is an appropriate period of time for a nurse to interview a family, and necessary material can be covered in this period. Entry skills are evaluated and prerequisite skills (including an introduction to simulation as a method of instruction) are given if needed. If the designer decides to do so, a pretest is devised and given. At this point, the designer might reexamine whether simulation is the most appropriate teaching method. If so, the family interview guide would be developed or located. (This step flows from the model.) A scenario and/or role information must be provided for each player. There are a number of alternatives available to the educator at this time including.

1. All players can be given the same scenario (**common simulation presentation**).

2. Different information or instructions can be given to different players (**parallel simulation presentation**).

3. Additional information can be revealed to players at critical points in the simulation (**serial simulation presentation**).

4. All players can start with the same information, with some players possessing "secret" information and additional information being presented to all players at prescribed intervals during the course of the simulation combinations.

> In a common simulation presentation, all learners are given the same scenario.

> In a parallel simulation presentation, different information or instructions are given to different players.

> In a serial simulation presentation, additional information is revealed to players at critical points in the simulation.

Boxes 3–1, 3–2, and 3–3 show some materials that could easily be developed for a family interview simulation. The scenario may be a written outline, a list of the sequence of events, or a general description of the flow of the simulation.

Box 3–1   Family Interview Simulation, Outer Envelope

Enclosed are four other envelopes, containing:

1. General directions
   One of the players is now to open the general directions envelope and read the directions aloud to the rest of the players.

2. Nine role cards
   After reading general directions aloud, open the role card envelope. Each person is to draw a card without reading it. Do not let others see your role card.

3. Timekeeper directions
   The person who draws the Timekeeper role card opens this envelope only when "time" has been called.

4. Recorder directions
   The person who draws the role of recorder opens this envelope which says:

Please return all materials to their appropriate envelopes so that others who follow you can use this simulation easily.

These directions are found inside a small envelope that is placed, along with the other envelopes, in the larger, outer envelope.

Box 3–2   General Directions for the Family Interview Simulation

---

General Directions

Read the directions that follow aloud to the group:

This is a simulation visit by the nurse to the Cronin family. Seven to eight players are required to complete the simulation adequately. The timekeeper may play two roles if he or she feels able to complete both tasks.

Now open the FAMILY ROLE CARD ENVELOPE. Place the role cards with FAMILY ROLE CARD side facing up on the floor or on a table. All players are to choose a card and read the direction to themselves only. Players are to say, "I'm ready to play" when they understand their roles. When all players have signaled their readiness, the timekeeper begins play. (The timekeeper will begin and end play and lead the post-simulation discussion.) Any questions that need further clarification should be directed to the instructor.

Note: Copyright 2006, Carolyn Chambers Clark

Box 3–3   Sample Role Card for Family Interview Simulation

Nurse Role

You are going to interview the Cronin family and make an initial assessment using the family interview guide.

You may refer to the guide as you interview the family. Begin the interview as if the family has come to the out-patient clinic for assistance with the youngest son's (John's) bedwetting. Seat the family in the circle and begin the interview.

Linda, a new nurse educator, took a workshop on using simulations with learners and was excited about trying the strategy. She knew a flow chart might help her plan the sequence of events, but she wasn't sure how to begin. She consulted with Rudolfo, a more seasoned nurse educator, who was very gracious with his time and showed her two flow charts he'd developed. He gave her a copy of both and offered to critique her attempts at a flow chart or help in any way he could.

A useful tool in designing simulations (and other learning experiences) is the flow chart. It allows the designer to plan the sequence of events and their relationship to one another. See Figure 3–1 for the flow chart for the family interview simulation.

The nurse educator chooses whether props, cues, materials, name tags, and so on are to be used and how they can be incorporated into the simulation. The sequence of interactions is decided upon, and a method for communicating the designed sequence to participants is planned. The post-simulation discussion (debriefing) is usually an open discussion between players and the nurse educator. The operation and structure of the model is discussed, and players analyze their strategies and relate them to behaviors of other players and to their real counterparts.

Personal feelings and reactions to the simulation are also encouraged. Questions to be focused on during debriefing can be verbalized by the nurse educator, written out, or placed on audiotape. The nurse educator may be available during the simulation to coach or direct. If the nurse educator decides not to be present, learners can be asked to audiotape or videotape the simulation, or one of the participants can be assigned the role of recorder and directed to take play-by-play notes of what has occurred. These records can then be used in debriefing, with or without the presence of the nurse educator.

Decisions about debriefing and the presence of the nurse educator are based on learner ability, simulation sophistication, specificity of directions, time constraints, a wish not to influence the flow of the simulation, or a wish to encourage learner responsibility for learning. Posttests can be developed based on whether productive or reproductive learning is desired. If the debriefing or simulation practice itself serves as sufficient evaluation, no posttest is given.

Figure 3–1 Flow chart for family interview simulation

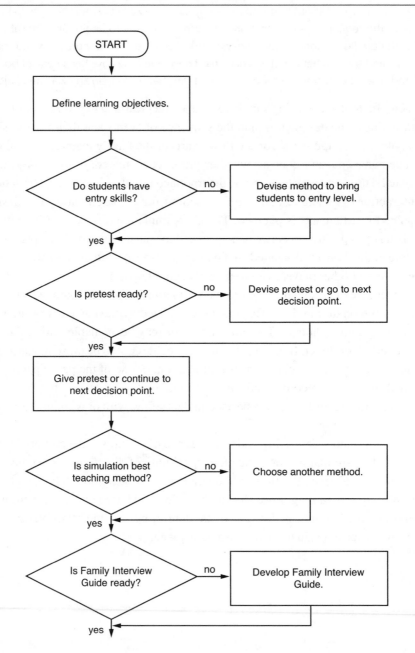

(continues)

Figure 3–1   Flow chart for family interview simulation (continued)

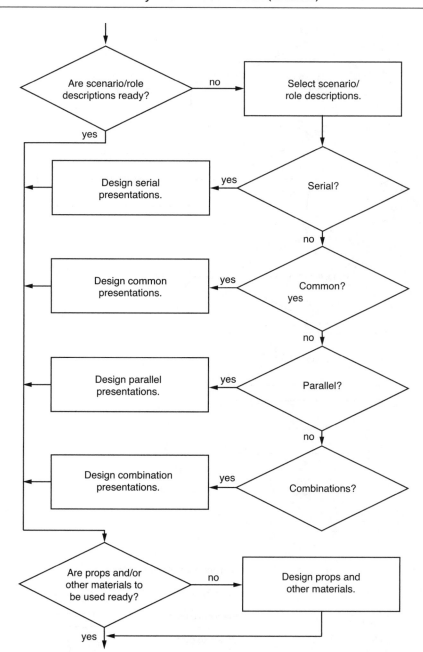

(continues)

Figure 3–1   Flow chart for family interview simulation (continued)

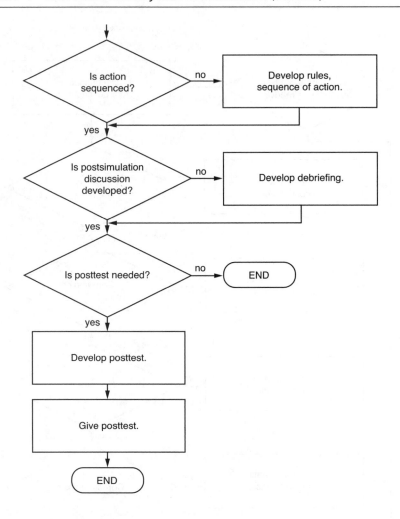

KEY:

Beginning and end of process	
Decision point	
Prescribed action	
Where to go next	

Instructor's Simulation Manual

In addition to developing instructions and materials for participants, it is wise to develop an instructor's manual. This can be used for the designer's own reference, by learners when no nurse educator is present, or by other nurse educators who wish to use the simulation but are inexperienced in its use.

An instructor's manual for a simulation usually contains the following information:

- Brief overview of the model
- Instructional objectives
- Nurse educator role(s)
- How to select and prepare participants
- How to introduce and conduct the simulation
- Debriefing directions and/or specific questions to use during discussion
- Bibliography

■ Nurse Educator Challenge

If you were developing a simulation, how could you divulge information to participants as the simulation unfolds? Give a rationale for your choice.

The overview often contains two or three sentences regarding the number of players involved, their general level of learning, the model upon which the simulation was based, and how the simulation can be integrated within the curriculum. Instructional objectives are stated in the instructor's manual, along with specific ways the simulation can help learners to attain them. In most simulations, the nurse educator plays the role of umpire.

At times, the nurse educator may serve as a resource person who supplies information at critical points in the simulation—for example, by entering with a simulated telegram or message from a prominent person or source. Simulations (and simulation games) use this kind of dramatic situation to add to the excitement and fun of learning. The nurse educator can also serve as a more conventional resource person who refers participants to available sources of information about the problem at hand. In some simulations, the nurse educator may play roles such as timekeeper, or more specialized roles such as client. In some simulations, the nurse educator is the dispenser of materials and evaluator of simulation play, while in others participants direct the action. The role the instructor is to play in the simulation is carefully described in the manual.

The instructor's manual can contain a statement to be read to the participants explaining what a simulation is and preparing them for the activity. For simulations that require specific prerequisite skills, these skills are listed in the manual, and suggestions are listed for bringing participants to entry level.

Pretests and their use are explained if applicable. A key to criterion performance on the pretest is also helpful. In some simulation situations, learners are chosen to play roles, in others they are assigned to roles, or their role is based on the chance draw of a card. The designer needs to think through the value of each assignment method and select the most appropriate one.

It is helpful to indicate the sequence of activities for the simulation. Some information to include is:

- When to pass out materials
- When new information is to be presented to the participant(s)
- What the main players are assigned to do
- What props or cues are needed
- What materials need to be copied or prepared prior to the beginning of the learning experience

The importance of debriefing is explained in the manual, and specific questions to use during that phase of the simulation experience are listed. Alternative suggestions for debriefing, such as asking learners to tape or write a record of the simulation, are also described. The role of the nurse educator or learner group leader in debriefing is explained as the person who reinforces instructional objectives and helps evaluate the effects of simulation.

A posttest is included if applicable and if it differs from the pretest, and suggestions for its use and scoring are included. A bibliography of materials used in the construction of the model includes relevant readings or references to other related simulations that can be used. The level of sophistication and depth of coverage of an instructor's manual depends on the designer. If the simulation is being published for a large audience of potential users, an in-depth coverage is suggested. If the simulation is to be used by the designer only, minimal coverage is probably needed. Figure 3–2 shows a flow chart for the design of an in-depth instructor's manual for a simulation.

Figure 3–2   Flow chart for an in-depth instructor's simulation manual

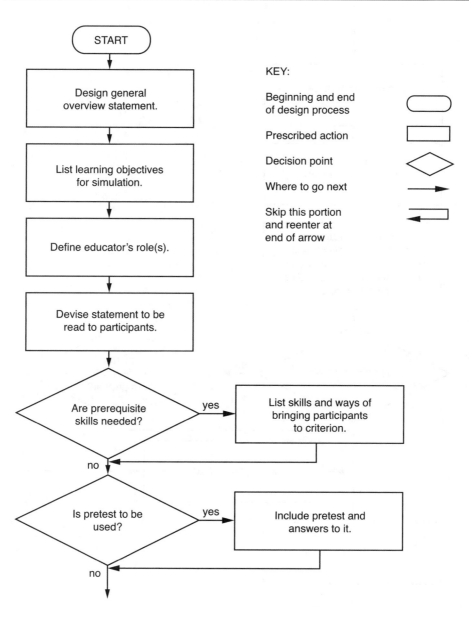

(continues)

Figure 3–2   Flow chart for an in-depth instructor's simulation manual (continued)

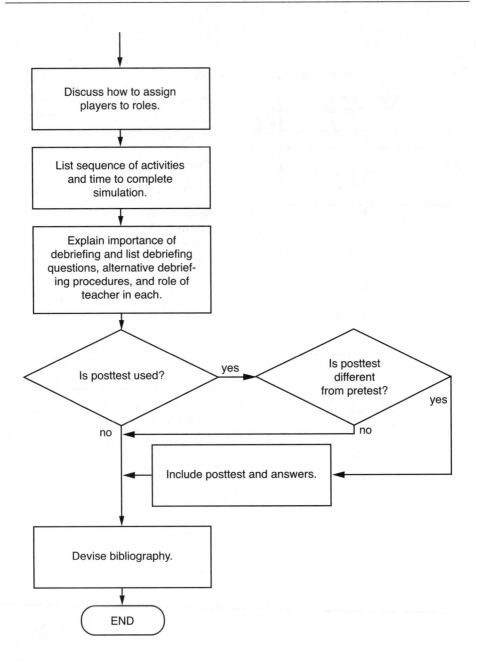

Tryout and Revision

Simulation tryouts and revisions are actually part of simulation design process because feedback from tryout and revision often produces changes that can result in clearer models and more playable learning experiences. Having learners enact the simulation will reveal gaps, omissions, and inconsistencies. The nurse educator needs to be prepared for the unexpected when a simulation is first tried out; what appeared to be understandable and useful in thought may turn out to be incomprehensible or useless in practice.

Feedback from players can be invaluable and should be encouraged. Once the nurse educator can pass the point of taking negative criticism personally, feedback can be used to improve the simulation. Many times players develop new insights or can suggest additional material that adds substantially to the depth and focus of a simulation. It may be wise to develop a feedback form and request that players complete it after having finished the simulation. Another way to collect information about needed revisions is to ask for reactions to the simulation materials and directions during debriefing. Figure 3–3 shows the process of development of a simulation. The next section describes working with simulation games.

> Agnes, a new nurse educator, had heard about simulation games and read about their use in business and other classes. She couldn't see how playing games was going to help anyone learn. In fact, she thought it was downright foolish until she attended a workshop and played a simulation game herself. That evening, she started to develop her own simulation game.

■ **Nurse Educator Challenge**

Explain why you think Agnes changed her mind? What is it about simulation gaming that is attractive to participants in the learning strategy?

Simulation Games

Simulation games combine the properties of simulations—an operating model that displays processes over time—with the properties of games—roles, goals, activities, constraints, and payoffs. Playing roles is an element of simulation gaming (and some simulations). In simulation games, roles are defined in interacting systems, and players are given instructions about constraints on their behavior and the rewards

Figure 3–3   Design process for a simulation

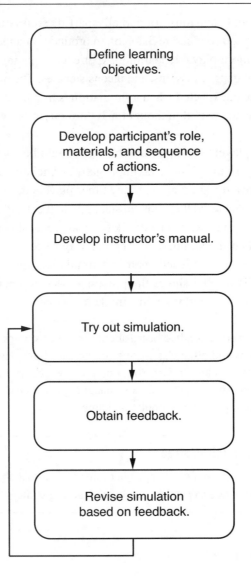

Note: The circular arrow means
        the nurse educator repeats
        the steps as needed.

or punishments (payoffs) they will receive for specific behaviors.

Simulation games differ from role playing in the degree of structure and direction in their emphasis on interaction processes rather than individual roles. Simulation games differ from simulations in that the former have constraints—such as time, mobility, available resources, rules to follow—payoffs—such as bonus chips or other symbols of winning or losing—options to skip a turn, and "fun." In most cases, chance is involved, such as accruing points as the result of the throw of dice or the draw of a card.

> Simulation games combine the properties of simulations with the properties of games, including constraints, rules, chance, rewards, and payoffs.

Simulation games often use game boards, score sheets, and various objects such as bonus chips, dice, playing cards, and manuals to direct play. Monopoly is an example of a game. Props are often used in simulation games. These can be real objects used in the referent situation or symbolic references, such as gold chips, that represent a million dollars.

Simulation games can have a competitive element when two teams or individual members compete for a prize, for a solution, or to win. There are also noncompetitive or cooperative games when a hospital staff, community agency personnel or faculty, and learners of a school of nursing might cooperate to achieve a joint goal. Some learning goals for cooperative games might be to increase communication and understanding of others. Simulation games can be used to teach cooperation and collaboration between a small number of individuals—a nurse and client, for example—or among members of very large groups, such as the staff of a hospital.

The nurse educator builds in competitive or cooperative aspects and decides how many players could minimally and maximally play the game. Whether a simulation game focuses on cooperative communication aspects or on maximizing learning of content, problem solving, or cognitive skills depends on the learning objectives.

Benefits of Simulation Gaming

There are well-documented reasons for using simulation games (Camino & Calcagno, 1995; Shepherd & Cosgriff, 1998; Livingston, 1999; Mercado, 2000; Ryan, 2000; Meligrana & Andrew, 2003). Simulation games have been shown to:

- Prepare learners for professional practice
- Encourage, stimulate, and motivate learners
- Engage learners in critical thinking

- Develop problem-solving skills
- Enable learners to understand issues from multiple perspectives
- Provide an experiential approach to learning
- Foster creativity, imagination, and better retention of theoretical ideas and concepts
- Assist learners in learning how to negotiate systems

Advantages of Simulation Games

Many claims have been made for simulation gaming as a total learning experience, and it is. The advantages of using simulation games in the classroom are:

- *Learners prefer simulation games*—they have fun playing them and learn from them (ExperienceBuilders, 2003; Randel, Morris, Wetzel, and Whitehill, 1992). This finding can be both an asset and a liability. Nurses who think learning must be a serious business can convey this attitude to learners; this nurse educator learning problem can result in a dissipation of learner concentration on the simulation game.

- *Learners learn in a new order*—the other major substantiated finding is that knowledge gained from simulation gaming experiences (experiential learning) proceeds in a reverse sequence from knowledge gained from information processing. In **information processing,** the learner receives the information, comes to understand the general principle, infers particular applications, and then acts by using the general principle in a particular instance. In **experiential learning**, the steps are acting, understanding the particular case, generalizing, and acting in a new circumstance.

> In information processing, the learner receives information, comes to understand the general principle, infers applications, and then acts.

> In experiential learning, the learner acts first, understands the particular example, generalizes, and acts in a new circumstance.

Information processing requires less time, but learners frequently complain that they cannot apply what they have learned. Such comments probably mean they do not really understand the principle and how to particularize. While the experiential learning that occurs in simulation games (and simulations and role playing) is time consuming, all three represent graphically the principles and consequences of one's actions.

For example, it is difficult to overlook the connection between acting in a simulation by choosing to delay a client's p.r.n. pain medication, and receiving feedback from the client about the delay. The consequences of learners' actions are immediately evident, forcing them to deal with the complaining client.

Experiential learning does not neglect the interpersonal aspects of problem solving that information processing experiences often do. Within the simulation game format, players need to think through plays or moves, but they also need to persuade teammates of the effectiveness of a particular action.

- *Being actively involved in creating simulation games yields maximum benefits* —Boocock (1994), one of the pioneering users of simulation games in education, found that the maximum benefits of simulation games are likely to occur when one takes an active role in their creation. This is one good reason to involve learners in the creation of a simulation game. Not only will it reduce the time the nurse educator spends developing the simulation game, but it will benefit learners who must use critical thinking skills to devise a game that matches the learning objectives.

  Motivation will be inherent if game creation is part of the learning objectives for the course and learners are graded on their efforts, and because of the sheer fun of development.

- *Simulation games can change players' attitudes or behaviors*—this only happens if the planned experiences within the games require them to employ knowledge or skills related to a particular attitude or behavior. For this reason, the design of simulation games as a learning system requires that objectives be closely tied to instructional experiences, and that game plays be tied to learning objectives. If simulation games can change attitudes, nurse educators' consideration of them as teaching methods is especially timely at present, when nurses' self-concepts are changing as nursing roles expand, nursing skills become more complex and demanding, and assertiveness with peers is stressed (Clark, 2003).

Simulation games provide a relatively safe, standardized practice environment. Learners need be less concerned about harming the (simulated) client or pleasing the nurse educator, and should concentrate on learning the task at hand. Well-designed simulation games that control and structure outcomes can also provide reliable evaluation tools for judging learner performance.

Disadvantages of Simulation Games

There are several disadvantages to using simulation games as a teaching strategy.

- *It may be difficult for nurse educators to operate in ways that run counter to many of their instincts*—one of the most difficult tasks is yielding control of the class to the rules of the game. Also, nurse educators may find it difficult not to help learners who request it, yet the game may call for ambiguity, and to help learners when they ask for it may be counterproductive to learning. Also, there is a temptation to explain thoroughly all the rules of the game prior to play; since the experience itself will clarify rules, this, too, can be counterproductive. Nurse educators may also feel a strong urge during the debriefing period to lecture participants about the meaning of the simulation game or to explain the experience (see Debrief/Discussion in the simulation section for ideas about how to debrief), rather than to assist them in interpreting and understanding the experience.

- *The largest obstacle may be that nurse educators may not know and understand how to use a simulation game*—they may balk at the idea of using it if they distrust its validity. They may complain that some games represent only a part of reality situations, or that chance and uncertainty should not be included. This objection may be based on a misunderstanding of game models; a model is a simplification and abstraction of elements the game designer decided are important. There are ways of modifying existing games or of designing new games that nurse educators may consider more representative of reality.

This book should begin to help nurse educators to overcome these practical problems, and become enthused about the many benefits this learning approach offers.

> Trudy, a seasoned nurse educator, had finally talked the dean into putting some money in the budget to purchase a simulation game. Once she had the money available, Trudy had to come up with a simulation game that met learning objectives for her courses.

■ Nurse Educator Challenge

What indicants did Trudy use to decide which simulation game would be best for her purposes? Give a rationale for your answer.

Evaluating Available Simulation Games

Available simulation games need to be carefully evaluated for their potential as teaching tools, especially in the areas of:

- Learning objectives and the model
- Game fit with existing curriculum
- Availability of pretests and posttest
- Playability
- Pragmatics

Fit with Learning Objectives

To decide whether a particular simulation game might meet learner learning needs, examine the relationship between learning objectives and the game model. Some questions to be asked in this area are:

1. Are the learning objectives stated in behavioral terms?
2. Are the learning objectives relevant to learner needs for learning?
3. Is there a one-to-one relationship between learning objectives and game plays?
4. Are all learners involved in game play all the time?
5. How relevant is the simulation game experience to the real world of the learners' clinical experience?
6. Does the debriefing session (or some other built-in mechanism) assist learners in drawing out and interpreting principles learned through playing the game?

Fit within Existing Curriculum

Simulation games should not be used simply as a time filler or novelty item. Yet, available simulation games may not lend themselves to instructional plans. Some questions to ask in this area are:

1. What is the theoretical model in the simulation game?
2. Does the model reinforce the existing curriculum?
3. Where in the curriculum can the simulation game be used to reinforce other learning experiences?
4. Is the game too long or too short to fit within classroom time constraints?
5. If the simulation game does not fit within curriculum or time constraints, can it be modified easily by changing rules or materials, or by using rounds of play rather than the entire game?
6. Can the game be used effectively as a homework or remedial assignment?

Pretests and Posttests

Simulation games can be used for learning as well as for evaluation purposes. Simulation games that include pre- and posttests may have an added advantage for the nurse educator. Some questions to be asked in this area are:

1. Is there a pretest included in the simulation game?
2. Is there a posttest included?
3. Does the pretest adequately tap learner learning prior to playing the game as spelled out in the objectives and as formulated in the game structure?
4. Does the posttest evaluate learner learning from playing the simulation game?
5. Does the posttest evaluate important aspects of learner learning?

Playability

A simulation game can seem to be challenging, interesting, and relevant according to its objectives, topics, and structure. When learners play the game, inconsistencies, unknowns, rule gaps, and irrelevant playing materials may be found. Questions to be asked in this area are:

1. Are clearly stated rules included with the simulation game?
2. Do the rules seem enforceable or unreasonable?
3. Are there inconsistencies in game plays?
4. Are there irrelevant or missing playing materials?
5. Has the simulation game been tested and revised with similar nursing populations?
6. Is there information included with the simulation game describing nursing educator and learner evaluations of the simulation game?

Pragmatics

In addition to theoretical issues, the nurse educator considers pragmatic issues when deciding whether or not to use or purchase simulation games. Some of these issues are:

1. Is the game available for preview and/or is specific information available from the author or publisher regarding theoretical issues?
2. What is the cost of the simulation game?
3. Is the cost prohibitive?
4. How easily can game materials be obtained?
5. If the game cost is high, is there a kit available to enable nurse educators to develop their own materials for the game?
6. How much playing space does the game require?

7. How many learners can play the simulation game at once?
8. How does the number of players required to play the game affect its various uses within the curriculum?
9. How portable is the simulation game; can it be played at home or in a car?
10. How many simulation games need to be ordered to be used efficiently for learner learning?
11. How much preparation prior to play does the simulation game require?
12. Are there sufficient directions for the nurse educator to run the game?
13. Is there a clear, specific instructor's manual that can be obtained for preview, even if the simulation game itself cannot be?
14. Are there specific debriefing questions included with the simulation game?

How to Run a Simulation Game

Trying an unfamiliar learning experience can be a frightening situation, especially in the case of a simulation game where action may be fast and the unexpected is apt to occur. A run of some simulation games may be noisy and seemingly chaotic. Even quiet games can be complex. It is therefore imperative to become familiar with all instructions, rules, and materials prior to attempting to run one. Sitting in while someone else runs the simulation game or being a participant can provide the familiarity needed.

Effectiveness of game play can be increased and learners will benefit if the nurse educator feels comfortable with parts of the game including game boards, artifacts, and any audiovisual equipment that are used as an adjunct to learning. Loose dice, signs, or score sheets may be lost, so it is helpful to have extra copies available.

■ **Nurse Educator Challenge**

What steps should a nurse educator take prior to running a simulation game? Give a rationale for your answer.

Preparing to Run a Simulation Game
Ways to prepare for running a simulation game include:

1. *Completing a run-through with colleagues*—a run-through is an excellent way of learning the mechanics of the game and also of anticipating any difficulties that might occur when running the game with learners.

2. *Talking with other educators who have run the game*—more experienced nurse educators can help provide important information such as advice about how to run the game, or discussing problems they encountered.

> Ramon, a new nurse educator, did not want to ask for help with running a new simulation game, even though he knew he needed it. When Cecily, a seasoned nurse educator, asked him how he was doing and to come to her office anytime if he needed assistance, he waited two weeks before taking her up on her offer. Ramon was glad he had swallowed his pride and gone to see Cecily because she gave him a lot of good advice not only on how to run a simulation game, but she volunteered information on how to integrate the game with his other course materials and told him she would be glad to be his assistant the first time he ran the game.

3. *Finding ways to integrate the game with other course materials in the curriculum*—prior to using the game with learners, it is useful to find ways to integrate the game with other course materials, including behavior objectives, goals, and content.

Some guidelines to be used in introducing a simulation game to learners are:

1. Have additional assistants available to run large or complex games, if possible.
2. Make a time schedule for the game run and refer to it often. Setting a clock to go off after a certain number of minutes may be a useful way to remind participants of when to stop a specific activity.
3. Decide whether to give out game materials or directions to players in advance of playing the game. The advantage of giving out materials in advance is that players may be better prepared to play their roles. The disadvantage is that players may not read the materials or forget to bring the materials to the scheduled class.
4. Arrive early to set up game materials, arrange furniture, and plan use of classroom space.
5. Decide whether observers or only active players are allowed to speak during game play.
6. Keep all explanations brief and simple.
7. Move quickly from talking about the game to demonstrating a cycle of play by touching and having learners touch the game materials as they are discussed.
8. Be aware that learners may be both confused and excited about playing a simulation game; tell them that game play will clarify directions and rules, and resist explaining the rules.

9. Describe the overall sequence of events: the play, major interactions, and when or whether debriefing will begin and end.

10. Use a chart or other media form to emphasize the meaning of symbols, resources, constraints, and payoffs.

11. Field questions by answering matter-of-factly and briefly, then move on to the next point in describing the sequence of play.

12. Consider having learner volunteers demonstrate a round (or part of a round) of a game to orient learners to play.

13. Rather than explaining game rules to learners several times, ponder the use of comments such as, "You can do anything in the game you do in the real world," or put the responsibility back on the learner, "I don't know. Get together with your classmates and see what you can figure out."

14. Set the game-playing tone by being facilitating, enthusiastic, impartial, a resource person, and a co-learner.

15. Pass out materials to game players.

16. Observe the process of the game for significant events, and then verbalize observations to players during debriefing.

17. Protect key resources and "secret" information to be revealed at critical points during the game or debriefing.

18. Avoid blaming players for their actions or trying to analyze their motivations.

19. Create an emotionally safe climate for learning.

20. Announce the time remaining for playing the game at various intervals during play.

21. Watch for game players who becoming increasingly uncomfortable in their role and reassign them to less demanding tasks.

22. Watch for game players who innovate by changing rules. If the changes do not disrupt play, do not intervene, but comment on the change in debriefing.

23. Allow adequate time for debriefing—at least twenty minutes.

24. Encourage players to express their thoughts and feelings about the game prior to discussing cognitive learning and the game model. This action will decrease the chance that emotion will interfere with learning.

25. After players have vented their feelings, encourage them to describe what they experienced in the game, to analyze the consequences of their behavior, and to draw conclusions about the use of what was learned for real-life situations.

26. Always give credit to the game designer, and do not replicate materials unnecessarily.

Simulation Game Design

Nurse educators may not be able to find a simulation game that suits their purposes. In that case, it may be necessary to design one. Designing a simulation game forces the nurse educator to think clearly and decide what elements of the real-life situation are relevant to learning.

The simulation game design process includes many of the same steps that simulation design requires:

■ Develop behavioral objectives
■ Present one model of reality
■ Determine entry skills and current level of learning (pretest)
■ Conceptualize the game structure and model

At this point, and at various points along the way, it is beneficial to generate alternative strategies to accomplish specified objectives before a design decision is made, such as: "Is this the most effective way to make the model concrete to learners?"

Input from others familiar with simulation game design can be helpful. Brainstorming with a group of peers or learners can also produce many ideas, some of which will usually be modifiable or directly applicable to the design process. As with any creative problem-solving quest, premature closure of possible strategies can result in a mediocre solution.

While designing a simulation game, the following issues must be explored: How many participants are required? How important will role playing be? Is a game board necessary? Is cooperative or competitive play to be encouraged? What is the sequence of play? How will debriefing and evaluation be implemented? What manuals and directions are necessary?

Each of these critical decisions will be discussed in turn. Discussion of topics in this order in no way implies they are considered in this linear fashion during the design process. Rather, design is the result of interactive decisions and refinements.

Number of Participants

An early question to ask is, "How many players are needed to represent this slice of reality?" Generally, small social systems, such as the nurse/client relationship, can be represented by two to four players. Larger social systems, such as families or groups, may require four to fifteen players. A simulated hospital unit or college faculty may require 15 to 50 players or more.

Role Playing within a Simulation Game

If it is decided that role playing is an essential element of the simulation game, specific role information for players is developed. One of the main advantages of using a simulation game format is that it requires players to learn the consequences of actions and to take responsibility for them.

In some simulation games, roles are imprecisely defined because the model is imprecise. In such cases, the player role may be to use spinners, dice, cards, and accompanying materials to compete or cooperate with other players.

When designing this type of simulation game, deciding on the choice of resources and materials players will use to achieve their goal(s) is the next logical step. Resources are translated into physical representations that can be purchased, exchanged, or won. For example, attaining a learning goal can be represented by a plastic or cardboard key (to the door of knowledge), and power or wealth can be expressed by using play money or chips. Decide what representative object is most likely to meet game objectives, enhance playability, and be cost effective.

Game Boards

The nurse educator decides whether a game board is necessary to serve as the focus of learning or as a symbol of moving forward in time or learning. If so, the board should depict essential symbolic focuses, and time, learning frames, or rounds should be visualized and sketched on paper. Size of the board and its potential mobility should also be considered.

Competition or Cooperation

The nurse educator decides whether competition, cooperation, collaboration, or a combination will be expressed during play, and how to build in the type of interactions

---

Nurse Educator Tip

Writing Role Descriptions

Write role descriptions without assigning attitudes and values. For example, you are a nurse about to begin a counseling relationship with a psychiatric client. Make all responses as a helpful psychiatric/mental health nurse would. An example of a role description that would not work is "You are an anxious nurse about to begin a counseling relationship with a paranoid client who hates nurses."

you desire. If participants compete against each other for a prize or score, competition is fostered. If participants are assigned cooperative or collaborative tasks or have a joint goal, cooperation and collaboration are fostered. If teams compete for a prize or score, cohesiveness and cooperative are fostered intra-group, and competitiveness is encouraged between groups. To decide which of these models is pertinent, the designer examines the reality slice being modeled and attempts to replicate essential aspects.

Sequence of Play

The sequence of play is designed so as to model the referent situation. Sequencing play is part of the design process that is especially related to other issues such as constraints, activities, payoffs, and chance.

Game Constraints

One constraint to be considered is time. Some questions to be asked in this area are: Is it important to limit player time to complete tasks? In the referent situation is time a factor?

> Simulation game constraints include such items as restricting time and limiting resources, mobility, or access.

If so, then some way of limiting time to complete tasks is built in to the sequence of play. For example, a timekeeper or an automatic timer can be used to simulate the pressures of time found in the real-life situation.

Other **simulation game constraints** that might be considered are:

- Limited information sources
- Physical or social condition and mobility
- The amount of power, money, or resources players start out with or can acquire
- Access to educational, political, social, or health institutions.

While considering these issues, it is important to formulate ideas about activities that could be sequenced to represent the referent situation, and how activities might fall into a hierarchy such as game rounds and payoffs.

Game Payoffs

Simulation game payoffs are designed based on the conceptual model being used. For

> Simulation game payoffs are items like fake money, points, and reward stars.

example, if winning and scoring are important aspects of the model, score sheets and directions for scoring are developed. Other possible payoffs are accruing fake money, points, reward stars, and related items.

Simulation Game Chance Factors

Chance can be added to simulation games by introducing chance cards, spins of a wheel or spinner, or
throws of a dice. Chance should be introduced only
if it corresponds to real-world chance factors—such

> Game chance factors
> correspond to real-world
> chance factors.

as flood, natural disaster, or genetic mutation, and not at the whim of the designer
or because no other strategy for sequencing is apparent.

Simulation Game Rules

As sequence of play begins to be formulated, ideas for
rules may occur to the designer. Rules always relate
to the sequence of play, but they could include for-
mulations such as: "No player can begin Round 2

> Simulation game rules
> always relate to the
> sequence of play.

until Round 1 has been completed," "Chance cards are to be drawn following the
occurrence of the simulated disaster."

> Herb, a seasoned nurse educator, usually had no difficulty creating a workable
> simulation game no matter what topic his continuing and community education
> director requested. For some reason, when she gave him his next assignment,
> he couldn't come up with one idea.

■ **Nurse Educator Challenge**

What advice would you give Herb about removing the blocks to his creative
process? Give a rationale for your answer.

Removing Blocks to Creating a Simulation Game

It is not unusual to become mentally blocked in the creative process of depicting the
referent situation. There are a number of techniques that can be used to remove
mental blocks including:

1. *Using transformations*—some questions to stimulate ideas are: How can I
    combine elements to depict reality? How can they be rearranged? Modified?
    Magnified? Minimized? Reversed?
2. *Using a thesaurus*—a thesaurus is a rich source of ideas. Look up the word
    connection for ideas like tie, bridge, tunnel, and clasp. One solution would be

to use tunnels as props linking concept representations, or concepts could be placed on cards and tied together to represent their connection.

3. *Using analogies and metaphors*—a simulation game is often an attempt to replicate a social system. When unable to think of a social system model, it is beneficial to think of physical or biological systems. For example, ask: How do biological systems deal with this problem? How would an animal deal with this problem? More specifically, if the problem is to demonstrate the concept of incorporation, ask: How does a bee take in pollen? How does a coffee pot take in water and ground coffee?

4. *Taking trips to stimulating places*—when unsure about how to use materials to represent a concept, it is often profitable to go to a variety, hardware, or art store where new ideas can be generated by looking at the diverse assemblage of materials and then deriving new ways to use or combine them.

5. *Participating in a pleasurable activity*—place the problem completely out of mind and become submerged in a pleasurable physical or social activity. Mental blocks sometimes disappear when this is done.

Debriefing Simulation Games

Debriefings are usually held following play of the game. Concepts and principles can be underlined during play through the use of programmed instructional manuals or in-game discussions about why certain players are acting in certain ways. As in simulation debriefings, some or all of the following are pertinent:

- Analysis of player strategies
- Cause-and-effect relationships revealed through the game model
- Relating the model to the referent situation
- Noting both accurate parallels and omissions, and personal reactions to playing the game

Posttests

Nurse educators decide whether more specific evaluation procedures are needed. If they are, a posttest is developed to focus on cognitive, affective, or perceptual-motor learning, depending on the model used to develop the simulation game. Posttests and pretests are the same test when reproductive learning is important.

Simulation Game Directions or Manuals

Participant manuals or direction sheets are developed to provide background information for participants. If the simulation game is packaged in a box, participant directions can be printed on the inside cover. If this is not feasible, directions can be placed on durable, preferably waterproof, material. Participant directions usually contain:

- An overview of the game purpose
- The reason for a simulation game being the method of choice for this purpose
- A brief statement of the range of participants who can play the game (for example, from five to eight players)
- Suggestions for using the game as a learning experience

Simulation Game Objectives

Learning objectives are stated. For some simulation games, objectives are placed on separate cards that correspond to the round being played. If there are rounds, there may be objectives for each round. The card for each round is read aloud by one designated player and is placed next to participants for ready reference. If there are no rounds, objectives can be stated on a separate sheet of paper.

Game Model

The next section of the participants' manual includes a brief but clear statement of the game model. It is here that the designer conveys to the user which part of the real-life situation the game seeks to simulate.

Player Roles

Players' roles can be stated in the manual or placed on separate role cards. Role cards are specific and may include specific statements to say at specific points in the game.

Game Resources

The manual specifies what resources are included. Resources will depend on the game model and could range from telegrams to politicians concerning health care legislation to nursing care plans. All game parts should be described in detail; a drawing or picture of materials can be helpful. The manual also includes an estimate of how long it will take to play the game and a list of game rules and scoring procedures, if applicable. If debriefing is part of the game, specific directions are included. Suggestions for repeated plays of the game or specific rounds can also be added.

Instructor or Game Runner Manual

The content of the manual will be influenced by the game model, but it should minimally contain an overview of the game and model, learning objectives, entry skills, pretest, scenario/role descriptions, game materials, sequence of play, rules, scoring procedures, debriefing procedures, and posttest (if applicable).

In addition, instructor anxiety can be decreased by adding additional structure. For instance, directions can be given about how the instructor can allocate time, perhaps by giving the instructor or game runner time estimates about how long it will take to train game running assistants, prepare materials, set up the game, introduce the game, and conduct the post-game discussion.

The manual should indicate if pre-game preparations are needed, like reproducing charts or other materials. Specific written instructions proposing words to use in introducing the game to participants are also helpful. Many of the suggestions for the design of simulations also hold for simulation game design, including the development of feedback forms to be used to evaluate the simulation game.

Tryout and Revision

> The external validity of a simulation game can be tested by how well the game models the real world.

> The internal validity of a simulation game can be measured by judging whether participant decisions over time conform to the environment of the simulation, or by testing whether better learners outperform poor learners.

Tryout and revision are important aspects of simulation game design. Most games cannot be claimed to be valid until the game has been played ten times, with the last three plays requiring no changes, although not everyone agrees with this rule of thumb. The **external validity** of a simulation game can be tested by how well the game models the real world. The **internal validity** of a simulation game can be measured by judging whether participant decisions in a simulation game over time conform to the environment of the simulation, or by testing whether better learners outperform poorer learners (Faria and Wellington, 2005).

Ethical and Mechanical Issues

While tryouts and revisions are being completed, the nurse educator begins to grapple with ethical and mechanical decisions. If the simulation game is designed while the nurse educator is a faculty member, it is important to clarify whether the copyright to the game belongs to the school or the educator. Many game designers are quite free in sharing their games; other sell their games to publishers or print them themselves. Designers who spend several years designing, perfecting, and using a simulation game must consider this issue.

Suggestions for the Use of Inexpensive Gaming Materials

It may be useful to explore the use of inexpensive gaming materials. Simulation games use game parts and unusual materials that are not easily copied, or that require more permanent construction than regular paper allows. Yet, more permanent materials often mean higher cost. These suggestions show how inexpensive yet relatively durable materials can be used.

1. Use 3 × 5" unlined index cards for role player descriptions. Information can be typed on the card and then a bar of paraffin wax can be run over it to provide fingerprint and waterproofing.
2. Purchase poker chips or chips from other games, or cut out circles of construction paper of different colors to represent power, money, status, and so on.
3. Tape together two small pieces of tag board (available in art stores) to serve as a fold-up game board. After painting (or drawing with a felt-tip pen) game routes, rounds, or whatever on it, a paraffin bar can be run over it for protection from spots or fingerprints.

Nurse Educator Tip

Dealing with Mechanical Considerations for Simulation Games

Mechanical considerations for simulation games include asking such questions as:

- Does the college have facilities for printing copies of the game?
- If so, how are these negotiated for?
- Are fees or charges to be permitted for allowing others to use the gaming materials?
- If so, are these to cover printing and developing costs only, or does the nurse educator expect to make a profit?

4. Purchase oilcloth or soft plastic and cut to size for a fold-up game board. Polyester paint, which is virtually nonremovable, can be used to paint on relevant information. It is suggested that the board be first sketched in pencil and then traced over with brush and paint.

5. Use large manila envelopes to hold smaller letter envelopes, which in turn are used to hold role cards, directions, assessments and other game materials. Again, paraffin wax protects the materials through many plays.

6. Find a box container company that makes various-sized boxes; one size may be the exact size needed to house simulation gaming materials, yet can be purchased in quantities at much lower cost than single boxes from a variety store.

7. Check out offset rates as opposed to copying rates; large quantities of score sheets or game directions can be offset by a college print shop.

8. Use soft materials to package simulation games if they are to be mailed. Burlap makes an attractive container for simulation game materials and is often lighter than a box. The burlap pouch can be placed inside a large padded mailing envelope and mailed safely and relatively inexpensively. Other soft materials can also be used, but all require sewing skills (two sides are sewn and a hook and eye used to hold the bag closed), special glue, or stapling equipment.

9. Use overhead transparency sheets or lightweight flexible plastic to protect game directions or manual covers. The sheets can be stapled to either side of a one- or two-page direction sheet, or they can be used as the front and back cover for participants' or instructors' manuals.

10. Browse through arts-and-crafts books. A local, general library collection usually includes many arts-and-crafts books that can supply ideas for inexpensive materials.

Special equipment (or an inexpensive facsimile) can often be found in variety, art, or hardware stores. Figure 3–4 shows a flow chart for a simulation game design.

This chapter presented a rationale for using role playing, simulation, and simulation gaming. Process simulation theory and chaos theory provided the underpinnings for the methods. Differences among the three learning strategies as well as specific directions on how to develop, implement, and evaluate results were provided. Chapter 4 focuses on peer learning and other group methods, including working with large classes.

Figure 3–4   Flow chart for simulation game design

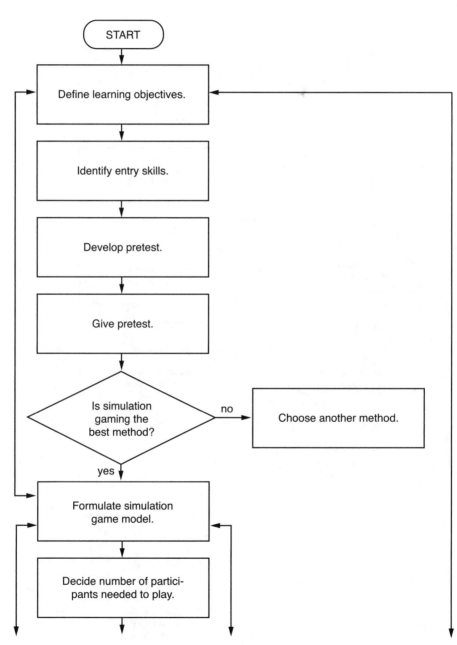

(continues)

Figure 3–4 Flow chart for simulation game design (continued)

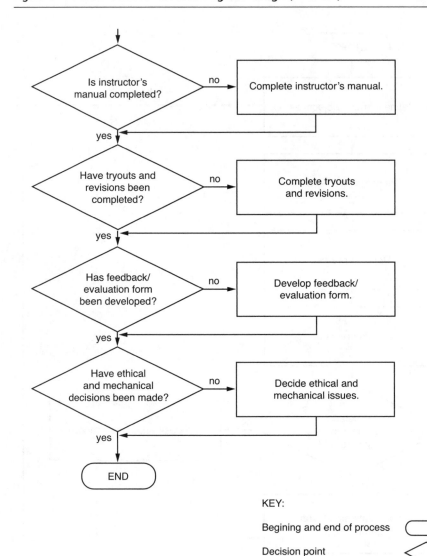

EXERCISES FOR NURSE EDUCATORS

1. Matching learning objectives to method
Write down the learning objective(s) you wish to achieve. Then write down which of three formats (role playing, simulation, simulation gaming) you plan to use to meet your objective(s). Then tell why you chose the particular format rather than another.

2. Simulation flow chart
Draw a flow chart for a 20– to 60–minute simulation. Refer to Figure 3–2.

3. Simulation design
Design the materials needed to conduct the 20– to 60–minute simulation you have chosen, including:
1. Pretest
2. Materials to be used, such as guide, assessments, etc.
3. Role descriptions/scenarios
4. Props and other cues, such as signs, name tags, etc.
5. Sequence of action
6. Debriefing questions
7. Posttest

4. Instructor's manual
Design an instructor's manual for the 20– to 60–minute simulation you have chosen.

5. Feedback for simulation design
Design a feedback form to use in tryouts and revisions of the simulation.

6. Learn more about simulation/gaming
Do one of the following:
1. Read the latest issue of *Simulation & Gaming.*
2. Adapt or use someone else's simulation or simulation game in a nursing class or with colleagues.
3. Have a focus group with 4–10 learners and get their ideas about using simulations and/or simulation games in class. Be sure to provide definitions of both prior to asking learners for feedback.
4. Attend a simulation gaming conference or an educational conference that presents simulation and/or simulation gaming.

7. Evaluating simulation games
Evaluate at least one simulation game using the criteria listed in this chapter.

8. Running a simulation game

Choose a simulation game and complete the following tasks:

1. Become familiar with the materials, sequence of play, and directions.
2. Complete a run-through with a group of peers or friends.
3. Devise a list of potential difficulties in using the simulation game.
4. Decide how the game could be integrated into a course.
5. Try out the game with a group of learners or faculty.
6. Prepare questions to use in debriefing (if the game doesn't include them).

9. Simulation game flow chart

Draw a flow chart for a 20- to 60-minute simulation game. Refer to Figure 3–3.

ADVANCED LEARNING EXPERIENCES

10. Simulation game design

Design the materials and make decisions about the design of the simulation game based on the flow chart you developed.

11. Process simulation theory

Devise three ways to use process simulation theory.

12. Journal writing

Use journal writing excerpts to develop a paper suitable for publication.

13. Manikin

Write a scenario for a manikin like the one Cindy observed.

14. Research

Devise a role playing, simulation, or simulation gaming problem statement for a research study.

References

Abramovich, E. (2006). Application of CBT in an inpatient setting: Case illustration of an adult male with anxiety, depression, and Axis II symptoms. *Clinical Case Studies, 5,* 305–330.

Arco, L., & du Toit, E. (2006). Effects of adding on-the-job feedback to conventional analog staff training in a nursing home. *Behavior Modification, 30,* 713–735.

Armstrong, J. S. (2000). Role playing: A method to forecast decisions. In J. S. Armstrong (Ed.), *Principles of forecasting: A handbook for researchers and practitioners.* Norwell, MA: Kluwer Academic Publishers. Retrieved September 26, 2006 from http://author.ecu.edu/csdhs/ah/upload/role_playing_byArmstrong.pdf

Barach, P., Satish, U., & Strenfert, S. (2001). Health care assessment using simulation. *Simulation & Gaming, 32,* 147–155.

Bender, T. (2005). Role playing in online education: A teaching tool to enhance student engagement and sustained learning. *Innovate, 1,* (4). Retrieved February 7, 2007 from http://www.innovateonline.info/index.php?view=article&id=57

Blatner, A. (2002). *Role playing in education.* Retrieved February 2, 2007 from http://blatner.com/dam/pdntbk/flplayedu.htm

Bodenman, G., Pihet, S., Shantinath, S. D., Cina, A., & Widmer, K. (2006). Improving dyadic coping in couples with a stress-oriented approach: A two-year longitudinal study. *Behavior Modification, 30,* 571–597.

Boocock, S. S. (1994). The John Hopkins Games Program. *Simulation and Games, 25*(2), 172–178.

Camino, E., & Calcagno, C. (1995). An interactive methodology for "empowering" students to deal with controversial environmental problems. *Environmental Education and Research, 1*(1), S9–74.

Cooper, E. O. (2004). Federal grant helps nursing students boost their cultural sensitivity. *Quest (Winter),* 1-4, 23. Retrieved February 9, 2007 from http://www.odu.edu/ao/instadv/quest/sensitivity.pdf

Currie, C. T., Hoy, D., Tierney, A. J., Bryan-Jones, J., & Lapsley, I. (2003). HipMod: Development of a multi-agent audit-based computer simulation of hip fracture care. *Health Informatics Journal, 9*(3), 183–191.

Dewey, J. (1963). *Experience and education.* New York: Collier Books.

Duke, R. D. (1975). The unanticipated consequences of modifying learning games for research on social behavior. In J. Elliot and R. McGinty (Eds), *Proceedings of the 14th Annual Conference of the North American Simulation and Gaming Association.* Los Angeles: University of Southern California Press, 117–120.

Earle, D. (2006). Surgical innovation: Surgical training and simulation lab at Baystate Medical Center. *Simulation & Gaming, 13,* 53–60.

ExperienceBuilders. (2003). *A comparison of simulation-based and conventional training methods.* Retrieved October 1, 2006 from http://www.experiencebuilders.com/eb/why/white_papers/simulationeffectiveness.pdf

Fagan, R. (2006). Counseling and treating adolescents with alcohol and other substance use problems and their families. *Family Journal, 14,* 326–333.

Faria, A. J., & Wellington, W. J. (2005). Validating business gaming: Business game conformity with PIMS findings. *Simulation & Gaming, 36*(2), 259–273.

Fisak, B. J., Oliveros, A., & Ehrenreich, J. T. (2006). Assessment and behavioral treatment of selective mutism. *Clinical Case Studies, 5,* 382–402.

Frank, A. I. (2006). Three decades of thought on planning education. *Journal of Planning Literature, 21,* 15–67.

Gebara, J., & Tashijan, H. (2006). End-of-life practices at a Lebanese hospital: Courage or knowledge? *Journal of Transcultural Nursing, 17,* 381–388.

Gibbs, G. R., Doggett, C., & Frost, S. (2005). Virtual learning environments for efficient health service practitioner education. Proposal for health services in West Yorkshire. Retrieved September 27, 2006 from http:// www.hud.ac.uk/hhs/teaching/nursingvle.htm

Haddad, A. (2006). Playing a standardized patient in an ethics course: What nursing students learn. Creighton University. Retrieved February 1, 2007 from http://chpe.creighton.edu/Chpe/snapshots/Haddad/nursing.pdf

Hecht, M. L., & Kreiger, J. L. R. (2006). The principle of cultural grounding in school-based substance abuse prevention: The drug resistance strategies. *Journal of Language and Social Psychology, 25,* 301–319.

Inglis, S., Sammon, S., Justice, C., et al. (2004). Cross-cultural simulation to advance learner inquiry. *Simulation & Gaming, 35,* 476–487.

Ip, A., Linser, R., & Jasinski, M. (2002). *The zen of being an effective "Mod" in online role-play simulations.* Retrieved February 7, 2007 from http://ausweb.scu.edu.au/aw02/papers/refereed/ip/paper.html

Jenkins, P., & Turick-Gibson, T. (1999). An exercise in critical thinking using role playing. *Nurse Educator, 24*(6), 11–14.

Kendall, K. W., & Harrington, R. J. (2003). Strategic management education incorporating written or simulated cases: An empirical test. *Journal of Hospitality and Tourism Research, 27, 143–165.*

Kirsh, B., & Tate, E. (2006). Developing a comprehensive understanding of the working alliance in community mental health. *Qualitative Health Research, 16,* 1054–1074.

Lee, M., Hajek, P., McRobbie, H., & Owen, L. (2006). Best practice in smoking cessation services for pregnant women: Results of a survey of three services reporting the highest national returns, and three beacon services. *Journal of the Royal Society for the Promotion of Health, 126,* 233–238.

Leigh, E. & Spindler, L. (2004). Simulations and games as chaordic learning contexts. *Simulation & Gaming, 35*(1), 53–69.

Livingston, I. (1999). Role-playing planning public inquiries. *Journal of Geography in Higher Education, 23*(1), 63–76.

Lotz, K. S. (2007). *Get real. Simulated patients and hospitals help boost not only the number of students reached, but how well they learn.* Retrieved March 12, 2004 from http://www.nurse.com.

Lovecraft, A., Chapin, W. D., Parker, D. C. W., & Sadler, D. (2006, February). *Simulations and role playing (S&RP) 1Track Summary.* Presented at the 2006 APSA Teaching and Learning Conference Track Summaries. Washington, DC.

Marks, M. & O'Connor, A. H. (2006). The round-robin mock interview: Maximum learning for minimum time. *Business Communication Quarterly, 69,* 264–275.

Mayo Clinic. (2006). *Teaching the art of compassion: Herberger College of Fine Arts and Mayo Clinic partnership.* Retrieved February 1, 2007 from http:community.uui.asu.edu/features.mayo.asp.

Meligrana, J. F. & Andrew, J. S. (2003). Role-playing simulations in urban planning education: A survey of learner learning expectations and outcomes. *Planning Practice & Research, 18*(1), 95–107.

Mannick, F. (2005). Preventing STDs in African American and Latina girls. *The American Journal of Nursing, 105*(8), 22.

Mercado, S. A. (2000). Pre-managerial business education: A role for role-plays. *Journal of Further and Higher Education, 24*(1), 117–126.

Miaskowski, C. & Maxwell, T. L. (2002). *The art and science of pain management: The nurse's role in teaming with the clinician and empowering the patient.* Presented to the Twenty-Seventh Annual Congress of the Oncology Nursing Society. Retrieved September 26, 2006 from http://www.cmecorner.com/macmem/ons/ons2002_12.htm

Nelson, D.L., & Blenkin, C. (2007). The power of online role-play simulations: Technology in nursing education. *International Journal of Nursing Education Scholarship, 4*(1), 1-12.

Peters, V. A. M., & Vissers, G. A. N. (2004). A simple classification model for debriefing simulation games. *Simulation & Gaming, 35*(1), 70–84.

Petranek, C. F., Corey, S., & Black, R. (1992). Three levels of learning in simulations: Participating, debriefing, and journal writing. *Simulation & Gaming, 23*(2), 174–185.

Pham, L. B., & Taylor, S. E. (1999). From thought to action: Effects of process-versus outcome-based mental simulations on performance. *Personality and Social Psychology, 25*(2), 250–260.

Raelin, J. A., & Coghlan, R. (2006). Developing managers as learners and researchers: Using action learning and action research. *Journal of Management Education, 30*(5), 670–689.

Randel, J. M., Morris, B. A., Wetzel, D., & Whitehill, B. V. (1992). The effectiveness of games for educational purposes: A review of the research. *Simulation & Gaming, 25,* 261–276.

Rohrbach, L. A., Grana, R., Sussman, S., & Valente, T. W. (2006). Type II translation: Transporting prevention interventions from research to real-world settings. *Evaluation and the Health Professions, 29,* 302–333.

Ryan, T. (2000). The role of simulation gaming in policy-making. *Systems Research and Behavioral Sciences, 17,* 359–364.

Schwartz, M. S., & Weber, J. (2006). A business ethics national index (BENI): Measuring business ethics around the world. *Business and Society, 45,* 382–405.

Shepherd, A. & Cosgriff, B. (1998). Problem-based learning: A bridge between planning education and practice. *Journal of Planning Education and Research, 17,* 148–357.

Staib, S. (2003). Teaching and measuring critical thinking. *Journal of Nursing Education, 42*(1), 498–508.

Taylor, S. E., Pham, L. B., Rivkin, I. D., & Armor, D. A. (1998). Harnessing the imagination: Mental simulation, self-regulation, and coping. *American Psychologist, 53*(4), 429–439.

Taylor, S. E., Pham, L. B., Rivkin, I., & Armor, D. A. (1998). Harnessing the imagination: Mental simulation and self-regulation of behavior. *American Psychologist, 53,* 429–439.

Teed, R. (2006). *How to teach using role-playing.* Retrieved January 22, 2007 from http://serc.Carleton.edu/introgeo/roleplaying/howto.html

University of New Mexico College of Nursing. (2006). *Teaching and learning strategies.* Retrieved September 27, 2007 from http://hsc.health.unm.edu/consg/critical/role_playing.shmtl.

FOUR

Group Methods and Peer Learning

■ INSTRUCTIONAL GOALS

Upon completion of this chapter and the nurse educator's learning experiences, the learner will be able to:

- ■ Explain the benefits of using group and peer methods of learning
- ■ Identify group phases
- ■ Employ discussion groups
- ■ Utilize small-group tutorials
- ■ Implement theme-centered groups
- ■ Plan ways to implement peer learning
- ■ Demonstrate ways to work creatively with large classes

Upon completion of this chapter, the more advanced nurse educator will be able to:

- ■ Devise a problem statement for a study comparing different types of peer and group methods of learning
- ■ Complete a small research project comparing peer group to discussion group results or small group tutorials to theme-centered groups, or examining the effect of working creatively with large classes

Key Terms

ARS	Narrative pedagogy
Brainstorming	Peer learning
Cognitive map	Peer review
Cohesiveness	Peer supervision
Concept mapping	Peer support group
Constructivist school	Sessional switch
Cooperative learning	Small-group tutorial
Debate	Socratic method
Group leadership	Task functions
Learner entry skills	Theme-centered group
Maintenance functions	

Introduction

Nurse educators are being faced with increasing numbers of learners to teach and supervise. The mere fact of large numbers of learners is not the primary stumbling block to providing effective feedback and supervision. The problem resides in the communication structure of many classrooms. Even when lectures are not used, one-way transmittal of information between educator and learners is often the norm. The principal disadvantage of this system is that the nurse educator cannot carry on a dialogue with more than one learner at a time.

Such instructional methods also do not follow our knowledge of how adults learn. Members of the **constructivist school** of learning have provided theoretical and empirical evidence that individuals do not learn by the passive association of ideas and symbols or responses to stimuli (the behaviorist model of learning), but by actively constructing knowledge and understanding in and through daily learning activities.

> The constructivist school of learning proposes individuals learn via active construction of knowledge and understanding.

This chapter focuses on group and peer learning, two active learning methods, which can enhance critical thinking by encouraging two-way communication. They offer the nurse educator unique opportunities to have learners teach one another, take responsibility for their own learning, give and take peer support, practice hearing from and giving information to a greater number of people other than just the nurse educator, practice taking risks, and learn how to review one another's practice (Bostock, 2000; Keppell, Eliza, Ada, and Chan, 2000).

Suggestions are made for using group methods with the beginning learner and with more advanced learners. Exercises for nurse educators appear at the end of the chapter for learners in both the masters and doctoral programs.

When nurse educators begin to work with small groups of learners, it is mandatory to understand how groups operate, to learn methods of intervening to help groups move forward, and to model appropriate group leader actions. Prior to examining group dynamics, the evidence supporting group learning as a viable teaching method is presented.

The Evidence Supporting Group Learning

A number of studies have shown the benefits of group methods on learners' critical thinking abilities. Magnussen, Ishida, and Itano (2000) sought to determine if inquiry-based learning (IBL) enhances critical-thinking ability as measured by the Watson Glaser Critical Thinking Appraisal (WGCTA). The WGCTA was administered to 228 nursing learners in the first semester and 257 learners in the final semester of their program. Results showed that inquiry-based learning as a teaching methodology was effective in developing critical thinking, but traditional teaching methods, such as lecture, were not.

Hoke and Robbins (2005) examined the effect of active, cooperative learning as a method of teaching critical thinking skills. They used a combination of faculty role modeling, learner interaction and group learning, and group testing within a didactic class. The researchers found the group who used active, cooperative learning scored higher clinical grades than those learners who had been taught using a lecture approach.

Khosravani, Manoochehrik, and Memarian (2005) used a quasi-experimental study to determine the effects of holding group-dynamic sessions in clinical training on critical thinking skills of baccalaureate nursing learners. Sixty learners were selected and randomly divided into two equal groups. Data collection included a demographic questionnaire and four forms of clinical reports based on nursing process. Learners in the experimental group discussed selected family health topics during 8-10 group-dynamic sessions. Learners in the control group participated in the routine educational program. T-tests revealed that learners who participated in a group that discussed selected topics on family health showed a significant increase in the following critical thinking skills over the learners in a routine educational program: diagnosis, clinical reasoning, clinical judgment, prediction, and creativity.

A randomized controlled trial examined small group teaching methods for learning musculoskeletal examination skills compared with the provision of written materials only or written materials plus a videotape (Lawry, Schuldt, Kreiter, Densen, and Albanese, 1999). Significantly higher scores were attained by learners taught in small group sessions. The researchers concluded that small group instruction with hands-on supervised practice is superior to more passive instructional methods for teaching musculoskeletal examination skills.

An interpretive phenomenological study revealed how **narrative pedagogy** encouraged more than the predominantly emphasized critical thinking forms of analytical thinking such as problem solving. Narrative pedagogy emphasizes how learners learn and experience thinking about clinical situations. Forty-eight nurse educators and eleven learners participated in a distance desktop faculty development study that was conducted to improve the learning climates in schools of nursing. Nurse educators were asked via interview to describe a time they had "tried something new." Learners were asked to reveal one time when one of their nurse educators tried something new with teaching. A team of four nurse researchers examined the data and supported their written interpretations with quotes or excerpts from participant responses. One example shared by a learner named Mae related how in post-clinical conference, her nurse educator invited learners to make their own clinical assignments and share what this strategy meant to them. As each learner shared, the nurse educator and learners collectively considered the account from multiple perspectives. This teaching device invited learners to consider the complexity of clinical accounts and the multiple ways any practice situation can be understood. The researchers concluded that when Mae's nurse educator asked learners to reflect on, share, and collectively consider the meaning of selecting their own client assignment, she created a place in post-clinical conference for learners to learn and practice interpretive thinking. The important aspect of learning in this case was not choosing their own clients, but the reflection and sharing and hearing from their peers about how nurses know and connect with clients (or fail to know and connect), how they answer clients' questions, and how they provide care (Scheckel and Ironside, 2006).

Group methods can also have a positive affect on learner enthusiasm and outcomes. In an Australian study, Jamrozik (1996) examined public health teaching and found that attendance at the course improved sharply, the perceived relevance of the materials learned increased, and learner feedback was very positive after the introduction of self-directed learning methods. Other findings included that the instructor

> Narrative pedagogy emphasizes how learners learn and think about clinical situations.

spent less time in front of the class and instead provided only mini-tutorials each day by presenting to small groups, and focused on the skills required to understand the published literature on the aspects of diagnosis, investigation, management, and prognosis of individual clients.

■ **Nurse Educator Challenge**

Which of the group studies described above has the strongest research design?

Advantages of Using a Group Learning Approach

One advantage of using groups for learning is that greater knowledge and fuller information can be elicited, and the variety of approaches and unique solutions increases. Group learning can provide an expansion in the number of ways of solving problems and ways of blending them into a workable whole. One group member's idea may set off a chain reaction of related ideas in other group members.

Another advantage of using groups is that tasks can be subdivided, with each person being given the responsibility for completing one aspect of the task. The more group members are involved in decision making and task completion, the more investment they will have in its implementation, and the more they will support it (Watson and Michaelsen, 1991). This is of special advantage in situations where the solution cannot be implemented without the help of a number of individuals.

> Group leadership consists of actions directed toward setting and attaining group goals, and of behaviors designed to improve the quality of interaction among members.

If tasks and functions are shared, leadership is shared. One view of leadership is that it is a set of influence functions. The philosophy of this book is that **group leadership** consists of actions directed toward setting and attaining group goals (**task functions**) and of behaviors designed to improve the quality of interaction among members (**maintenance functions**) to build closeness in the group, and to free individual competencies for group benefit. If leadership is defined in this manner, participation in effective groups can lead to the enhancement of leadership skills for each group member, a decided advantage of learning using this format.

> Task functions are group behaviors directed toward setting and attaining group goals.

> Maintenance functions improve the quality of interaction among group members.

As learners work together in groups on various aspects of a project, the potential for understanding other learners and their opinions and feelings grows. This advantage allows learners to become more sensitive to another's needs. This same skill is useful when working with clients or teaching other learners.

When working in a group setting, individual learners view problems in process and identify how other group members deal with the problems and with each other. This kind of experience can help group members grow as individuals because they learn a variety of ways of communicating about, thinking about, and reacting to group problems. When a group climate is open and trusting, group members can receive support from one another for their actions, thoughts, and feelings.

Potential Disadvantages of Group Learning

There are several potential disadvantages of group experiences, although some negative forces can be turned into positive forces should they develop, including:

- *Pressures within groups,* such as the desire to be accepted, to please others, or to attain status can lead to conformity. (When disagreement and novel ideas are encouraged and accepted as group goals, conformity is not a problem.)

> Dr. Jacobsen, a new nurse educator, looked forward to her first meeting with her clinical group. The pre-conference went well. After an incident on the clinical unit involving an unexpected death of one of the patients, the post-conference discussion took on a chaotic atmosphere; it buzzed with anxiety, anger, and argument about who or what had caused the death. Dr. Jacobsen remembered something she had learned from one of her teachers and said, "This is an upsetting event. We don't really have all the facts yet, but we can discuss what happened, even if we don't all agree. Rather than arguing, if you disagree with something someone else said, just say, 'I disagree, here is what I observed, or here is how I see what happened.' That way we can gather more information for discussion." After that statement, the group calmed down and put more energy into problem solving.

- *Extensive disagreement and arguing* can be disruptive to a group, especially when it is in the early developmental stages when trust and acceptance are important issues. In learner groups disrupted by arguing, nurse educators must intervene by modeling effective ways of disagreeing or by providing learning experiences for learners to disagree constructively. Learners who have empathy skills at level three will be able to acknowledge disagreements without attacking other group members. Comments that could be used in such a situation are: "I hear your point, but I disagree," or "Your viewpoint as I understand it is . . . I'd like you to hear mine now." Disagreement and argument are often due to:

- A lack of ability to hear or understand the other's viewpoint,
- An inability to compromise,
- An attack of others' personal attributes or behavior rather than a critique of their ideas, or
- An insufficient knowledge or experience with ways of solving the problem.

Depending on the source of the difficulty, the nurse educator intervenes to provide group members with practice in paraphrasing, compromising, giving "I" messages ("I think . . .," "I feel . . .," "I observed . . .") or providing needed information or resources.

- *Monopolizing and scapegoating* can be problematic. Situations where one or two group members monopolize the conversation (monopolizing) or where one or more group members seem always to be blamed for what occurs (scapegoating) seem especially prone to occur in group settings.

    > About halfway through the post-conference, Dr. Jacobsen noticed that two students were monopolizing the conversation and derided comments from other learners. Dr. Jacobsen intervened by asking for comments and suggesting that other group members make at least one positive comment to the speaker before disagreeing or criticizing.

- *Problem solving or solution finding* in a group takes time. The group can be assisted to come to decisions more effectively by having one or more group members provide feedback to the group concerning its progress. Some statements to use to facilitate the process are:

    1. "We're off the topic."
    2. "Let's get back to suggesting solutions."
    3. "As I see it, the problem is . . ."
    4. "Let's start writing down possible solutions on the chalkboard. Ginny, would you write down our ideas as we say them? So far we've talked about . . . but we need to explore . . ."
    5. "It seems that most of us agree with the second solution."

Nurse Educator Tip

Dealing with Learners who Monopolize Group Discussions

If one or more group members monopolize the discussion:

1. Give group members specified amounts of time to present their opinion or reaction to the group. Have a student timekeeper keep time and ring a bell or interrupt when two minutes remain.
2. Say to overly talkative members: "Thanks for your opinion, now let's hear from some of the other members of the group."
3. Ask quieter members to give their views.
4. Direct the group that is "scapegoating" a member to express their anger more openly rather than direct it at that person.

■ *Consensus in decisions,* rather than majority rule. Even though consensus takes time, it can prove a more effective solution. Decisions that are made by coercion, emotional pleas, attacks, or a premature vote are often the result of insufficient time or knowledge on the part of the group to reach a constructive consensus.

Group Warm Ups

Taking five to ten minutes to warm up and relax the group can reap benefits later on during the hour (Clark, 2003). Some examples include:

1. *Group back rub*—ask participants to rate themselves on a scale from 1–10 with 1 being bored, distracted, or stressed out and 10 being calm, energized, and ready to learn. Tell the group that tension can lead to tense muscles and an uncomfortable body. Ask every other person in the group to give a back rub to the person to the right. After three minutes, ask participants to switch roles then record a second rating.
2. *Soothe the savage beast*—play some soothing music or sounds (running water, ocean waves, etc.) and ask group participants to draw whatever images are brought forth. Optional: After 3–5 minutes, ask participants to discuss their drawings.

3. *Relaxation exercise*—play a relaxation tape or ask the group to kick off their shoes, loosen tight clothing, close their eyes, and let their breathing slowly move to their center, their abdominal area. Ask them to breathe in a healing color on each inhale and breathe out anything it's time to let go of, perhaps as a different color. Remain silent for the next few minutes, observing your own breathing in and out of colors.

■ **Nurse Educator Challenge**

Which of the three warm-ups would be the best choice? Give a rationale for your choice.

Phases of Groups

Nurse educators need to be aware of the phases their group is in so they will know the meaning of the behavior and how to intervene. A classroom or conference group develops systematically by passing through developmental stages or phases. At first, members are concerned about emotional issues of belonging and trust (Clark, 2003).

Members try to determine what is expected of them in the group and how they can be accepted; at the same time, decisions must be made regarding tasks to be accomplished. Patterns of teaching and learning begin to develop even while emotional issues of trust and acceptance are being resolved. The climate of the classroom is enhanced when members are free to focus on their stages of development as a group.

Conflict and frustration are expected happenings along the way to learning in a group. Early in groups there is a lack of unity as some group members resist

---

Nurse Educator Tip

Examining the Group Process

To help learners examine their group process, ask:

1. "Where are we now in this discussion?"
2. "Where are we going?"
3. "What are we doing to get there?"

collaboration and fear loss of individuality. In groups where learners are expected to assume responsibility for group direction, there may be expressions of resentment and pleas for the nurse educator to decide or direct.

> Dr. Jacobsen noticed that about halfway through the clinical rotation, learners in her post-conference group grumbled or whispered to each other when she asked for volunteers to discuss an event that exemplified a concept from one of their assignments.

■ Nurse Educator Challenge

If you were Dr. Jacobsen, what would you do? Give a rationale.

Educators who react to these feelings and pleas by taking over responsibility do not teach the group how to move to higher levels of responsibility and group functioning. Rather than counterattacking, withdrawing, or taking over, educators can model how to express feelings ("I'm upset too. It's scary to know that could happen here.") and then move on to the learning tasks, ("Let's talk about how what we observed relates to your reading assignment for this week."). In addition, educators can provide information and specific written or verbal directions and/or simulated or role-playing situations that demonstrate how to proceed to assist the group during this phase.

If the group is unable to move to problem solving, it may be helpful to go around the group and ask each person to take two minutes to express their feelings. If the group is still unable to move forward, the nurse educator can suggest that the members discuss their feelings in their peer support group.

> Cohesiveness is the attraction for the group and its work held by group members.

With direction, group members can learn how to solve group problems and move onto a phase where differences of opinion can be tolerated, where attraction for the group and its work (**cohesiveness**) increases, where members feel accepted and secure, and where they are able to solve learning problems. Some indicators of increasing cohesiveness within the group are:

- Group members will more frequently use plural pronouns like "we," "us," and "our."
- Learners will spontaneously offer to help and accept help from one another.

- Members take pride in the completion of learning tasks and in the work environment.
- Learners become flexible in their ability to change work groups, take other roles, and fill in where they can be helpful.
- Learners will continue in-class discussions after class by spontaneously planning to continue to work on a project during coffee or lunch, or planning to study together or meet later to complete a task (Jung and Sosik, 2002; Williams, Duray, and Reddy, 2006).

To increase cohesiveness in a learner group:

- Obtain feedback from learners regarding how each feels about the group, and

- Divide the class into groups of four and assign tasks that encourage them to get to know one another (Clark, 2003).

Observing Classroom Groups

Group events can provide useful information for the nurse educator. Some questions to ask when observing groups appear in the Nurse Educator's Tip that follows.

Nurse Educator Tip

Questions to Ask When Observing Classroom Groups

Preparing the Group
1. Are learners prepared for group discussions or activities?
2. How can I assist learners to be better prepared?
3. Do learners seem to know what the group goals are?
4. How can I assist the group in clarifying its goals?
5. Are there clear rules for the group to follow to meet its goals?
6. What materials should I prepare to assist learners to define or use already stated rules? Some rules to consider when preparing such materials are:
   - Only one person is to speak at a time.
   - Everyone is to listen to others' comments prior to commenting on them.

(continues)

Nurse Educator Tip *(continued)*

- Each person is to use the pronoun "I" when speaking.
- Group members are responsible for their own actions in the group.
- Prior to giving a negative criticism, present at least one, and preferably two, positive criticisms.

Group Member Knowledge and Actions

7. Do learners seem knowledgeable about how to reach group goals?
8. What materials do I need to prepare to guide the group toward its goals?
9. Are learners listening to one another's ideas and reactions prior to responding?
10. How can I provide experiences that will help learners become more skillful listeners?

Group Member Problems

11. Which learners seem uninvolved or silently angry?
12. How can these learners be engaged in the discussion?
13. Who usually breaks silences first?
14. What ways of prolonging productive silences can be used? (One way is to ask learners to remain silent for longer than usual and to write down their reactions as the silence proceeds. The nurse educator can ask later what learners learned about themselves during the silence.)
15. How do different learners deal with conflict and disagreement?
16. How can I use learning experiences to increase learner ability to deal constructively with conflict?

Group Leadership

17. Which learners perform most leadership functions? (see Box 4–1)
18. How can I build in structure so that other learners will learn to perform most leadership functions?
19. Which learners demonstrate untapped potential or need for skill practice in performing leadership functions?
20. Which learners use gestures or body posture that cancel out their verbal messages?

(continues)

Nurse Educator Tip *(continued)*

21. How can the nurse educator assist learners in giving more consistent messages? (One such comment might be, "You're saying you approve, but you're shaking your head.")
22. Which learners use blaming messages such as "You didn't . . ."?
23. How can the nurse educator or other group members guide blaming learners to take responsibility for their own behavior by using "I" messages?
24. Which learners have skills as group mediators, compromisers, or negotiators?
25. How can the nurse educator encourage learners who have these skills to use them for the benefit of the group?
26. How are decisions made?
27. How can the nurse educator develop learning experiences that encourage effective decision making?
28. Are dissatisfactions worked through with the group, or are they denied and overlooked?

Group Problem-Solving

29. How can I help group members to examine dissatisfactions, decide which are solvable, and work to improve the learning climate?
30. Are there opportunities for learners to practice group skills recently acquired?
31. How can this practice be provided?
32. Are learners learning to think and talk about how their group skills will apply to their future behavior as nurses?
33. How can learners be assisted to examine this issue?

In general, groups will be effective if some member or members ensure that both task and maintenance functions are met. Box 4–1 shows examples of task and maintenance functions and ways of fulfilling them.

Role playing, simulation, and simulation gaming are all teaching approaches that can be adapted for use with groups (see Chapter 3). Some types of groups that will be considered here are the discussion group, the small-group tutorial, the theme-centered group, and concept mapping groups. Each of these groups has different goals.

Box 4–1   Task and Maintenance Functions of Groups

Task Functions—keep the group on task	Maintenance Functions—help with the emotional aspects of group work
Start the group working on the task. Example: "Today we're to work on . . ."	*Give support and encourage group members.* Example: "That's a tough problem."
Keep the group focused on the goal. Example: "Let's get back to the problem."	*Relieve tension.* Example: "Let's not argue. I suggest we take a break."
Clarify unclear statements Example: "Explain what you mean."	*Encourage directness.* "You two work that out between you."
Suggest solutions to problems Example: "I suggest we divide up the task, and each work on part of it."	*Voice group feeling.* Example: "I sense we're all a little frustrated with this task."
Point out movement toward solution or goal. Example: "I think we're moving closer to a solution to the problem."	*Agree with others and accept their input.* Example: "That's a good idea. I like it."
Restate or summarize at intervals. Example: "Let's summarize what we've learned so far."	*Help the group evaluate itself.* Example: "Let's evaluate what we've learned."
Refocus discussion or focus on workable subtasks. Example: "Let's work on the first part of the problem until we have a better idea of where we're going."	
Give information. Example: "I looked up the topic, and this is what I found . . ."	

Discussion Groups

Group discussion stimulates the extension of knowledge and the critical evaluation and discrimination of ideas, although discussion groups are not specifically suited to initial learning of knowledge. Group discussions can help the nurse educator evaluate learner abilities to solve problems, make decisions, and use critical thinking.

When nurse educators participate in group discussions, they have an opportunity to question learners to find out their thinking process and the rationale they used for arriving at decisions.

Types of Discussion Questions to Use

It is useful for an educator to think about the type of questions to use. Three levels of questions evoke answers that range from simple to complex:

1. Low-level questions ask for facts. ("Name one stress management procedure." "What are three signs of myocardial infarct?")
2. Mid-level questions clarify and explain. ("Discuss the stages of the grief process and observations you would make as a nurse for each stage.")
3. High-level questions evoke critical thinking processes. ("Compare and contrast Selye's theory of stress with Lazurus's theory of stress and coping." "Describe the rationale for one approach to ADHD and discuss alternate approaches and their rationales."). (Oermann & Gaberson, 1998)

When using the discussion group approach, the nurse educator is involved in group work, as well as with the course content. For this reason, knowledge of group process, group development, and group dynamics is imperative. The following format can be used when working with discussion groups:

1. *Define group roles for learners.* Learners are given a written description of roles and sequence of role use. The roles, in order from the beginning to the end of discussion, are:
   - Initiator of discussion ("It's nine o'clock. Let's get started.")
   - Giver of and asker for information from others ("Let's have one person speak at a time." " What do you think about that?")
   - Giver of and asker for reactions to what was presented ("What do you think about what Tim just said?")
   - Re-stater ("If I heard you correctly, you think we should go around the group and each give an example"), example giver ("Sarah just told us about

her grief. Does anyone else have anything to add?"), and confronter ("Your statement is not entirely accurate."), and

■ Clarifier-synthesizer-summarizer ("Today we focused on anxiety and what to do to relieve it with clients.").

Throughout a group discussion, learners can be assigned by the nurse educator to assume one of the following roles:

- *Expeditor* who ensures that all group members speak ("Betsy, would you keep track and make sure everyone has a chance to say something today?"),
- *Timekeeper* who keeps to the budgeted time for a topic ("Julie, would you make sure we only spend ten minutes on each topic?"),
- *Evaluator* who gives a verbal statement regarding how the group is progressing toward its goals ("Ben, every fifteen minutes, would you make a statement about how the group is progressing toward its goal?"),
- *Standard setter* who reminds the group of its agreed-upon contract ("Karen, would you make sure the group stays on the assigned topic?"),
- *Encourager* who gives praise and encouragement to other group members ("Tommy, I want you to say well done or good point when someone makes a good point."),
- *Tension reliever* ("Terrie, I want you to tell the group 'let's stand up, take a few deep breaths, and swing our arms and shoulders to relieve our tension', and don't forget to demonstrate."), and
- *Active listener* who focuses intently on whoever is speaking ("The rest of you can take active listener roles and listen intently to whoever is speaking.").

The nurse educator can also help learners reflect on their group and team skills by asking questions at the end of class. Some suggested comments and activities appear in the Nurse Educator Tip box that follows.

2. *Provide the group with a cognitive map* for each learner to use when preparing for and conducting a discussion on assigned readings. The order of preparing and conducting a discussion can follow the same **cognitive map** or sequence of activities.

A cognitive map provides a general theme and subtopics to use to sequence a discussion.

Educators can direct learners to write down words or terms related to the readings that they do not understand. Next, learners can be asked to write down the general theme and subtopics presented by

Nurse Educator Tip

Questions to Ask at the End of Class/Conference:

- "Give me two examples of active listening behaviors you observed in your group (team) today."
- "Here's an observation form I filled out on your group (team) today; what implications do the findings have for your group (team)?"
- "I'd like you each to fill out an evaluation of what happened today and then we'll discuss what the findings mean to you and to the group."
- "I'd like you each to come up with a written plan for how you can improve your group (team) skills." (Ledlow, 1999)

the assignments as well as make a list of questions they wish to ask during the discussion, and finally to give their opinions of how what was studied can be related to other past, present, and future learning experiences.

3. *Ask group members to use the cognitive map as a guide* during the discussion. The nurse educator can write out specific directions regarding how to proceed. The following suggestions are only one method that builds on the learning process from concept to principle to more complex practice in applying, integrating, and problem solving. During the first part of the discussion, group members define terms and concepts, clarify misunderstandings about what was read or studied, and state the author's main points.

   Once specific subtopics have been agreed upon, the group decides how much time to allocate to each. The group then proceeds to discuss themes and subtopics, and to verbalize and answer questions raised by each group member. Next, the group tries to relate the information discussed to past, present, and future learning by stating how it contradicts, substantiates, or clarifies some other learning, or how it might be used in the nurse/client relationship. Finally, group members volunteer or are called upon to comment on their performance as a discussion group. The group can be requested to refer to their list of group roles and discuss which were or were not filled, why they think they were or were not, and what can be done to facilitate more effective role-taking.

   In this model the role of the nurse educator is to circulate among the small discussion groups (or sit back in a post-conference) and assist or answer questions when needed. The nurse educator should refrain from interrupting the group(s) or from taking over as leader.

When using this group method, as when working with any learning group, the nurse educator uses knowledge of group phases. For example, early complaints about this method may be related to member dependency and can be a reaction against being asked to take responsibility for directing their own learning. Likewise, early requests for assistance must be carefully monitored and divided into two categories: those that arise from incomplete directions concerning how to proceed and those that are due to anxiety, dependency, or a wish to have the nurse educator be an authoritarian leader.

> Dr. Jacobsen decided to use a cognitive map in the classroom with her students. She wrote out specific directions and provided them to the class. Then she sat back and waited for them to start discussing. When learners made faces and began to whisper to each other rather than discuss the planned topic, she wasn't sure what to do.

■ Nurse Educator Challenge

What advice would you give Dr. Jacobsen? Give a rationale.

In the case of the former, the nurse educator should provide (or develop and then provide) more complete directions. If the requests are due to learner anxiety or dependency, redirect group member(s) to their written directions and neutrally tell them that with practice, they will be able to direct their own group.

The educator should be aware that frustration and conflict are expected occurrences in early (and sometimes in later) group sessions and are not a cause for alarm unless the group task is ill-defined, or the group needs further skills or information to proceed. If there are too many small groups for the nurse educator to reach during class time, one learner in each group can take the role of recorder and present excerpts or questions from the recording of each small group to the whole class when it convenes. It is not wise for the nurse educator to allow small groups to proceed for more than one session without obtaining feedback regarding difficulties encountered, since learners may justifiably complain that they are not receiving sufficient direction.

As with other learning experiences, the nurse educator may ease into the method by conducting a mini-demonstration with several learners to model effective group discussion behaviors and/or preparing sample preparation sheets for group discussion. It may also be useful for the nurse educator to designate a leader for each group discussion whose major role is to ensure that the group follows the sequence of discussion as planned by the nurse educator. When this method is used, it is helpful if the leader role is rotated for each discussion group session so more learners have a chance to practice being the leader.

■ Nurse Educator Challenge

Knowing what you know now, what additional advice would you give Dr. Jacobsen? Give a rationale.

The above format may be most useful when introducing learners to discussion group experiences. Once learners become more skilled in directing their own group sessions, they may complain of feeling hampered by the method. When they have demonstrated that they are able to fulfill all roles and can move from concepts to problem solving, the nurse educator can consider using a more flexible discussion format. Learner suggestions and input regarding the format are also appropriate at this time.

4. **Cooperative Learning** *is another type of group discussion activity.* In cooperative learning, each group is given a task or problem within a packet of information. Each member of the group learns or solves one piece of the problem and then teaches the other members of the group what was learned. The nurse educator identifies a problem or task for the group to work on, divides it into equitable subtasks, and designs packets of information to give to learners (University of New Mexico, 2005).

> Cooperative learning occurs when each member of the group learns or solves one piece of the problem and then teaches the other members of the group what was learned.

■ Nurse Educator Challenge

If you were going to use a cooperative learning exercise with a class or conference group, what problem would you choose? How would you divide the problem into equitable subtasks? Give a rationale.

---

5. **Concept mapping** helps learners identify relationships between concepts. Concept mapping allows learners to compose a pictorial arrangement that links key concepts with directional arrows and annotations to show how they are related. The concept map develops as learners collect assessment data either through case studies or their clinical assignments (Clayton, 2006). For example:

- A skeleton diagram of the client's health problems from assessment data is analyzed and categorized.
- Relationships between nursing and medical diagnoses are indicated.
- Client goals, outcomes, and nursing interventions for each nursing diagnosis are charted.
- Client responses to each nursing intervention are provided (McHugh, 2002).

Concept maps have been used several settings. Koehler (2001) reported using them in group work, and Ignatavicius (2004) used concept maps in class discussions. Concept mapping was shown to be an effective tool for improving the academic performance of sophomore-level BSN nursing students in an introductory nursing research course. This study used an experimental group and compared results to a comparable control. Results included that students in the experimental group reported the course was informative, fun, and helpful for learning content (Rooda, 1994).

Daley (1996) constructed concept maps after interviewing students and faculty and adding it to information obtained in a course syllabus for a unit on oxygenation. The purpose of the study was to determine the amount of difficulty new associate degree nursing students had in linking concepts of the nursing process to basic science.

Gaines (1996) used concept maps as a teaching strategy for juniors in a BSN pharmacology course. The students worked in small groups to develop concept maps for certain drug categories. Gaines compared exam grades with grades on concept maps and found that concept maps can help students attain success in courses and nursing programs.

Caelli (1998) examined the use of concept maps as a way to move nursing students toward health promotion practice. Beginning nursing students constructed concept maps related to developing a positive concept of health. In their small group discussion, they debated appropriate linkages, concepts, and positive states of health. At the end of the learning unit, students completed a final concept map. The researcher concluded that concept mapping can play an important role in assisting nurses toward health promotion practice.

Daley, Shaw, Balistrieri, Glasenapp, and Piacentine (1998) evaluated critical thinking in BSN students during the final semester of their senior year. The researchers used a random sample of three students from each of six clinical groups and compared first and last maps for hierarchical organization and differentiation of concepts. They found a significant improvement in student ability to conceptualize and think critically. Concept mapping information showed that students who were unable to verbally discuss concepts had a better understanding than more outspoken students whose maps demonstrated misperceptions and gaps in knowledge.

■ **Nurse Educator Challenge**

Develop a concept map for one client. Make note of the obstacles, questions, and comments that arise as you work. They will come in useful when you teach the strategy to learners.

It is always useful to use a post-discussion reaction sheet. Learner comments will provide useful feedback about your teaching methods and about student learning. See the following Nurse Educator Tip.

The contents of one or more post-discussion sheets can be used as feedback to group members or as data upon which to base changes in group membership or discussion group rules.

Nurse Educator Tip

Develop a Post-Discussion Reaction Sheet

In collaboration with learners, the nurse educator can develop a post-discussion reaction sheet that can be used to evaluate:

- The results of the discussion
- The organization of the discussion
- The lack or provision of leadership functions
- The preparation of discussants
- The presence or absence of restrictions to express viewpoints
- The members' feelings about working with each other.

Small-Group Tutorials

The discussion group method is often nurse educator-centered and nurse educator-planned, but the **small-group tutorial** is learner-centered and learner-planned. The small-group tutorial is an approach used for complex learning activities. Learning is individualized and problem-based within the group context. Learners set their own goals and progress at their own rate.

> A small-group tutorial is a problem-based, learner-centered, and learner-planned approach used for complex learning activities.

Concepts from several disciplines are integrated as learners attempt to think and work out complicated problems. Memorization of facts and content is deemphasized. A group of learners decides to work on a selected learning problem. They may proceed from a set of prescribed learning objectives, or they may be assisted in developing their own. The group may decide to focus on a particular clinical problem encountered through reading or through specific nurse/client interactions.

■ **Nurse Educator Challenge**

Pretend you are a nurse educator about to use a small-group tutorial for the first time. Would you use a set of prescribed learning objectives or help learners to develop their own? Give a rationale for your answer.

The group can be given written directions regarding how to proceed. The first step is to direct learners to pose the questions for study and to identify related issues. (This is the reverse of a common teaching situation in which the nurse educator defines the problem and directs learners to answer specified questions about it.) The common situation is not problem solving, but a sophisticated question-and-answer game.

The group tutorial approach, on the other hand, teaches learners to ask pertinent questions, to collect data and search out information related to various aspects of the problem, and then to formulate the problem based on the synthesis of available data. Once the group has researched and formulated the problem, the learners proceed to plan how to manage the problem. This includes identifying various approaches and solutions to the problem, choosing one, trying it out, and evaluating the results. The group also evaluates individual member and group performance.

The group tutorial is a very flexible learning approach. Group members act as stimulants for one another's learning. They also serve as sources of peer support and feedback. Nurse educators play the roles of catalyst and resource person. Although they may be subject matter experts in the problem chosen for learners, they should avoid giving lectures or speeches on the topic. Rather, they should serve as facilitators who assist learners in finding the information or solution.

■ **Nurse Educator Challenge**

A learner has asked you for the definition of a term. What is your response? Give a rationale for your answer.

For example, when asked for assistance, a nurse educator who tells learners simply to "look it up" is not helpful. Some facilitating comments that could aid learners to locate information are:

- "What specific kind of information do you need?"
- "Where do you suppose you could find it?"
- "How do you suppose a nurse practitioner or nurse faculty member would go about researching that?"
- "How might you find out?"
- "Where could you look to find that out?"
- "Whom could you consult for information in that area?"

No matter what group strategy is used, a group can become blocked. **Brainstorming** could help. As in other creative efforts, tutorial groups may run into roadblocks. Brainstorming is particularly useful when this happens. Facilitate group movement through the block by suggesting the group use the brainstorming technique. If learners are unfamiliar with it they can be provided with the brainstorming directions that appear in the Nurse Educator Tip that follows.

> Brainstorming is a method for identifying the maximum number of solutions or ideas about a problem.

The role of the learner in the group tutorial is active and responsible. It may not be an approach to use with beginning learners, as it requires a high level of cognitive complexity and self-direction. It may be more appropriate for a masters degree student toward the end of the program and/or doctoral level learners. When using this method, the nurse educator is a co-learner more

Nurse Educator Tip

Brainstorming

1. Brainstorming is a technique for identifying the maximum number of solutions to or ideas about a problem. Quantity, not quality, is important.
2. The most important rule in brainstorming is to write or weigh as many solutions or ideas as occur without censoring them for reasonableness.
3. Someone in the group volunteers to write down all the ideas so everyone in the group can refer to them and have further ideas or solutions occur to them by examining the list.
4. Group members are to continue listing ideas and solutions without commenting on any contributions.
5. No criticism of others' ideas is allowed.
6. In addition to contributing ideas of their own, group members may suggest how others' ideas or solutions could be combined or expanded.
7. Only after the group has exhausted all ideas and solutions is the group to begin to decide which of them to try.

than a nurse educator. The success or failure of the group is dependent on the cooperation and collaboration of the nurse educator and the group. Each person is responsible for other group members' learning. A successful group tutorial experience can provide learners with valuable self-directed leadership, collaborative problem solving, and research skills.

The Theme-Centered Group

The **theme-centered group** reflects a concern for individual autonomy, a respect for the learner's personal experience, and a recognition of the complex relationship among the learner's experience, the classroom group, and a theme or focus of inquiry. This kind of group is based on the group psychotherapy model that group forces are powerful determinants of the learner learning experience. Group activity and group culture are viewed as interwoven with an individual's experience, classroom phenomena, and a theme or focused area of academic inquiry.

Ackerhalt (1977) reported on a theme-centered group experience that was designed to give graduate nursing learners an opportunity to explore group leadership principles. One part of the session focused on the preplanned theme: Does being female influence leadership behavior? The sequence of events that followed was:

> A theme-centered group reflects a concern for individual autonomy, a respect for the learner's personal experience, and a recognition of the complex relationship among the learner's experience, the classroom group, and a theme or focus of inquiry.

1. The nurse educator discussed the tasks of small-group leaders as structuring the focus of discussion and interacting with organizations that sponsor the group.
2. The nurse educator pointed out that female group leaders frequently have difficulty performing these tasks.
3. The nurse educator raised the question: "Might not this difficulty be due to the fact that the tasks are discordant with the female role conception of women as nurturing rather than instrumental?"
4. Several learners responded to the nurse educator's question with comments about how naive nurses are and how insurmountable this problem is. (The nurse educator classified this in her mind as a sub-theme, entitled "The Plight of Women" or "Ain't It Awful.")
5. One learner shared an experience she had as a child, when her mother took a job as a bus driver when her father died. The learner wondered whether her experience of observing her mother might have influenced her current ability to lead groups without difficulty.
6. Other learners shared reminiscences of relationships with significant women and how these experiences may have affected their self-image as group leaders.
7. The nurse educator called attention to her own failure to keep the group focused on the topic and questioned whether group members' fatalistic outlook might have been a solution for a conflict between their aspirations as group leaders and their views of how women should act.

This exercise illustrates how a group facilitator blended skills with elements of the learners' own unique histories to examine a theme from a unique perspective. This approach is in line with Cohn's conceptualizations: When nurse educators try to make learners learn facts or opinions from the nurse educator's viewpoint, there is no consideration for the learner's uniqueness or historicity. Cohn compares force-feeding food to children as analogous to force-feeding facts to learners; both disappear, but may come out undigested and may result in a poisoned, angry, or conforming child or learner (Cohn, 1971).

This method attempts to combat the learner's sense of isolation and depersonalization. It differs from group therapy, which has only one theme: I want to feel or function better. Theme-centered groups can deal with any theme that individual learners are concerned with. According to Ackerhalt (1977), the nurse educator's roles in theme-centered groups are:

1. Identifying a theme that corresponds to the overall purposes of the learner group.
2. Preparing and/or acquiring resources required to facilitate group exploration of the theme.
3. Clarifying participants' tasks and roles and rules.
4. Stimulating group member involvement in the theme.
5. Maintaining the interest of the group in the theme.
6. Drawing relationships among individual learner experiences, group processes and the identified theme.

■ **Nurse Educator Challenge**

You are planning to begin a theme-centered group. What would be your first steps in developing such a group? Give a rationale for your answer.

Group members can be primed or prepared for a theme-centered group session by being asked to think about the theme, to read a pertinent passage or book, to view a film, or to write their reactions to the theme or their goals for the session. Nurse educators are not only knowledgeable about group dynamics; they have peer learning skills as well.

Peer Learning

In classrooms where peer relationships are not supportive, considerable tension can develop, leading to decreased learning. In many classrooms, tension and distrust may be reinforced by a competitive race for grades. Learners may think, "I can't help my classmates, or they'll get a better grade than I will." At the same time, while learners may be fearful of letting down their guard with peers, they may also struggle with a sense of isolation, loneliness, and superficiality in their personal relationships (Callaghan, 2006; Cottrell, 2002; Ekstein and Wallerstein, 1971).

Meanwhile, the novice nurse educator may be thinking: "How can I divide myself so that I can teach and be supportive to so many learners?" With large groups, ongoing personal contact with the nurse educator may not be feasible; even if it were, nurse educators ought to begin to question why they should be the center of learning and support (Callaghan, 2006; Cottrell, 2002; Ekstein and Wallerstein, 1971).

In the real-life work world (the referent situation), nurses learn from their peers, conduct peer reviews, and share lunch and social time with peers. Because the referent situation is filled with peer learning, a good solution to the problem of having to spread nurse educator/learner time too thinly is to structure learning experiences in such a way that learners teach each other, supervise and review one another's work, and provide support for one another. This is called **peer learning.** Such structuring requires initial planning and modeling behavior by the nurse educator. After observing the nurse educator, learners are gradually directed toward learning experiences where they supervise and provide support for one another.

> Peer learning occurs when students learn from their peers.

Evidence for Peer Learning

What is the evidence supporting peer learning as a teaching method? One study used Bandura's social learning theory for the framework to investigate the effects of peer teaching on baccalaureate nursing learners' clinical performance. It was hypothesized that learners who were taught by peers would achieve significantly higher improvement scores than learners taught by nurse educators alone, and would rate their preference for peer teaching equal to or higher than instructor teaching. The experimental design involved 50 volunteers on two surgical units—one for peer teaching and one for instructor teaching. The researchers collected data from pre- and post-psychomotor and cognitive tests of a surgical dressing procedure, and from a clinical teaching preference questionnaire. Learners taught by peers achieved significantly higher psychomotor and cognitive scores than learners taught by nurse educators alone, and learners rated their preference for peer teaching equal to or higher than instructor teaching as hypothesized (Iwasiw and Goldenberg, 1993).

In a less-structured approach, nurse academics at a Sydney university paired first- and third-year learners for clinical skills practice sessions. The nurse educators linked the Australian Nursing Council Inc. (ANCI) standards of practice to skills acquisition. Results included an increase in understanding of the relevance of competency standards to practice (for third-year learners). Evaluation of the peer learning approach indicated that all learners valued the experience (Goldsmith, Stewart, and Ferguson, 2006).

In a qualitative study by Loke and Chow (2006), undergraduate nursing learners were invited to join a peer-tutoring approach. Fourteen learners in their third year were recruited to serve as peer tutors, and 16 learners in the second year in the same program participated as tutees. Peer tutors attended a training workshop and received guidelines for performing peer-tutoring tasks. They were asked to provide a total of 10 weekly tutoring sessions throughout the semester on a one-to-one basis with their tutee. Focus groups and individual interviews were conducted at the middle and end of the semester to evaluate learner experiences in the tutoring process. Content analysis of focus groups showed that peer tutoring enhanced learning skills/intellectual gains and personal growth. Negative experiences included frustration from dealing with mismatched learning styles between tutors and tutees, and the required time commitment. Nurse educators who plan to use peer teaching might benefit from matching learning styles between tutors and tutees and building in extra credit for required time commitment.

■ **Nurse Educator Challenge**

For novice educators: How would you use peer learning with your population of learners? Give a rationale for your answer.

Advantages of Peer Learning

Major advantages of the peer learning model are:

- Learning to take responsibility for one's own learning,
- Learning to give and take support and negative criticism,
- Practice hearing a number of viewpoints,
- Gaining a sense of ownership of the assessment process, improving motivation,
- Learning that mistakes are opportunities rather than failures,

- Practicing transferable skills, especially evaluation skills,
- Experiencing deep rather than superficial learning, and
- Learning to review one another's practice (Brown, Sambell, and McDowell, 1998; Bostock, 2005).

Such a model teaches learners to be flexible in moving among the roles of learner, novice nurse educator, and peer. It would seem a fine vehicle for introducing learners to the real-life situation of independent practice and peer review. The model also has implications for reducing the teaching/learning problems of relating to authority figures and overidentification with the nurse educator (Callaghan, 2006; Cottrell, 2002; Ekstein and Wallerstein, 1971).

Another advantage of peer learning is that learners who teach others frequently learn as much or more than the learners they teach (Clark, 1975). Peer learning is also an inexpensive teaching/learning method. Few materials or expensive audiovisual equipment are needed. Interaction among peers is the vehicle by which learning occurs. Because there are many learners, learning can be self-paced and feedback can be immediate.

Disadvantages of Peer Learning

A potential disadvantage of the peer learning model for novice educators is that they must abdicate the safe and potentially reassuring role of expert or idol (Callaghan, 2006; Cottrell, 2002; Ekstein and Wallerstein, 1971.) It is not unusual for learners to comment to the nurse educator (Clark, 1975) after a peer learning experience, "I learned as much from the other learners as I did from you."

Another disadvantage for educators is that peer learning situations require careful planning and structuring prior to its implementation (Bostock, 2005) and during class (Fagen, Crouch, and Mazur, 2002). Nurse educators must also devote a great deal of time to thinking about ways in which peer learning can be introduced into the curriculum. It is important to keep in mind that learning models that use more structure, such as programmed instruction and/or intensive step-by-step directions, and those that relate to simpler tasks are best used early in a curriculum. Experiences that require more complex learning, such as peer supervision and learner-run games and simulations, are best scheduled later in the course.

No matter where peer learning is placed in the curriculum, some learners and faculty members may resist the idea. Learners at low levels of cognitive complexity may find it most difficult; for them, a gradual introduction and maximum modeling and specific direction will be needed.

Researchers examining peer instruction (Fagen, Crouch, and Mazur, 2002) found that 10 percent of respondents reported that their colleagues were skeptical of the benefit of learner discussions that take away lecture time. Another disadvantage of this method of learning is that the nurse educator may need to be continually present, at least during early peer learning experiences. See the following Nurse Educator Tip for ideas on dealing with faculty resistance to peer learning.

Nurse Educator Tip

Dealing with Faculty Resistance to Peer Learning

To reduce resistance from faculty members who believe only the nurse educator is an expert, and who fear loss of status, prestige, or even their jobs should learners prove themselves capable of teaching one another:

- Compare achievement of learners taught with and without peer teaching methods on identical exams.
- Ask skeptical colleagues to sit in on a class, take the assessment tests, or listen to positive learner feedback about the method (Fagan, Crouch, and Mazur, 2002).

Another disadvantage of the peer learning model is the risk of nonconstructive learning. Peer learning is an experience that requires that the nurse educator take certain risks and endow learners with maximum responsibility for their own learning. Without careful planning and monitoring, nonconstructive learning can occur. For example, learners may give each other negative criticism, miss important learning points, or give incorrect information to each other. For these reasons, the nurse educator provides handouts to guide peers, and circulates through the classroom during learner-led group discussions to encourage learners and observe for any problems (Fagan, Crouch, and Mazur, 2002).

Learners may also resist taking responsibility for their own learning, possibly because they are unaccustomed to active participation and may consider discussions a waste of time. See the following Nurse Educator Tip for suggestions about what to do when learners resist peer learning methods.

Nurse Educator Tip

When Learners Resist Peer Learning Methods

- Persist with the peer learning approach because learners who may be initially skeptical or resistant to the idea usually warm up to it once they find the method helps them learn.
- Present class-averaged data on learner performance to the class to motivate participation in peer learning (Fagan, Crouch, and Mazur, 2002).

Peer Supervision and Review

Peer supervision is a variant of peer learning. Peer supervision refers to the interpersonal process between two (or more) learners who review each others' nursing practice or learning activities. Baccalaureate nurse learners may not be ready to participate in peer supervision unless they participate in more structured experiences such as a simulation game first (Clark, 1975). Nurse learners near the end of their clinical experience may be ready to be peer supervisors, depending on their level of cognitive complexity.

> Peer supervision occurs when learners supervise each other's practice or learning activities.

Examples of Peer Supervision in Nursing

Nehren and Larson (1968) first reported the use of nursing students as supervisors for other learners. In their model, the nurse educator was continually present. The supervisory group consisted of the nurse educator and four learners in the graduate psychiatric nursing program.

Learner A was assigned to supervise Learner B, Learner B was assigned to supervise Learner C, Learner C was assigned to supervise Learner D, and Learner D was assigned to supervise Learner A. Eventually all learners supervised and observed others being supervised, in addition to being supervised themselves. Process recordings were used; each learner was allotted thirty minutes to report the nurse/client encounter and to receive supervision from the assigned learner supervisor. Following this 30-minute period, the nurse educator and other learners who listened to the presentation made suggestions and provided positive feedback. In this peer supervisory model, the authority remained vested in the nurse educator.

■ **Nurse Educator Challenge**

Critique Nehren and Larson's model. Give a rationale for your response.

Burnside (1971) developed her peer supervisory model based on Nehren and Larson's model. Again, nursing learners in a graduate psychiatric program were the target population. Burnside expanded and loosened the model in some ways. For example, although she was present during the oral presentations, learners were allowed to decide whether or not they wished to read process recordings for their presentations. Also, learner supervisors negotiated with learner supervisees concerning all their written work.

Burnside used various forms and guides to help the learner-supervisor evaluate classmates' written work. Both supervisee and supervisor comments were turned in to Burnside, who in turn returned a carbon copy of her reactions to the supervisor's comments to each pair of learners; the instructor made no direct supervisory comments to the supervisee. In this way, learners came to know communication issues from different perspectives: from a peer-learner stance (when supervised), from a supervisory stance (when supervising) and from a learner-peer stance (when writing and reading a supervisor's comments).

Burnside structured the supervisors' behaviors by asking them to examine how they related to supervisees (e.g., the process of supervising—were they overly harsh or overly apologetic?) as well as how they evaluated the supervisee's work (e.g. , the content— did the supervisee use a theoretical framework, were papers well organized and easily read, were gaps in thought noticeable, and were assumptions made with too little data?).

Burnside stated that the original goal was to prepare the learner supervisor for a new teaching role. The supervisee also benefited. An unexpected outgrowth of the learning experience was the development of unplanned conferences called and directed by learner-supervisors and supervisees. The learners devised the criteria for peer supervisory behavior. It was agreed that the learner supervisor would:

1. Maintain goal direction in the relationship.
2. Provide consistent negative and positive feedback.
3. Be responsive to the learner's needs.
4. Individualize the supervisory process.

5. Be accessible to the supervisee.

6. Utilize feedback from the supervisee.

These criteria were used as guidelines for supervision and for midterm evaluations of the supervisors (Burnside, 1971).

■ Nurse Educator Challenge

Critique Burnside's model. Give a rationale for your answer.

Lamberton and colleagues (1977) developed a peer supervision model they referred to as **peer review**, which they defined as "an encounter between two individuals equal to one another in education, abilities, and qualifications, in which one person critically reviews the practice that the other has documented in a client's record" (p. 47).

They used their model throughout four courses in the family nurse clinician program at the School of Nursing at the University of Pennsylvania. At each course level, instructors decreased direction and increased input from learners, as well as the complexity of the peer review practice and its similarity to the referent situation.

> Peer review includes reviewing a peer's client documentation.

First, the instructor encouraged cohesiveness by asking learners to write autobiographies and distribute a copy to each member of the class. The authors pointed out that since learners are apt to interpret negative feedback as lack of support, nurse educators taught learners how to state their observations without judging or valuing them.

During this first course, nurse educators led seminars and appraised one another's sessions, making both positive and negative comments on the presentation and on faculty and learner input. In this way, they served as role models for constructive criticism. Learners then followed suit, and at some time during the second course they were able to give more accurate critiques of each other's performances.

In the third clinical course, learners brought copies of records from the chart of their client. The researchers noted a swing from totally positive reactions to the learning method, to totally negative reactions, to a blend of the two extremes as learners become more accustomed to making peer review comments and as they felt they could trust and learn from one another.

In the fourth clinical course, learners carried out peer review independently, and faculty became involved only when asked to do so. Learners choose their peer reviewers so as to have their practice critiqued twice during the course by two different reviewers. Each observer submitted a brief written account to the faculty, but no content discussion was included.

■ Nurse Educator Challenge

Critique Lamberton and his colleagues' model. Provide a rationale for your answer.

Another peer supervisory model was developed at the Lienhard School of Nursing at Pace University–Westchester by Clark (2003). Learners who took the course, Group Dynamics, received structured peer supervisory and peer support experiences. In the course, learners opted to lead or observe a support or teaching group for six to eight sessions. Once their group was under way and they had met a criterion level for written process recordings of group interactions, they learned to give oral presentations to their peers.

The first step in the process was the completion of selected readings and gaining familiarity with two guides (see Boxes 4–2 and 4–3).

Box 4–2   Peer Group Supervisee's Guide

Peer group supervisees' presentation guide and evaluation of supervision

Name of person(s) supervising: _____

Name of person(s) being supervised: _____

I. You have 20 minutes to present data on one or more group sessions you have led. Be sure to cover all four areas below in the allotted time. You may wish to write your presentation on this guide.
 A. Group themes:
 B. Group problems (e.g., monopolizing, scapegoating, anxiety, conflict):
 C. Transferences and countertransferences:
 D. Problems you need help with:

II. When you have completed your presentation, listen to the supervisor's comments and then write down in this space your evaluation of the supervisor's assistance. Include specific examples of how the supervisor was and was not helpful. Make suggestions for how the supervisor could have been more helpful to you.

Box 4–3   Guide for Evaluation of Supervisees' Written Process Recordings

Read the supervisees' written process recordings of the group session. Compare them with the sample process recordings and your textbook. Evaluate the recording by answering the following questions in the space provided.

1. What statements were made that were supported by data that you can congratulate your peer on?

2. What assumptions were made without sufficient data to support them?

3. What theories (or concepts) were applied to observations that you can congratulate your peer about?

4. What additional theories or concepts did you note that you can tell your peer about?

5. Was it easy to read and follow the recording? If yes, then congratulate your peer on that effort.

6. Did you find any areas that were difficult to follow or read in the recording? Please inform your peer of those areas.

7. What noticeable gaps in observation or thought did you note? Please inform your peer of those areas.

8. What specific alternative actions were stated and were they stated as specific behaviors or goals? Please congratulate your peer on those actions.

9. Were alternative actions missing and how would you state them as specific statements or behaviors? Please inform your peer of your ideas.

10. What other positive comments or additional suggestions do you have to make to your peer(s)?

Learners were also expected to form small groups outside of class to provide support, supervision, and feedback. Any assigned papers were to be evaluated in these groups before handing them in. The nurse educator monitored the groups only to ensure they were operational and that all learners were members of one or another small group. It was important to assist learners who did not readily become involved with a group because they might be playing the role of isolate or scapegoat. The nurse educator served as a resource person to the groups and could choose at any time to request feedback from the group.

At first, nurse learners verbalized difficulty evaluating their peers. Learners asked to supervise peers may initially feel overwhelmed and think they will be unable to help others. When given specific guidelines and a written form for evaluating another learner, and after watching the nurse educator demonstrate the skill, learners will usually take on the role of helpful supervisor.

Peer supervising learners also reported fearing that they must prove themselves, but after a positive experience with peer supervision, they soon reported enjoying learning from one another. They also reported that the most difficult part of the supervisory role was to give an oral or written evaluation of the supervisee, especially if a portion of the learner's grade was dependent on that evaluation. Learners had some difficulty with this evaluation, but commented that it forced them to think through the process of grading and evaluating their peers (Clark, 2003; Burnside, 1971).

■ Nurse Educator Challenge

Critique Clark's peer supervisory model. Provide a rationale for your comments.

Peer teaching and supervision is not only applicable to graduate levels. It has been tested and found effective at elementary school levels in hundreds of studies (Kalkowski, 2001). Why is peer tutoring and peer supervision so effective? Kalkowski (2001) found it was because the peer who supervises or teaches is not far removed from the novice party in authority, knowledge, and instructional competence. Such differences affect the nature of discourse between peers, and place both in less passive roles as well as offering a freedom to express opinions, ask questions, and risk untested solutions.

Many methods can be used in peer learning. Simulations, simulation games, and role playing can be used as peer teaching vehicles (see Chapter 3). Pretests, posttests, and programmed teaching manuals allow learners to teach one another without having an instructor present.

Howard, a new nurse educator, was eager to provide peer learning experiences for a group of community learners. He spent many hours devising peer learning materials and felt confident he had developed learning situations that were not only helpful, but were based on theory. The first day of class, learners took out their notebooks and pens and sat ready to take notes from his lecture. When he told the class they were going to be peer learners, he received many negative comments and requests to "just give us a lecture."

■ Nurse Educator Challenge

What would you do if you were Howard?

Devising Peer Learning Situations

Learners not used to peer learning situations may have to be eased into the model. The following suggestions may serve to direct nurse educators in its use:

1. *Assess environmental constraints.* It is futile to try to implement peer learning where sanctions take the place of incentive. Voluntary cooperation of learners is mandatory.

2. *Review principles of effective learning systems* and apply them to this learning experience.

3. *Gradually move learners to a point of taking more responsibility* for their own learning.

4. *Provide mini-peer learning experiences,* where learners teach each other definitions or describe an article they have read.

5. *Explore the use of peer learning with simple tasks,* such as bed-making, temperature-taking, ace-bandage-wrapping, and so on. Once learners have met the task, they can be watched once as they supervise another learner; then they supervise other learners without being directly observed. Students are monitored through occasional visual observation, or by requesting written or verbal feedback about the peer learning session.

6. *Assign learners readings* that explain peer learning and peer review, or write up and give out a written explanation of what they are and why they are important in nursing.

7. *Begin using peer learning with a small group of learners,* perhaps a clinical group or small continuing education adult learning group, where problems

with its implementation might be less complex. It may also be useful to role play peer learning with a trusted colleague to demonstrate for the class exactly what is expected. If a colleague cannot attend the class, you could make a video in advance to show to learners.

8. *Decide on a method of pairing learners for peer learning experiences.* Depending on the learning objectives, some possible methods are:

   a. *Random assignment*—learners draw slips of paper that contain other learners' names. This method may or may not simulate the real-life work world where nurses may or may not have any say in who supervises them. An advantage of this method is that the nurse educator cannot be blamed by learners for poor group assignments.

   b. *Interpersonal choice*—some learners may choose others with whom they work well and from whom they derive support. Others may be drawn to work with learners with whom they feel they will be able to work, but then they may become locked in an interpersonal struggle over power, authority, responsibility or whatever. Implementing this method conveys to learners that they are responsible for the consequences of their actions. It also provides the option of helping learners develop strategies for working through teaching/learning problems.

   c. *Learning preferences*—consider using Figure 1–3 (Assessing Learner Preferences) for pairing learners. This method operationalizes how learners perceive themselves, and, as such, may or may not be a true indication of how they really act. The method does convey to the learner that the nurse educator believes that in the ideal situation, a peer should be chosen in a systematic manner, based on styles of learning.

   d. *Sessional switch*—by this method, peer learners switch peer nurse educators or supervisors each session of class. This decreases the possibility of learners becoming locked into an inescapable encounter, where one learner perceives the relationship to be a bad one. When using this method, decide how to re-pair learners; one of the above methods or a combination could be chosen. Use of this method conveys to learners that no action is immutable, that learners can move out of impossible situations and that they can learn from more than one or two other people.

   > Sessional switch means learners switch peer nurse educators or supervisors each session of class.

9. *Decide where the peer learning will occur* either in class, out of class, in the clinical area, in a group, in pairs, and so on.

10. *Plan a modeling or demonstration* of what peer learning, peer supervision, or peer review is.

11. *Devise a system for evaluating* **learner entry skills**. Some skills to be considered are: ability to empathize, ability to give effective feedback and constructive criticism, knowledge of subject matter or perceptual motor skill, knowledge of peer learning or peer review procedures, and familiarity with monitoring and evaluation tools.

> Learner entry skills for peer learning include the ability to empathize and give effective feedback and constructive criticism, knowledge of subject matter or perceptual motor skill, knowledge of peer learning or peer review procedures, and familiarity with monitoring and evaluating tools.

12. *Devise a system for teaching requisite skills* based on entry pretest or evaluation.

13. *Develop evaluation tools* for learner supervisor and supervisees. (Refer to Boxes 4–1 and 4–2.)

14. *Decide how frequently and directly the nurse educator will monitor supervisor and supervisee progress,* based on complexity of task, learner ability, and instructor freedom and philosophy.

15. *Decide whether the peer learning experience will be graded,* and if so, whether the nurse educator is responsible for a portion of the grade. Consider the idea that the grade itself may not be as significant as what the learner gleaned from examining the process of grading and deciding how to evaluate others' work. Such an experience may be particularly relevant for learners who plan to be nurse educators themselves.

16. *Prepare to be accessible to learners,* should they require additional assistance.

Peer Support

Merely because learners can learn from one another, it does not follow that they will feel comfortable with one another or learn to be more empathic or supportive. While it is inevitable that nurses will be pressured to provide peer review for one another, it is less likely that nurses will be provided with the structure and direction to implement their own **peer support group**.

Once in the work situation, the knowledge and experience gained from being part of a supportive peer group can translate into positive gains and can

> Peer support groups help learners adjust to changes in life, school, or work.

provide an antidote to feelings of isolation and lack of autonomy. Peer groups can also help their members find jobs, identify resources needed to accomplish goals, create positive change in work situations, and gain personal and social satisfaction.

The future work world is certainly one useful focus for peer support groups. Nurse learners in various phases of their education have different needs that could also be filled by one or several support groups. Early in their nursing education, learners are struggling with whether they wish to be nurses or not, fear of failure, cultural shock, and other professional and social identity issues. Later on in their program, they often have strong needs to become involved and then to become less involved with clients. As they start to master beginning nursing skills, they may again question whether they want to be nurses and which specialty area they want to concentrate on should they continue in the field. Throughout their education, they probably require support concerning family or dating pressures (or lack of them), personality clashes with educators (within or outside nursing) and clients, and various personal issues. Toward the end of a nursing program, they struggle with issues of separation, grief, fear of failure in the work situation, and more widely based social, professional, economic, and political issues.

Learners could profit from the experience of a structured support group or a series of them throughout their nursing program. The support group is not group therapy; it is a leaderless group in the sense that there is no designated leader and the focus is on support, not on diagnosing or changing behavior. Nurse educators could structure peer support groups in the initial nursing course by using directions similar to those in Box 4–4. The same group could meet throughout the nursing program, or learners could be given experiences with several different ones. Box 4–4 provides directions for learners about forming peer groups.

The peer support group serves as a vehicle for learning, and especially affective (emotional) learning, but there is no attempt to discuss these changes. The peer support group can enhance cooperation and collaboration among learners in school and can be encouraged as an experience to be continued after graduation. If this is not feasible because of geographical or other considerations, learners ought to be taught how to develop their own work support groups once they have graduated.

Women in business have been using the power of support groups and networking, which men have always known about. Nurses might begin to use the same kind of peer support groups to decrease divisiveness within nursing (Sawatzky, 1998; Brykczynski, 1997; Fitzpatrick, 1995)

When classes are very large, it may be necessary to divide the group into smaller groups. This may necessitate a new room arrangement including small tables with

Box 4–4   Peer Group Formation: Directions to Students

Each of you is expected to join with 4–10 other class members to form a group that will be maintained throughout the semester. The purposes of this group are to:

1. **Provide support for one another.** You are to form these groups immediately and begin to plan how you will help each other. A first step is to get to know one another a little more personally. How you do this is up to your group. This experience can increase your empathy skills and cooperative ability as well as decrease feelings of isolation and competitiveness.
2. **Help one another learn.** You are to meet outside of class time to help one another prepare and critique assignments. Research has shown you can learn as much or more from teaching one another as you can from your instructor. This experience will increase the number of teachers and positive inputs available to you. Work to provide constructive criticism and positive feedback for each other.

You may also wish to use your peer group for in-class activities. Or, you may wish to opt to expand your horizons and learn to work with others in the classroom. Your only obligations to the instructor are:

a. Let the instructor know if by the third week of class you have not found a group to work with.
b. Bring learning problems and concerns to the peer group first. If the problem seems unsolvable, then go to the instructor immediately.

Note: The author is indebted to Dr. Judith Ackerhalt for her ideas concerning peer support groups.

chairs around them. If smaller groups are not possible, there are still measures nurse educators can take to enhance critical thinking.

Working with Large Classes

Many methods can enhance learning when working with large classes. All of them promote active learning. Some of the methods that can be incorporated into lesson plans are the Socratic method, oral presentations and debates, combining lecture with other methods, and electronic response systems.

Socratic Method

The **Socratic method** includes **systematic questioning** and drawing comparisons.

> Systematic questioning involves a series of open-ended questions that leads learners along predetermined paths that allow multiple responses that lead to comparisons and generalizations.

During the systematic questioning phase, the nurse educator designs a series of open-ended questions that leads learners along predetermined paths, but that offers multiple possibilities for responding and avoids questions with only one correct answer. In the second part of the method, the nurse educator encourages learners to draw comparisons and generalizations from the situation being analyzed (Oermann and Gaberson, 1998; Overholser, 1992).

Karen, a seasoned nurse educator, listened while one of the participants in her class bemoaned the lack of participation and poor results from a learning approach. The goal of Karen's questions was to understand the meaning the learner attached to her experiences and to hint at possible theories or concepts that might be helpful, as well as help examine the advantages and disadvantages of maintaining her viewpoint. Specific questions Karen asked were "Which is most troubling to you, the lack of participation or the poor results?" When the learner indicated the latter, Karen asked, "What are the activities with poor results?" "What does (name of theorist) have to say about the activity?" "What activities did you feel a sense of pleasure or accomplishment about?" "What does (name of another theorist) have to say about that?" "Is it possible to engage in (name of activity) and try (specific activity) along with it?" "What might be the consequences of engaging in (name of both activities) to this degree?" "What is your plan now to deal with the lack of poor results with this activity?" Karen then moved on to deal with the lack of learner participation.

Although this may seem like a long time to take to deal with one learner's complaint, the nurse educator is modeling for the class how to think about problems which can have long-term effects. The nurse educator is probably also aware that if one learner had a problem with activities, chances are more did (or will), too. Taking the time necessary to teach this invaluable process is well worth the effort.

Paul (1993) suggested several ways to involve large classes of learners in the Socratic method:

- One-third of the class sits in a circle and discusses an issue or controversial topic. The rest of the class positions themselves around the circle and critiques the discussion from a critical thinking perspective. This format can also be used with simulations, role playing, and/or simulation games.
- Learners write summaries or raise questions or new perspectives after hearing a 10-minute lecture or watching part of the class discuss an issue.

Elise, a seasoned nurse educator, found that when the class engaged in the Socratic method, at least two, and sometimes more, learners argued about their perspective on an issue. As a result, Elise decided to try a debate in the classroom to see if that ended arguments, but also enhanced learners' ability to present a position without arguing.

Debate

Debate is a method especially effective in determining learner ability to analyze problems and issues in depth in front of an audience. In a debate, learners must develop an argument for or against a particular position or stand on an issue. Debating provides practice in critical thinking and in presenting well-thought-out information in a professional manner. To debate effectively, learners must be able to:

> In a debate, learners develop an argument for or against a particular position on an issue.

- Consider alternate points of view and formulate a position,
- State with clarity and enthusiasm the main point of a position,
- Define clear terms and concepts,
- Use logical reasoning to support the chosen position using facts and evidence,
- Evaluate alternate positions, and
- Rebut alternate positions in a focused, convincing, and interesting way (Oermann and Gaberson, 1998; Nitko, 1996).

Asking two or more learners to debate both sides of a nursing issue is an excellent way to keep learners involved in a large lecture class and enhance critical thinking skills. The other participants in the class can use the debate time observing their classmates' presentations, writing evaluations, and suggesting alternate ways to debate the issue. Nurse educators can reserve 15 minutes of class time to debate an issue and evaluate and revise arguments.

■ **Nurse Educator Challenge**

What possible obstacles might be encountered when using the debate method in class? Give a rationale for your answer.

Oral Discussion/Presentations

Asking learners to discuss what they've learned or make small presentations to the rest of the class are other way to provide active learning in large classes. Although learner attention and comprehension decreases during a lecture, at least one study provided evidence that peer instruction in a cooperative learning environment not only promoted critical thinking, problem solving and decision-making skills, but also yielded higher scores on quizzes related to the presented content. This is not unexpected. Learners must talk about what they are learning, write about it, relate it to past experiences, teach it to others, and apply it in their daily lives to really learn the material (Rao and DiCarlo, 2000). Some ways to use oral discussion/presentation in class include developing test items, finding an error in statements, learner presentations, game show formats, newspaper clippings, and cartoons.

Bowles (2006) described a preassigned written task that can be applied by nurse educators. The method included:

- Asking each learner to produce a multiple-choice test question related to the topic for discussion that day, and including a rationale for the correct response. (This step can be assigned as an out-of-class or in-class activity).
- Learners present their question to the class until a learner comes up with the correct answer and provides the correct rationale.

This format can be used in several ways: to assess class understanding, to review for a test, or to provide some or all of the questions for an exam with another group of learners. For example, the questions and answers devised by one class of learners can be used as a test for another group and vice versa. This method would be especially useful for a nursing education class that includes test development.

Bowles (2006) also described an activity she called, "Find the Error." In this activity, the instructor prepares a set of 10–25 one-line statements. Each statement requires higher-ordered thinking, contains an inaccuracy, and is related to the day's assigned material. For example, if the day's focus is on diabetes, the first statement might relate to a definition of a term related to diabetes, while the 10th or 25th statements might include a comparison between two theories with relevance to diabetes. In both cases, a slight inaccuracy would be included.

Once learners receive the one-line statements, they can be asked to study each statement for a specified period of time by themselves, while pairing up with another learner, or in a small group. After 10–15 minutes, the whole class comes together and the nurse educator uses Socratic questioning to further learner knowledge; help analyze the question and its correct response; and infer, interpret, and explain the correct meaning of the statement.

Another method that has proven successful with large classes is to organize a 50–minute class into three to four learner presentations of 12–20 minutes. The nurse educator may choose to conduct a brief discussion or question period following each presentation. When class periods are divided up this way, understanding is facilitated, as evidenced by improved performance on exams (Rao and DiCarlo, 2000).

Improved performance on quizzes can occur when the nurse educator pauses for at least two minutes on three separate occasions during a lecture to allow for discussion. Learners in big lecture classes did significantly better on free-recall quizzes and comprehensive tests when their instructor paused in this way. Even with only short pauses of a couple of minutes during a lecture, the inevitable monotony of lecture was reduced, and analysis and synthesis of concepts as well as sharing of knowledge among classmates was enhanced (Bonwell and Elson, 1991; Ruhl, Hughes, and Schloss, 1987).

One study showed that learner ability to solve problems was always enhanced by discussion, especially when it was discussion with peers (Bonwell and Elson, 1991). Even though nurse educators may believe they must cover a certain amount of content by lecturing, this study showed that peer instruction enhanced the quantity, depth, and detail of material covered. As an added benefit, minimal extra time is required for this active approach. As Mazur (1998) pointed out, peer instruction can greatly improve the level of understanding with relatively little effort, time, or money.

Bowles (2006) described using an active learning strategy she called "What's My Line?" A panel of 4–8 learners sits in front of the room and the rest of the class serve as contestants. Each panel member portrays a specific condition related to one of the readings for the day and is provided with a cue card with accurate information on it. Class members ask yes/no questions of the panel until they guess the condition or health problem. This activity promotes the critical thinking skills of analysis, inference, and interpretation.

Kelsky (2006) suggested bringing in newspaper clippings related to the course content, reading them aloud, and asking the class what they would do to solve the problem. Articles on domestic violence, murder, learning, nutrition, illnesses and more are readily available in daily newspapers. Providing case histories or clinical problems from the nurse educator's own practice can also be an effective way to engage learners in discussing how they would handle the problems and justifying their answers.

Bowles (2006) suggested using cartoons because the humor provided a release and also humanized the nurse educator. Additionally, cartoons can be chosen that represent important concepts such as middle age, obesity, alcohol intake, sleep deprivation, vegetarianism and more. To use this method, the nurse educator must ask how the condition can best be represented in terms of lifestyle changes, diagnosis, teaching needs, and family dynamics.

Using cartoons meets other goals. Learners must use the critical skills of analysis, inference, and interpretation. Explanation is demonstrated when learners write a five-minute essay about their conceptualization and/or experiential knowledge base related to the message of the cartoon (Bowles, 2006).

> Jessie, a new nurse educator, wanted to try a game show format and cartoons to encourage critical thinking, but she was afraid learners might find such activities non-professional.

■ Nurse Educator Challenge

What would you tell Jessie? Give a rationale for your answer.

If nurse educators worry learners will not get needed content, handouts of crucial information can be provided, leaving precious class time for discussion, analysis, feedback, and peer learning. Kelsky (2006) suggested using overheads extensively to provide vocabulary and definitions. Learners quickly learn to copy down information from the overheads, and the nurse educator can use the information as a stepping stone to discussion with learners about important issues, providing examples of concepts and, most importantly, asking learners to provide examples. Kelsky (2006) also suggested giving five-minute quizzes on the readings each week at the beginning of class to ensure learners come to class prepared to discuss critical information.

Nurse Educator Tip

Sources of cartoons include:

- Daily newspapers.
- Web sites including:
    http://www.nurstoon.com
    http://www.nursinghumor.com

Audience Response Systems

It can be difficult to know the extent of learner knowledge unless they take an exam. An alternative way to judge learning is the use of **audience response systems (ARS)**. These systems allow each person in a large group to submit answers to multiple-choice questions by clicking on a handset with buttons 0 to 9 to indicate their answers. The machine then tallies responses and presents the results as a bar chart.

Most of these systems include learner input devices (inexpensive keypads that are either infrared or radio frequency or more expensive two-way, Web-based computer devices), operating system software on the instructor's classroom computer, and a classroom projection system to display nurse educator questions and learner responses (Lowery, 2005). An example of a newer Audience Response System is available at http://www.iclicker.com.

An ARS system decreases or eliminates embarrassment or anxiety about speaking in front of the class, or being identified by the instructor as having a negative reaction

> Audience response system (ARS) allows each person in a large group to submit answers to multiple-choice questions by clicking on a handset with buttons 0 to 9 to indicate their answers.

Nurse Educator Tip

Audience Response Systems

A brief primer for Audience Response Systems (ARS) users can be found at the Center for Education Research and Evaluation Web site at:

http://library.cpmc.columbia.edu/cere/web/facultyDev/ARS_handout_2004_tipsheet.pdf

to a lecture. Learners need only push a button to have their response recorded. Some of the systems—for example, the clapometer—allow the nurse educator to display questions while continuing to lecture (e.g., "Are you confused by the current topic?" "Are you bored by the current topic?").

Obtaining information about learner response can allow the nurse educator to prepare the next lecture or discussion so it meets learners' needs as tabulated by the ARS. Learners can also go to a central database to find:

- Questions indexed by lecture, and
- How other learners responded to questions raised by the lecturer.

Some of the advantages of the ARS method are that they increase:

- The lecturer's knowledge of learner understanding,
- The learner's knowledge of their own understanding,
- The learner's knowledge of lecturer's expectations,
- The learner's understanding of difficult material, and
- The learner's attendance (when responses are tied to grades), comprehension, active participation, and peer learning.

Other benefits of ARS are:

- It requires learners who didn't answer during the lecture to do so in order to download the group response.
- The nurse educator can set the system to flag the correct answer, or not, as desired.
- Each question can be a starting point for a Web-based discussion forum.
- Selective viewing of the data is possible—for example, it can be set to show only responses generated by a particular clinical group, a group that is not doing well, or some other subgroup.
- Learners can re-vote on an issue once a peer discussion has ended.

To obtain maximum results with an ARS systems, the nurse educator should:

- Allow significant time for dialogue,
- Give learners access to material before the teaching session,
- Be firm about setting a limit that learners are to come to class prepared, and
- Enter the classroom with only an outline for the session, fully expecting that important information will be identified through dialogue with learners (Cutts, Kennedy, Mitchell, and Draper, 2004).

The Evidence for Using ARS Systems

A study of health care providers using ARS systems found that the response system has potential as a teaching tool because it made the presentation more fun, helped learners be more attentive, and allowed them to learn more than in traditional lecture formats (Latessa and Mouw, 2005).

Tips for Using ARS Systems

Robertson (2000) suggested the following tips for using an ARS system:

1. Keep questions short to optimize legibility.
2. Never use more than five answer options.
3. Don't use overly complex questions; offer only two choices.
4. Build in more time than you think you'll need for discussion.
5. Allow plenty of time to test out the system and rehearse the presentation prior to using it in the class.
6. Provide clear instructions for the audience.
7. Use the ARS system only when the subject matter lends itself to such an approach.

Once this information is available it can be provided in class, in a self-directed study unit, online, or can be used to discuss (in person or via e-mail) how to implement needed approaches with clinical faculty.

Nurse Educator Tip

To find out what learners need to and want to learn to feel equipped to use classroom information to function as a professional in clinical situations, ask them. Take a few minutes at the beginning or end of class and ask them which of the following things (or others) are important to them to cover in class.

- Best ways to prepare for a clinical experience.
- Ways to reduce anxiety when being evaluated in the clinical area.
- Examples of best/worst nurses' notes.
- How to put a client at ease prior to a procedure.
- How to talk to/get along with other staff on the clinical unit.

Assigning written papers is one tactic that has been used to prompt critical thinking. Unfortunately, time is usually not allotted for feedback, discussion, and learning from what was written. Allotting time for these activities is crucial for learners to learn from their mistakes. Correcting wrong multiple-choice answers and asking for a rationale about why each choice was selected could be a way to retain the format, but the nurse educator should add critical thinking activities (Walsh and Seldomridge, 2006).

EXERCISES FOR NURSE EDUCATORS

1. Implement peer learning
Design, try out, and evaluate a peer supervisory learning experience for learners that includes:

a. Objectives,
b. Pretest, entry skill measurement, or specifications,
c. Materials to teach entry skills or information about peer learning,
d. Materials to use as guides, assessments, and so on,
e. A procedure to pair learners together,
f. A mini-demonstration of the peer learning experience,
g. Evaluation tools for learners,
h. Monitoring procedures,
i. Grading procedures,
j. Ways to be accessible to learners, and
k. Ways to use what was learned from this project.

2. Implement peer support groups
Devise a system to implement peer support groups to function inside the class-room, outside the classroom, or both. Give a rationale for the system you choose.

3. Identify group phases
Observe your own or another's classroom. Identify the following processes and suggest ways to use the information you gather:

a. Behaviors that indicate concern for belonging and trust,
b. Conflict and frustration and their sources,
c. Cohesiveness,
d. Listening skills,

e. Monopolizing,
f. Scapegoating,
g. Uninvolved learners,
h. Silent learners,
i. How learners and nurse educators deal with conflict and disagreement,
j. How leadership is handled,
k. Body gestures and accompanying verbalizations,
l. "I" and "You" messages,
m. How decisions are made,
n. Lack of knowledge about group goals,
o. Lack of preparation for group discussion,
p. Lack of rules for learners to follow to meet goals,
q. Learners sharing responsibility for learning,
r. How verbalized dissatisfactions are handled,
s. Opportunities for learners to practice group skills,
t. Opportunities for learners to discuss how group skills apply in the referent situation, and
u. What the nurse educator learned from this project and how it can be applied in the classroom.

Optional: If group observation and facilitation are new concepts, obtain a copy of Suzanne C. deJanasz's Teaching Facilitation: A Play in Three Acts (*Journal of Management Education. 25*(6), 685–712). It provides a highly interactive simulation and supporting materials and activities that provide an effective means for enhancing group skills.

4. Use discussion groups
Devise, try out, and evaluate a learning system using the discussion group method that includes:

a. Objectives,
b. Written group roles for learners and the nurse educator,
c. A cognitive map for learners to follow in preparing and presenting the discussion,
d. Written information for learners on ways of evaluating their participation and the nurse educator's assistance (or lack of it), and
e. Ways to implement in the classroom what was learned.

5. Use the small-group tutorial
Devise and try out a plan for a small-group tutorial. Consider asking for learner input in the development of written directions and evaluation of the tryout in the following areas:

a. Information about the purpose and definition of the group tutorial,
b. How to pose questions for study and related issues,
c. How to collect data and search out related information,
d. How to formulate the problem for study,
e. Strategies for planning how to manage the problem (such as brainstorming),
f. How to try out and evaluate the results of the problem, and
g. How the nurse educator will assist the group.

6. Use the theme-centered group
Plan and implement the theme-centered group method in the classroom, being sure to consider the following aspects:

a. How to present information to learners about the purpose, meaning, and usefulness of the method,
b. An appropriate theme,
c. Rules for interaction during the session,
d. Objectives for the group session(s),
e. Information about the nurse educator's role in the group, and
f. How to obtain helpful feedback from learners about the method and its use.

7. Devise methods for working with a large class
Plan at least three ways to work with a large group other than lecture or that combines lecture with other methods. Try out your methods and obtain learner feedback on:

a. Which method was most challenging,
b. Other ways to combine methods to enhance learning, and
c. Ways the nurse educator can provide support and learning for every learner.

8. Group Warm-ups
Try out the group warm-ups with three small groups. Evaluate the findings in terms of ease of use and learner reaction effect on learning.

9. Problem Statement
Devise a problem statement for a study comparing different types of peer and group methods of learning. Obtain feedback from at least two other learners.

10. Research Questions
Refer to the Nurse Educator's Tip on Questions to Ask when Observing Classroom Groups, and generate at least three research questions.

11. Research Project
Complete a small research project, perhaps developing a short checklist for learners to complete, comparing peer group to discussion group results or small group tutorials to theme-centered groups, or examining the effect of working creatively with large classes. Share the findings with at least two other learners.

References

Ackerhalt, J. (1977). *A teaching model: The theme-centered interaction method.* Unpublished paper. Teachers College, Columbia University.

Bonwell, C. C., & Elson, J. A. (1991). *Active learning: Creating excitement in the classroom.* Washington, DC: George Washington University Press.

Bostock, S. (2000). *Learner peer assessment.* Retrieved October 13, 2006 from http://www.Keele.ac.uk/depts/aa/andt/lt/docs/bostock_peer_assessment.htm

Bowles, D. J. (2006). Active learning strategies . . . not for the birds! *International Journal of Nursing Education Scholarship, 3*(1), 1–11.

Brown, S., Sambell, K., & McDowell, L. (1998). What do learners think about assessment? In S. Brown, (Ed.), *SEDA Paper 102.* Birmingham, AL: SEDA.

Brykczynski, K. A. (1997). Holism: A foundation for healing wounds of divisiveness among nurses. In Phyllis Beck Kritek (Ed.), *Reflections on healing: A central nursing construct* (pp. 234–241). New York: NLN Press.

Burnside, I. M. (1971). Peer supervision: A method of teaching. *Journal of Nursing Education, 11*, 15–22.

Caelli, K. (1998). Shared understandings:Negotiating the meaning of health via concept mapping. *Nurse Education Today, 18,* 317-321.

Callaghan, G. M. (2006). Functional analytic psychotherapy supervision. *International Journal of Behavior and Consultant Therapy, 2*(3), 416-443.

Clark, C. C. (1975). Struggling (a poem). *Perspectives in Psychiatric Care, 13*(2), 72.

Clark, C. C. (2003). *Group Leadership Skills* (4th ed.). New York: Springer.

Clayton, L. H. (2006). Concept mapping: An effective, active teaching-learning method. *Nursing Education Perspectives, 27*(4), 197-203.

Cohn, R. C. (1971). Living-learning encounters: the theme-centered interaction method. In L. Blank, G. Gottsegen, & M. Gottsegen (Eds.), *Confrontation encounters in self and personal awareness.* New York: Macmillan.

Cottrell, S. (2002). Suspicion, resistance, tokenism, and mutiny: Problematic dynamics relevant to the implementation of clinical supervision in nursing. *Journal of Psychiatric and Mental Health Nursing, 9*, 667-671.

Cutts, Q., Kennedy, G., Mitchell, C., & Draper, S. (2004). *Maximising dialogue in lectures using group response systems.* Retrieved November 6, 2006 from www.dcs.gla.ac.uk/~quintin/papers/cate200r.pdf

Daley, B. J. (1996). Concept maps: Linking nursing theory to clinical nursing practice. *Journal of Continuing Education in Nursing, 27*(1), 17-27.

Daley, B. J., Shaw, C. R., Balistrieri, T., Glasenapp, K, K., & Piacentine, L. (1999). Concept maps: A strategy to teach and evaluate critical thinking. *Journal of Nursing Education, 38*(1), 42-47.

Ekstein, R., & Wallerstein, R. (1971). *The teaching and learning of psychotherapy* (2nd Ed.). New York: International University Press.

Fagan, A. P., Crouch, C. H., & Mazur, E. (2002). Peer instruction: Results from a range of classrooms. *The Physics Educator, 40*(April), 206-209.

Fitzpatrick, J. (1995). *Annual Review of Nursing Research.* Vol. 13. New York: Springer Publishing Company.

Gaines, C. (1996). Concept mapping and synthesizers: Instructional strategies for encoding and recalling. *Journal of the New York State Nurses Association, 27*(1), 14-18.

Goldsmith, J., Stewart, L., & Ferguson, L. (2006). Peer learning partnership: An innovative strategy to enhance skill acquisition in nursing learners. *Nursing Education Today, 26*(2), 123–130.

Hoke, M. M., & Robbins, L. K. (2005). The impact of active learning on nursing learners' clinical success. *Journal of Holistic Nursing, 23*(3), 348-355.

Ignatavicius, D. D. (2004). From traditional care plans to innovative concept maps. In M. H. Oermann & K. T. Heinrich (Eds.), *Annual review of nursing education, Volume 2,* (pp. 205–216). New York: Springer Publishing Company.

Iwasiw, C. L., & Goldenberg, D. (1993). Peer teaching among nursing learners in the clinical areas: Effects on learner learning. *Journal of Advanced Nursing, 18*, 659–683.

Jamrozik, K. (1996). Clinical epidemiology: An experiment in learner-directed learning in Western Australia. *Medical Education, 30*(4), 266-271.

Jung, D. I., & Sosik, J. J. (2002). Transformational leadership in workgroups: The role of empowerment, cohesiveness & collective-efficacy on perceived group performance. *Small Group Research, 33*(3), 313–336.

Kalkowski, P. (2001). *Peer and cross-age tutoring.* School Improvement Research Series. Portland, OR: Northwest Regional Educational Lab.

Kelsky, K. (2006). *Clicking with large classes.* Teaching effectiveness program, University of Oregon. Retrieved September 24, 2006 from http://tep.uoregon.edu/workshops/nurseeducatortraining/largeclasses/engaginglearners/buildingrelationships/clicking.html

Keppell, M., Eliza, A., Ada, M., & Chan, C. (2006). Peer learning and learning oriented assessment in technology enhanced environments. *Assessment and Evaluation in Higher Education, 31*(4), 453–464.

Khosravani, S., Manoochehrik, H., & Memarian, R. (2005). Developing critical thinking skills in nursing learners by group dynamics. *The International Journal of Advanced Nursing Practice, 7(2)*, 1–17.

Koehler, C. J. (2001). Nursing process mapping replaces nursing care plans. In A. J. Lowenstein & M. J. Bradshaw (Eds.), *Fuszord's innovative teaching strategies in nursing* (3rd ed., pp. 303–316). Gaithersburg, MD: Aspen.

Lamberton, M., Keen, M., & Adomanis, A. (1977). Peer review in a family nurse clinician program. *Nursing Outlook, 25*(1), 47–53.

Latessa, R., & Mouw, D. (2005). Use of an audience response system to augment interactive learning. *Family Medicine, 37*(1), 12-14.

Lawry, G. V., Schuldt, S. S., Kreiter, C. D., Densen, P., & Albanese, M. A. (1999). Teaching a screening musculoskeletal examination: A randomized, controlled trial of different instructional methods. *Academic Medicine, 74*(2), 199-201.

Ledlow, S. (1999). *Strategies for helping learners develop team skills.* Retrieved April 17, 2007 from http://clte.asu.edu/active/teamskills.pdf.

Loke, A. J., & Chow, F. L. (2006). *Learning partnership—The experience of peer tutoring among nursing learners: A qualitative study. International Journal of Nursing Studies,* Retrieved April 17, 2007 from doi:10.1016/j.ijnurstu.2005.11.028.

Lowery, R. C. (2005). *Teaching and learning with interactive learner response systems: A comparison of commercial products in the higher-education market.* Presented to the Annual Meeting of the Southwestern Social Science Association and its affiliates, March 23–26, 2005, New Orleans, LA. Retrieved September 3, 2006 from http://people.uncw.edu/lowery

Magnussen, L., Ishida, D., & Itano, J. (2000). The impact of the use of inquiry-based learning as a teaching methodology on the development of critical thinking. *Journal of Nursing Education, 39*(8), 360-364.

Mazur, E. (1998). *Peer Instruction: A user's manual.* Upper Saddle River, NJ: Prentice Hall.

McHugh, P. (2002). *Concept mapping: A critical-thinking approach to care planning.* Philadelphia: FA Davis.

Nehren, J. G., & Larson, M. L. (1968). Supervised supervision. *Perspectives in Psychiatric Care, 6*(1), 25–27, 32–43.

Nitko, A. J. (1996). *Educational assessment of learners* (2nd ed.). Englewood Cliffs, NJ: Prentice Hall.

Oermann, M. H., & Gaberson, K. B.(1998). *Evaluation & testing in nursing.* New York: Springer Publishing Company.

Overholser, J. C. (1992). Socrates in the classroom. *College Teaching, 40*(1), 14–19.

Paul, R. W. (1993). *Critical thinking: How to prepare learners in a rapidly changing World.* Santa Rosa, CA: Foundation for Critical Thinking.

Rao, S. P., & DiCarlo, S. E. (2000). Peer instruction improves performance on quizzes. *Advances in Physiology Education, 24*(1), 51–55.

Robertson, L. J. (2000). Twelve tips for using a computerized interactive audience response system. *Medical Nurse Educator, 22*(3), 237–239.

Rooda, L. A. (1994). Effects of mind mapping on students achievement in a nursing research course. *Nurse Educator, 19*(6), 25-27.

Ruhl, K. L., Hughes, C., & Schloss, P. (1987). Using the pause procedure to enhance lecture recall. *Nurse Educator Education and Special Education, 10*, 14–18.

Sawatzky, J. E. (1998). Nurse perceptions of changes impacting nursing practice. *Concern, (*November), 1–5.

Scheckel, M. M., & Ironside, P. M. (2006). Cultivating interpretive thinking through enacting narrative pedagogy. *Nursing Outlook, 54*, 159–165.

University of New Mexico. (2005). *Jigsaw.* Retrieved September 19, 2006 from http://hsc.unm.edu/consy/critical

Walsh, C. M., & Seldomridge, L. A. (2006). Critical thinking, one step back. *Nurse Educator, 45*(6), 212–219.

Watson, W., & Michaelsen, J. (1991). Member competence, group interaction, and group decisionmaking: A longitudinal study. *Journal of Applied Psychology, 76*(6), 803–809.

Williams, E. A., Duray, R., & Reddy, V. (2006). Teamwork orientation, group cohesiveness, and student learning: A study of the use of teams in online distance education. *Journal of Management Education, 30*(4), 592-616.

FIVE

Value Clarification, Perceptual Exercises, Journal Writing, and Poetry

■ **INSTRUCTIONAL GOALS**

Upon completion of this chapter and the nurse educator's learning experiences, the learner will be able to:

- Identify areas where values clarification is the appropriate learning method
- Invent one values clarification exercise for use with learners
- Choose learner situations where value hypotheses may be useful
- Devise one value hypothesis exercise for learners
- Identify areas where a perceptual exercise is an appropriate learning method
- Invent one perceptual exercise for use with learners
- Identify situations when journal writing is an appropriate learning method
- Devise one way of using journal writing to enhance learning
- Identify situations when poetry writing could enhance learning
- Create a poem based on a learning experience

Upon completion of this chapter, the more advanced learner will be able to:

- Try out one of the following with at least three learners and write up the results: Value clarification, perceptual exercise, journal writing, or poetry writing
- List problem statements for value clarification, perceptual exercises, journal writing, and poetry writing
- Devise a research design for one of the listed problem statements

Key Terms

Alliteration	Onomatopoeia
Autonomy	Perceptual exercises
Heteronomy	Poetry writing
Holonomy	Value hypothesis method
Journal writing	

Introduction

Most nursing programs include in their terminal objectives statements about the learners' need to become more self-aware. There is certainly a basis for these objectives. Nurses must learn to be helpers and so must nurse educators. Both must learn to take on, and in, certain character attributes. In this sense, education is a character training process (Maslow and Lowry, 1998).

The knowledge explosion and the number and type of changes to which nurse educators must adapt in the work setting add to the need to be able to trust their own inner resources and problem-solving process and their ability to handle novel problems creatively. Learners grow in this ability not only through examining their work with clients and other learners, but through analyzing and tying these outer processes to their inner feelings; this tie can result in an integrated whole.

Self-realization leads to more effective decision making, value judgments, and ethical decisions (Maslow and Lowry, 1998). It is perhaps for these reasons that program objectives hope to assist the learner in achieving this awareness and integration.

Samantha, a new nurse educator, cannot figure out why many learners in her class overlook their emotional reactions to learning situations, making it impossible for them to function in a professional manner. Samantha decided to talk with a more seasoned psychiatric/mental health nurse educator to share ideas.

With the exception of psychiatric mental health courses, there may be few structured activities to bring about self- and other awareness. Even psychiatric mental health nursing experiences may not bring about the effect planned, or they may focus more on verbal analytic and diagnostic skills with clients. When learners are asked to present data from nurse/client discussions, they often experience anxiety and may immediately decide that the process is too uncomfortable. Too much discomfort leads to decreased learning, and the learners who could perhaps benefit the most from self-discovery are cut off from it even though they may feel the need for it.

Educators must also believe that self-awareness is important, or it would not appear so often in their lists of objectives. Nurse educators may not feel comfortable with this aspect of teaching and learning, and may not have the requisite skills as a facilitator of self-awareness activities.

Samantha wanted to become more proficient in the use of one or more structured exercises to aid learners to become more self-aware. The two things she did not want to do were expose learner inner thoughts and feelings, or increase their anxiety. Even with these two limitations, she was able to find several learning methods.

■ Nurse Educator Challenge

What structured exercises do you think Samantha chose?

Some conceptual frameworks and exercises designed to provide a systematic way of viewing experience without undue exposure are discussed in this chapter. They include:

- Value clarification,
- Value hypotheses,
- Perceptual exercises,
- Journal writing, and
- Poetry creation.

A common denominator for all of these is the use of information already known by the learner. This is in contrast to educational experiences built on the premise that only an expert—usually the educator—has reliable knowledge. In the exercises discussed in this chapter, it is assumed that participants come with a backlog of experience that is pertinent to the current learning situation. The purpose of many exercises is to help learners clarify and realize what they already know about the topic or skill; with this approach, learners are more likely to feel less threatened and to experience increased levels of self-esteem. The first structured learning experience to be discussed is value clarification. For more theory and concepts related to ethics and morality, see Chapter 1.

Values Clarification

Owen, a nurse educator, wanted to make sure learners took on professional values. From past experience, he found lecturing about values and their importance didn't work. He talked to some other colleagues, and one of them suggested he investigate values clarification. Owen discovered that values consciously guide behavior, but beliefs can program behavior with virtually no examination of underlying rationale. Beliefs can also limit perception, cause undervaluing, and hinder creativity. Owen not only wanted to inculcate values, he wanted learners to have a rationale for action, which was why he chose values clarification.

■ Nurse Educator Challenge

What this a wise choice? Give a rationale for your answer.

In the past, it may have been feasible to teach values by stating what the appropriate action was in a given situation. Today, nurses are faced with so many complex choices and alternative responses that they may face confusion and conflict concerning the value of health, death, family, sex, work, friendship, leisure, salary, aging, drugs, instructions, learning, rules and authority, physical appearance, and lifestyles.

Some of this confusion may be a function of the complexity and sophistication of the times. Some may be the result of experiences with clients, peers, and educators that evoke value questions. Because of this, beliefs can limit perception, cause undervaluing and hinder creativity (Simon, Howe, and Kirschenbaum, 1995).

Traditionally, nurse educators used moralizing or indoctrination to teach values. In some situations, and for some general rules, this type of value teaching works. A teacher who is moralizing or inculcating might say, "From my experience, I have learned that confidentiality is a rule to follow for the following reasons."

The implication in this kind of comment is that the nurse educator does not want learners to have to go through the pain of discovering for themselves that confidentiality is a rule that has distinct advantages. Rather, learners should be told what to do and are expected to act as told. This kind of statement has a definite authoritarian ring to it and is apt to result in a low level of moral development. Although some learners will follow this kind of directive, others will not.

If the nurse educator allows learners to develop professional values entirely on their own, other difficulties may arise. Learners will still be bombarded with stimuli and confronted with pressures and forces to act in particular ways, yet they will have no basis upon which to decide appropriate action. Ignoring ethical and moral dilemmas will not make them go away.

One way to deal with the issues of ethics and morality is for the educator to model appropriate behavior and to live out a set of values. The difficulty with this approach is that learners come in contact with many role models. Some exemplify consistent, well-thought-out approaches, while others do not. The result may be that some learners imitate the nurse educator and others may imitate other role models. The value clarification approach gives learners a conceptual framework and a set of skills to clarify and develop values, and problem solve whether or not the educator is present (Simon, Howe, and Kirschenbaum, 1995).

There are five important "value indicators" including:

- Attitudes,
- Aspirations,
- Purposes,
- Interests, and
- Activities.

By examining learner statements or actions in some or all of these categories, the nurse educator can help to clarify what is valued. Values are not personal and fully developed until the learner has gone through the steps of prizing, choosing, and acting (Simon, Howe, and Kirschenbaum, 1995).

Methods of Values Clarification

Verbal and written exercises are used to encourage learner consideration of alternative modes of thinking and acting, of the consequences of the various alternatives and of whether their actions match their stated beliefs. Such activities also offer suggestions for how to bring the two into closer harmony.

Values clarification exercises also give the learners options for their use in and out of class. Choice is important because only when learners begin to choose and evaluate the consequences of their choices will they being to develop their own values (Simon, Howe, and Kirschenbaum, 1995).

Options for Using Values Clarification

Some options that might be pertinent to nursing educators are the choice of whether to:

1. Share the valuing process with learners.
2. Participate in value clarification exercises. If the nurse educator decides to use this method in class and to have learners choose whether they will participate verbally or in writing, those who choose not to participate can be told that while it is all right not to participate, it is important that they remain quiet so as not to distract other learners. Making this kind of statement often has a paradoxical effect; once learners are told they will not be forced to participate, they often decide to participate.
3. Have learners complete value clarification exercises by themselves (dialogue with self) or to clarify values with peers and/or other nurse educators (dialogue with others).

Depending on the objective of the exercise, time available, cohesiveness of peer relationships, and learner/teacher levels of trust, the nurse educator might opt for the dialogue-with-self method or the dialogue-with-others method. For learners who are especially wary of exposing their views to others, or for whom introspection is an undeveloped skill, dialogue with self may be preferable. For learners who feel comfortable in and work well with groups, and with exercises that demand group action, dialogue with others might be preferable.

Samantha was not sure whether to provide a dialogue-with-self exercise for a learner shy about presenting his view to others in the class or whether to develop a dialogue-with-others exercise.

■ **Nurse Educator Challenge**

If you were Samantha, which would you choose? Give a rationale for your choice.

Values Clarification Processes: Helping Learners Develop Values

Values clarification exercises are developed to relate to one or more of the six processes of valuing. In addition to the nurse educator learning the six processes, it is helpful to teach learners the processes by listing them on paper and by stating that in order for learners to develop their own values, they must complete all six processes. The choice of when and how learners complete the processes may be left somewhat up to them, or any of the educator/learner contract methods described in Chapter 2 may be used. The tools by which to complete the process should be made available to learners by the nurse educator.

The steps of value clarification and their attendant processes follow (Simon, Howe, and Kirschenbaum, 1995). By using the boxes that appear in this section (or using them as a template), nurse educators can assist learners to develop appropriate values.

Prizing

Prizing is the first step in value clarification. It includes two processes: (1) Prizing and cherishing, and (2) clearly communicating one's own values and actively listening to others'.

1. *Prizing and cherishing*—in this process, learners set priorities, become aware of what they are for or against, begin to trust their inner experience and feelings, and examine why they feel as they do. See Box 5–1 for an example of a value clarification exercise exemplifying prizing and cherishing that can be used with learners to help them put this process into action.

2. *Clearly communicating one's own values and actively listening to others'*— in this process, learners are encouraged to make their values known to others, while at the same time prizing others' rights to communicate their values. At first, opinions could be disclosed to self, then to a trusted peer or teacher, to a small group and finally to the class, personnel in a clinical setting, or public administrators or officials. Box 5–2 illustrates a value clarification exercise exemplifying this step. It can be used as an exemplar to teach learners to develop this process.

Box 5–1   Issues Surrounding Being a Nurse Educator: A Self-Inventory

A value clarification exercise that examines feelings about and attitudes toward being a nurse educator.

Objective:
To examine the strength of one's feelings about issues surrounding being a nurse educator

Instructions:
Circle the response that most closely indicates the way you feel about each item:

SA = Strongly agree
AS = Agree somewhat
DS = Disagree somewhat
SD = Strongly disagree

This exercise will stimulate questions and ideas that you may wish to record on the last page.

Item Response

1. Nurse educators serve as role models for effective feedback.	SA	AS	DS	SD
2. Learners should be trusted to be self-directed.	SA	AS	DS	SD
3. Nurse educators should reveal themselves as people.	SA	AS	DS	SD
4. Nurse educators set legitimate limits and expect learners to convey humanism.	SA	AS	DS	SD
5. Nurse educators help put learners in touch with their feelings	SA	AS	DS	SD
6. Nurse educators teach learners to achieve level 3 or higher empathy	SA	AS	DS	SD
7. Nurse educators assess learner preferences.	SA	AS	DS	SD
8. Nurse educators structure learning experiences in the direction of higher levels of moral reasoning.	SA	AS	DS	SD
9. Nurse educators strive to make classroom exercises correlate with real life experiences.	SA	AS	DS	SD
10. Nurse educators are managers of classroom learning.	SA	AS	DS	SD

Box 5–1   Issues Surrounding Being a Nurse Educator: A Self-Inventory (continued)

11. Learners are active participants in structured
    classroom activities.   SA   AS   DS   SD
12. Nurse educators structure classroom
    experiences so they help learners develop
    a professional and/or personal identity.   SA   AS   DS   SD
13. Nurse educators develop effective
    learning systems.   SA   AS   DS   SD
14. Learners are motivated because classroom
    material is meaningful.   SA   AS   DS   SD
15. Nurse educators help learners use coding
    system to store long-term memory information.   SA   AS   DS   SD
16. Nurse educators set learning tasks that
    guarantee success.   SA   AS   DS   SD
17. Nurse educators provide a variety of contexts
    within which to apply what has been learned,
    increasing generalization.   SA   AS   DS   SD
18. When learners fail to learn, the nurse educator
    examines the direction, evaluation, content
    and sequencing, method and constraints of
    learning systems.   SA   AS   DS   SD
19. Learning objectives are based on Bloom's or
    Mager's theory.   SA   AS   DS   SD
20. Exams should differentiate between learners
    who have fulfilled the terminal objectives
    and those who have not.   SA   AS   DS   SD
21. Evaluation tools used are both reliable and valid.   SA   AS   DS   SD
22. Classroom experiences include specific strategies
    for solving problems in the referent situation.   SA   AS   DS   SD
23. Role playing situations can increase empathy;
    allow learners to experience strong feelings
    in a structured environment; fuse cognitive,
    affective, and perceptual-motor learning;
    and discuss sensitive issues in a relatively
    safe environment.   SA   AS   DS   SD

(continues)

Box 5–1   Issues Surrounding Being a Nurse Educator: A Self-Inventory (continued)

24. Simulations increase ability to function in a complex and reactive environment, apply behavior in a variety of contexts, and experiment.   SA   AS   DS   SD
25. Simulation games provide intrinsic motivation, can change learner's attitudes, and provide a standardized and safe learning environment.   SA   AS   DS   SD
26. Peer learning helps learners take responsibility for their own learning.   SA   AS   DS   SD
27. Nurse educators have a good grasp of classroom group dynamics.   SA   AS   DS   SD
28. Discussion groups, cognitive maps, concept mapping, and small group tutorials can be structured to individual learning and involve learners in setting their own goals.   SA   AS   DS   SD
29. Theme-centered groups reflect concern for individual autonomy and provide an opportunity to understand the complex relationship between learner experience and a theme or focus of inquiry.   SA   AS   DS   SD
30. Value clarification exercises allow learners to understand their values and consider alternative modes of thinking and acting.   SA   AS   DS   SD
31. The value hypothesis is helpful because it allows learners to read works by prominent authorities that present opposing views.   SA   AS   DS   SD
32. Perceptual exercises are helpful because they assist in learning from past and future experiences.   SA   AS   DS   SD
33. Journal writing allows learners to reclaim parts of themselves that have been denied or discarded, allowing a wholeness and forward developmental movement.   SA   AS   DS   SD
34. Poetry writing can help learners understand a powerful and moving experience.   SA   AS   DS   SD
35. Individualized and self-instructional methods encourage learners to organize their experience and learn how to learn, achieve success, problem solve, and develop critical analysis abilities.   SA   AS   DS   SD

Box 5–1   Issues Surrounding Being a Nurse Educator: A Self-Inventory (continued)

36. Computer learning is helpful because it can
    telescope time, serve as a learner or client
    for practice, help nurse educators manage
    learning by administering tests, analyze test
    results, prescribe remedial instruction, identify
    the most effective paths and modes of instruction,
    point out weaknesses in instructional content,
    maintain learner progress records, allow for
    choice of instructional materials, and provide
    an alarm system for the nurse educator when
    a learner is identified as having difficulty learning.   SA   AS   DS   SD

Questions and Ideas

1. The more SA chosen, the more in tune you are with the teachings of this book.
2. The more SD chosen, the less in tune you are with the teachings of this book.
3. Examine each SD item and ask, "What is it I disagree with about this item?" Go back and read the section in the book this item pertains to. Find at least one other research or conceptual/theoretical article that backs up your stand. If you can't find an article, consider changing your stand on this item.

Write about your reactions to this value clarification exercise.

Self-Evaluation:

1. Now that I've completed this exercise, I notice these changes when I think about myself as a nurse educator:

2. If I were developing this exercise, I'd add:

3. Add that component here and evaluate its effect on your image of you as a nurse educator.

Box 5–2   Controversial Issues Exercise

A value clarification exercise to assist learners to communicate their values and to prize others' value choices.

Objective:

To communicate feelings about a controversial issue and to allow others to communicate their feelings.

Instructions:

1. Read the controversial issue statement below.
2. Do not sign your name, but make one comment illustrating how you feel about the statement or issue (Part A).
3. Route this paper around the class; each student is to read every other student's comment without judging it; the idea is to communicate your feelings and allow others to do the same.
4. If you wish, record your reactions to the exercise itself (Part C).
5. Reroute the paper, read other students' reactions to the exercise, and decide whether you feel the same or different about the issue now; give a rationale for your feeling (Part B).

Controversial Issue Statement:

Whenever a doctor writes, "Do not call code 99" for the client, the nurse should not call the cardiac arrest team for that person.

Part A: My reaction to this statement is:

Part B: Now that I have read others' reactions, I feel the following way about the issue (try to give a rationale for your reaction):

Part C: My reactions to this exercise are:

Choosing

Choosing is the second step in the value clarification process. It includes the processes of (1) choosing freely, and (2) choosing thoughtfully.

1. *Choosing freely*—during this process, learners examine values their parents, teachers, peers, or significant others have imposed on them. By being given the chance to choose, learners can begin to learn to make responsible choices. (See Box 5–3 for an exercise to teach learners how to choose freely.)

Box 5–3   Derivations of Sexual Value

A value clarification exercise to assist learners to begin to choose values freely.

Objective:

To examine some of your values concerning sex and sexual behavior.

Directions:

Read the statements below and circle the response that most closely indicates the way your parents, friends, or teachers have told you to act.

After circling all responses, go back and write an alternate view of how else you might respond if someone had not told you how to act.

1. My parents told me premarital sex was wrong.   Yes   No
   Alternate view:
2. My teachers never discussed sexual matters with me.   Yes   No
   Alternate view:
3. My clinical nursing instructor would tell me to prevent
   clients from having sexual intercourse in the hospital.   Yes   No
   Alternate view:
4. My teachers acted as if I would never have sexual
   feelings for a client.   Yes   No
   Alternate view:
5. My peers pressured me into sexual situations before
   I was ready.   Yes   No
   Alternate view:

(continues)

Box 5–3 Derivations of Sexual Value (continued)

6. My parents never talked with me about
   contraceptive methods.   Yes   No
   Alternate view:

7. My parents told me masturbation was wrong.   Yes   No
   Alternate view:

8. My parents acted as if touching and body pleasure
   did not exist.   Yes   No
   Alternate view:

9. My teachers described sex in a clinical, technical way. Yes   No
   Alternate view:

10. My peers are often embarrassed by and have incorrect
    knowledge about sex.   Yes   No
    Alternate view:

Evaluation:

1. If I were developing this exercise, I would add:

2. Add that component or statement and answer it with a Yes or No.

3. Evaluate the effect of this addition to your perception of sexual value:

2. *Choosing thoughtfully between alternatives*—during this process, learners are encouraged to consider all possible alternative choices, to examine the process by which they choose, and to consider the possible consequences of each choice. (See Box 5–4, which can be used as it stands or as a template for assisting learners to choose thoughtfully between alternatives.)

Box 5–4   Values and Classroom Situations

A value clarification exercise to assist learners to choose thoughtfully between alternatives.

Objective:

To examine alternative ways of acting in various classroom situations.

Instructions:

1. Read each example below and briefly tell what you would do in the situation and why.
2. When you have written down how you would respond, meet with several other learners and share responses to each situation.
3. Work in the small group on one situation at a time; decide which is the best solution. Be sure to weigh the pros and cons of each solution. More specific directions for small-group work are found in Part B.

Classroom Instructions: Part A

1. Several of the more verbal members in the class are hostile and negative about classroom activities. You don't agree with their behavior, but you don't want to seem like the teacher's pet. What would you do? Why?

2. You are interviewing a family in a classroom simulation. The nurse educator has stepped out for a moment to take a phone call. A stranger steps into the classroom and brandishes a knife in the air. What would you do? Why?

3. One of your fellow learners, to whom you find yourself attracted, asks you out. You know this person is involved with another learner in the group. What would you do? Why?

(continues)

Box 5-4   Values and Classroom Situations (continued)

4. The nurse educator stated in the course syllabus that learners would be graded based on achievement of learning objectives. After the midterm, it is evident that the class was graded on the curve. What would you do? Why?

Small Group Work Instructions: Part B

Working in your small group, have each person read aloud what he or she would do in Situation 1 and why. Now discuss the consequences of each solution. After the group has considered the consequences, each person is to reevaluate his/her solution. As a group, decide the one best solution, given the pros and cons of each one. Then, proceed to the next situations and complete the same process.

Acting

Acting is the final step in value clarification. It includes the processes of (1) trying out the value choice, and (2) developing a pattern of action.

1. *Trying out the value choice*—during this process, learners are aided in developing a plan of action and trying it out. Contracts may be drawn up between the learner and self or others.

2. *Developing a pattern of action*—this process is a continuation of trying out the valued choice.

Learners evaluate what happened when they acted, note inconsistencies between their affirmed values and their actions, and make plans to reinforce actions that will support the value (see Box 5–5, which can be used with learners or as a template to develop another values clarification exercise to assist learners to develop a pattern of action).

Box 5–5   Acting on Values

A values clarification exercise to assist learners to develop a plan of action and carry it out consistently.

Objective:

To develop a plan of action and carry it out consistently.

Directions:

1. From the topic list below, choose a topic that interests you and on which you have a strong point of view.

2. Define one issue you wish to work on related to the topic you have chosen.

3. Write down the first steps needed to begin informed action on the issues by choosing from the action list below.

4. In one month, examine your actions on the issue in terms of the following: movement toward the goal, inconsistencies between value and action, and need for a plan to reinforce actions that will support the valued act.

Topics

Health	Physical appearance
Aging	Abortion
Sex	Family relationships
Handicapped people	Friendship
Rules	Euthanasia
Salary	Drugs
Lifestyles	Learning
Work	Institutions
Leisure	

I choose the following topic:

(continues)

Box 5–5   Acting on Values (continued)

Actions

Call a meeting	Write a letter
Attend a meeting	Learn a new skill
Start a discussion	Picket
Take an interview	Get on radio, TV,
Organize a petition drive	or into the newspapers
Ask others to become informed	Become a delegate
Become informed	Distribute brochures
Go on a diet	Stop smoking
Raise money	Send a telegram
Start exercising	Get on an influential committee
Conduct a house-to-house campaign	Provide a service
"Walk in their shoes" for one day	Plan ways of providing health
Wear a button	

From the list of actions and/or my own ideas, I choose to pursue the following steps:

1.

2.

3.

4.

Follow-up: It is now one month later; my evaluation of my action is:

Situations Especially Pertinent to Values Clarification

Situations that lend themselves to values clarification include:

- Crossroads,
- Decision points, and
- Transition periods that learners might encounter.

If values clarification does not seem appropriate to learner needs, value hypothesis may provide a better way to clarify values.

Value Hypothesis

Samantha tried out values clarification with a learner group, but some of the participants questioned that they should be developing their own values and focused more on what they had learned from their religions and families than they did on the exercise she developed. To overcome this obstacle, Samantha decided to use value hypotheses.

■ Nurse Educator Challenge

Was value hypothesis a good choice? Give a rationale for your choice.

Another way of clarifying values is the value hypothesis (Phenix, 1974). In this approach a hypothesis is developed—for example, that euthanasia should be allowed. The learner reads works by prominent authorities on the issue who are proponents of opposing and/or different views. Then the learner develops a short essay, examining the ramifications of each view.

The learner examines the economic, social, psychological and political effects of each view. Such an approach helps the learner examine an issue in an orderly, problem-solving fashion, based on awareness of the total situation, rather than on the basis of emotion, pressure to decide, or others' views. According to Phenix (1974), there are three sources of values: **heteronomy** (imposed, traditionalist, authoritarian, absolutist), **autonomy** (inner, liberal, nonconforming), and **holonomy** (presupposes that one has looked at all alternatives insightfully; free within limits of responsibility).

> Heteronomy is a source of values that is imposed, traditionalist, authoritarian, and absolutist.

> Autonomy is a source of values that is inner, liberal, and nonconforming.

> Holonomy is a source of values that presupposes that one has looked at all alternatives and is free within limits of responsibility.

The **value hypothesis method** attempts to aid the learner in arriving at a whole, overriding heteronominous view of the issue. Some value hypotheses that could be assigned by learners to:

- Pregnant women over forty years of age should be counseled to have amniocentesis.
- Life-support systems should be withdrawn from clients whose existence without them would not meet current definitions of living.

- Dying clients should be allowed to decide on the amount and frequency of pain medication they receive.

> **The value hypothesis method attempts to aid the learner in arriving at a whole, overriding view of the issue.**

- Any woman who does not want to complete a pregnancy should be given an abortion.
- Work tasks should be distributed equally among personnel.
- Sterilization should be compulsory/voluntary.
- Sexual relationships between clients should be limited.
- Homosexual individuals should not be allowed to teach heterosexual learners.
- Learning should be voluntary.

Perceptual Exercises

Perceptual exercises can help learners clarify what they have learned from their past experiences and how this learning will affect present and future relationships. Perceptual exercises tap perceptions of past experience: what one was thinking, feeling, saying and doing. Perceptual exercises are especially effective in assisting learners to learn from highly-charged situations. It is in those kinds of situations that the learner is apt to have a global, general reaction, often of a negative sort. Some of the more primitive, disorganized reactions, such as dread, rage or panic, can occur when the learner is faced with overwhelming situations. Some perceptual exercise situations that can be assigned to learners are:

> **Perceptual exercises assist with learning in highly-charged situations.**

- Facing crises,
- Being asked to perform a task that is in opposition to the learner's values,
- Being placed in an unsafe situation,
- Working with dreaded learners or educators, and
- Participating in role-induction procedures.

At such times, if anxiety levels are high enough, the learner is likely to have a generalized reaction of "this is horrible." Perceptual exercises allow the learner to break the situation down into its component parts, so it can be dealt with in a rational, problem-solving manner. Perceptual exercises can be used for a number of different purposes including:

- *To set an atmosphere of looking at oneself without feeling threatened.* This kind of exercise is developed in a matter-of-fact format that conveys to the learner that it is expected that some nursing situations result in strong nurse reactions. By focusing the learner's attention on these situations, the educator communicates the idea that these can be examined and dealt with constructively. Because perceptual exercises can help to set this tone, they can be used as warm-ups for workshops or at the beginning of a class or learning system. They help learners to center their attention on inner experiences and perceptions, and they set the mood for the learning experiences that are to follow. For example, Box 5–6 is an illustration of a perceptual exercise that has been used to set a tone of comfort and to focus participants on group experiences. It can be used prior to, during, or after an in-class group experience.

Box 5–6   Being in a Group: Focused Recollection Exercise

This perceptual exercise has been used to center learners' focus on their past group experiences. This exercise is used prior to discussing with learners how they will function as future group leaders.

Objective

To help recognize threads of continuity and change underlying personal experiences with all types of groups.

Directions

List 10–15 of the most significant groups to which you have belonged during the various phases of your life. These organizations of individuals may include family and marital, peer, or friendship groups. Groupings created for the accomplishment of work, educational, military, or political activities should also be considered. Remember groups that have developed because of common sentiments or emotional needs. Include short-lived, spontaneously emerging collections of persons and long-term encounters that may have been planned.

You may begin the recollection process by arbitrarily dividing your life into three time periods:

- The initial period, which begins at birth and ends with high school graduation.
- The period between high school graduation and what you would characterize as the most recent period.
- The most recent period.

(continues)

Box 5–6 Being in a Group: Focused Recollection Exercise (continued)

1. Imagine this most recent time of your life. Let the most significant groups to which you currently belong appear before your mind's eye. List them as they present themselves to you.

2. Do the same, focusing first on the initial period of your life and then on the intermediate period. Let the most significant groups present themselves to you, and continue to record them. List no more than 10–15 groups.

Initial Period	Intermediate Period

3. Select one group from each phase. Picture yourself as you were when you were in each group. How old were you? What did you look like? Picture the details of the environment. Who else was present? What was the situation you recall? How did it feel to be you, then? Take a few moments to describe each situation. Writing these details down will help you to remember feelings and events you have forgotten.

Recent Group	Initial Period Group	Intermediate Period Group

What similarities do you notice in terms of your experience in each of the three groups? What differences are noted? What was most satisfying about each group? Most dissatisfying or upsetting?

Note: Used with permission of Judith Ackerhalt.

■ *To clarify terms that will be used and to tie the learner's knowledge of related experiences to a conceptual model.* For example, DeFabio (personal communication) combined a list of stressful life events and their correlated stress values with directions to the learners to search their memories, and list which of the life events occurred to them in the recent past. By combining a conceptual framework with their own experience, learners already begin to note how stress can influence them and others.

This kind of personal tie to theory can have a greater effect on learners than merely telling them that all people experience stress. In addition, when used at the beginning of a learning system on crisis, the exercise focuses all learners at the same point in time and centers them at the same entry skill level.

By using a matter-of-fact approach, the learner is told indirectly that it is expected that individuals undergo stress and that it is in fact a universal human condition. This kind of message is in keeping with a humanistic approach to nursing education. It can begin to unearth learner empathy by tapping the level of human experience that relates all human beings to each other.

A related kind of exercise ties the learner's past experiences with helping people to present and future experiences as a helping person (see Box 5–7). This approach demystifies the helping process and assists learners to clarify what they have learned from past role models. By moving from what learners already know from observing helpers to more complex helping skills and discriminations, inductive reasoning and integrated learning are fostered.

In the exercises shown in Box 5–7, an additional purpose can be met through the use of discussion questions that serve to focus small-group discussions. Through this process learners can learn about helpful behaviors they have not encountered by listening to other learners, and they can feel they are not alone in feeling satisfied or dissatisfied in their relationships with others. Group support provides the vehicle for examining experiences that all learners probably find threatening or satisfying.

Box 5–8 is a perceptual exercise that helps the learner to focus on highly charged situations. In the "Ideal Patient/Dreaded Patient" exercise, learners may become aware of how their expectations and past experiences can color present and future nurse/client relationships, yet this is done in a non-threatening way that learners can relate to easily.

Preparing learners for a new role is another purpose perceptual exercises can serve. For example, in "Picturing Oneself in a New Role" (see Box 5–9), the novice teacher or learner nurse can prepare for future teaching situations by analyzing perceptions of past situations and picturing hypothetical future situations.

Box 5–7 Helping

Perceptual exercise regarding helping skills.

Objectives:
1. Name situations in which you have been helped.
2. Identify what happened in situations that were satisfying.
3. Identify what occurred in situations that were unsatisfying.
4. Recognize what situations had the most impact on how you learned about helping.
5. Analyze what level of empathy, respect, and concreteness were present in each experience.

The Exercise:
1. Think back to your childhood. Picture the first time you remember your parents helping you. Describe what it was like. How did you feel about their help?

2. Picture your high school years. Think of one or two people—teachers, friends, family members—who helped you. Describe what it was like. How did you feel about their help?

3. Think of your nursing education and—if applicable—your working time after graduation. Think of one or two people who helped you. Describe what it was like. How did you feel about their help?

Self-Evaluation:
1. Describe how this exercise has helped you perceive your helping skills and where they came from:

2. If you were developing this exercise, what question(s) would you add?

(continues)

Box 5–7   Helping (continued)

3. Add those questions below this line and answer them:

_____

4.

5.

6.

Evaluate the result and whether the questions you added enhanced your understanding of your helping skills.

Box 5–8   The Ideal Client—The Dreaded Client*

This perceptual exercise shows learners how their expectations can potentially affect nurse/client relationships.

Objectives:
1. Recognize when you are anxious.
2. Identify what kinds of clients make you feel anxious.
3. Analyze why certain clients make you feel anxious.
4. Identify how anxiety influences your perceptions of the client.
5. Recognize how anxiety influences your communication with the client.
6. Identify how anxiety influences the interventions you plan for the client.

*This exercise can be adapted to be used as Ideal Learner-Dreaded Learner
or Ideal Nurse-Dreaded Nurse or even Ideal Classmate-Dreaded Classmate.

(continues)

Box 5–8   The Ideal Client—The Dreaded Client* (continued)

The Exercise:

The Ideal Client

1. Think of three clients you like or with whom you'd like to work. Write the first name of each, then write several words or phrases that describe what each client is like.

2. What comes to mind that best describes how you relate to each?

3. How does each relate to you?

4. What is most gratifying about working with these clients?

5. How did they make you feel?

The Dreaded Client

6. Think of three clients with whom you have dreaded or do dread working.

7. Picture a typical encounter with each. Write down a key word or phrase that will identify the encounter. Write down what were your thoughts, feelings (including feelings about yourself and the client), and physical reactions.

8. How did you handle your discomfort in these situations?

9. How did you respond in each encounter?

Box 5–8   The Ideal Client—The Dreaded Client* (continued)

---

10. Was the response a usual one for you?

11. What comes to mind that best describes how each relates to you?

12. Identify why each client is dreadful to you.

Note: Developed by Susan DiFabio and used with permission.

Box 5–9   Picturing Oneself in a New Role

This kind of perceptual exercise is useful in helping learners to prepare for a new role. The attempt to picture oneself in a new role sets into motion a wide range of inner concerns.

Directions:

Answer the questions below as a way of preparing yourself for your new role.

1. Are there times when you have found yourself imagining what it will be like to be teaching a class? What do you picture?

2. Have you found yourself imagining situations that are dreadful, or have a dreadful outcome? Describe a hypothetical dreadful situation.

3. What are some of your recent memories of teaching/learning situations?

(continues)

Box 5–9   Picturing Oneself in a New Role (continued)

4. Do you frequently feel pressured to find ways of motivating, teaching, or evaluating learners or clients? Do you note a sense of urgency within yourself to help students cope with their chaos? To get organized?

5. Do you find yourself eager to acquire knowledge and skill about teaching?

6. Do you tend to watch role models carefully so that you might emulate them?

7. Do you feel somewhat mechanical when you are teaching or imagining viewing yourself teach? What exactly happens?

8. Do you find yourself thinking about how other faculty or nurses might judge your performance, rather than on teaching/learning? What are your thoughts?

9. Do you derive pleasure or pride from the status that being an educator affords? What is pleasurable or prideful about teaching?

10. Besides teaching, what other role could you see yourself in? What do you picture?

11. Do others seem to view you as a born teacher or educator? How do you know this? How might your answer affect your teaching ability?

Box 5–9   Picturing Oneself in a New Role (continued)

---

12. How would you describe the following groups' image of the status of nurse educators?

Nursing students

Nurses

Doctors

Clients

Other faculty

Your family

Community-at-large

Note: Used with permission of Judith Ackerhalt.

Perceptual exercises can be prepared in a number of formats. A written format is useful in meeting many objectives. Asking learners to draw what they are feeling or to use a drawn symbol to convey their wishes, aspirations, or motto will frequently tap perceptions at a deeper level than well-written words. Also, the idea of drawing conveys a sense of a fun time, a time to be creative; it can considerably increase group cohesiveness once initial anxiety about drawing is decreased. To do this, the nurse educator can stress that artistic talent is not important—what is important is to reach down and express a feeling, thought, or action.

Four learners in Samantha's class were involved in a violence in the workplace situation. She knew she wanted to use a perceptual exercise, but she wasn't sure whether the exercise should involve writing or drawing.

■ Nurse Educator Challenge

Which type of perceptual exercise would you choose? Give a rationale for your choice.

Another consideration when developing perceptual exercises has to do with the behavioral objectives to be met. The nurse educator might ask the following questions when beginning to design a perceptual exercise:

1. What is the end goal of the exercise?
2. What format (written, drawn, verbal, visual, tactile) would best meet the end goal?
3. What component of experience is to be tapped (thoughts, feelings, words, actions, or a combination)?
4. What time frame will best meet the end goal (tapping chronological, long past experiences, recent experiences, current experiences, or a combination)?

Another type of structured exercise is journal writing. This learning tool is covered in the next section of this chapter.

Journal Writing

Journal writing is dialogue with self. Flow writing (stream of consciousness) is the basic form of writing used. Writing flows from the connection between the responding mind and the writing and back again. Because writing produces a permanent record, it provides the data base for return at various points during a life for renewal and reappraisal. Learners often have a sense that something is wrong, but are unable to put their finger on the source. Journal writing can help learners focus on a portion of life experience, uncover major concerns, and begin to plan solutions.

> Journal writing is dialogue with self.

Journal writing allows learners to reclaim parts of themselves that have been denied or discarded. Being able to perceive parts of themselves they are not yet comfortable enough to reveal to others is a necessary part of growth and integration (Mayo, 1996)

Research Base for Journal Writing

DasGupta and Charon (2004) reported on the use of journals or reflective writing with medical students to help them become more self-aware personally and professionally, while Kok and Chabeli (2002) found that journal writing in clinical nursing education promoted reflective thinking and learning.

Pennebaker and colleagues investigated journal writing as a healing tool. Their work is based on research showing that inhibiting the expression of emotion can undermine the body's defenses. Confession in writing can neutralize the effects of inhibition and enhance the immune system (Davison, 1999; Pennebaker, 1997)

Hall (1990) reported the use of journaling with learners. Results included an enhanced ability to accept their potentialities and manage conflict.

Who May Benefit from Journal Writing

Some specific individuals who may benefit from journal writing include those faced with downsizing (Spera, Buhrfeind, and Pennebaker, 1994), and secrets they fear disclosing (Cole, Kemeny, Taylor, and Visscher, 1996).

> Dr. Rutherford decided to asked learners to write in their journals after several of them were unable to express their feelings aloud about the unexpected death of a favored teacher.

■ Nurse Educator Challenge

Did Dr. Rutherford make a wise choice? Give a rationale for your answer.

Learners may benefit from journal writing during some of these turning points:

- Entry into an educational program,
- First contact with learners,
- Crisis situations such as death, emergency, or error,
- Inability to verbally express feelings that are interfering with work,
- Movement from orientation to working phase in a program or group,
- Movement to terminate a relationship,
- Decisions about what area to work in,
- Upcoming job interviews, and
- Graduation.

Box 5–10 shows one learner's daily log entries at the beginning, middle, and end of a learning component.

Box 5–10 Daily Log

The daily log can provide a sense of continuity and achievement when out-wardly no change seems to have taken place.

1/23/07   *First meeting with new class. I was scared. I have so many things I want to learn, teach, and do. I'm worried I may not be good at this. As I read this over, I see how anxious I am about this.*

3/12/07   *As I look back at earlier entries I see how incompetent and anxious I felt. I also see how idealistic I was. Now I'm trying to work with the class rather than compete with them.*

5/10/07   *Despite the hustle-bustle of exams and rotations, I feel sad about leaving the class. I have mixed feelings about ending a frustrating, but satisfying, relationship with learners.*

Directions:

1. Complete a daily log of changes in your life for three days:

   Day 1:

   Day 2:

   Day 3:

Box 5–10   Daily Log (continued)

2. Go back and read over your entries. Write about how they have helped you understand changes over the three days.

3. If you were developing this exercise, what would you add?

4. Add that component or question here and answer it.

5. Evaluate the effect of your addition here.

Entries at the end of a clinical component, set of learning experiences, semester, year, or program can be used to help learners to integrate that period into their life. A format used with learners for this purpose, called "Looking Back," is shown in Box 5–11.

Whenever the learner has a particularly difficult, important, or gratifying relationship with a peer, teacher, or client, journal entries can be used to assist the learner to work it through. Box 5–12 shows an exercise to use called Me-to-You.

The learners' work can be seen as taking on a professional or other work role. Learners can be encouraged to use journal writing as a way to evaluate and integrate work experiences (see Box 5–13).

Whenever a particularly difficult experience is anticipated, journal exercises can prepare learners to be empathic and also to fit their life experiences to the life experiences of clients. An exercise might be used to prepare learners to work with children, families, or clients who have body changes, who need sex counseling, or who are dying.

Petranek, Corey, and Black (1992) found another use for journal writing. They conducted a study and found that journal writing significantly extended the analytical learning process by requiring each participant to organize the material and debrief on an individual basis. Although they used journal writing as an additional learning method with simulations, there is no reason why it cannot be used to enhance classroom discussions and all of the other learning methods discussed. The next section provides specific suggestions for using journal writing.

Box 5–11 Looking Back

Journal entries made at the end of a specific time period can help integrate those experiences into your life.

Objective:

To assist you to examine the meaning of this part of your life.

Directions:

Think about the period of time that has just elapsed. Do not force the answers to the following questions, but write them down as they occur to you.

1. This period in my life has been:

2. This period began:

3. Particular events that stand out about this period are:

4. Angers, satisfactions, involvements I remember:

5. Inspirations, dreams, or ideas I had were:

6. Good and bad luck that happened to me:

7. Work and activities that have been important to me during this time are:

8. Beliefs, attitudes, or values that were called into question were:

9. Things I have avoided saying about this period are:

Box 5–11 Looking Back (continued)

---

10. Things I want to forgive myself for during this period are:

11. Self-evaluation: now that I think about that time, I feel _____.

12. This exercise has been helpful because:

13. If I were developing this exercise, I would add:

14. Add that component right here:

Box 5–12 Me-to-You

Me-to-You is a journal exercise that can aid understanding and help integrate a relationship with a significant other.

Objective:

To conduct a written dialogue with a person who has been important to me recently.

Directions:
1. Write the name of the person with whom you are going to conduct the dialogue.
2. Think for a moment in silence about your relationship with that person.
3. Let responses to the comments in the Exercise Section flow from your inner thoughts.

(continues)

Box 5–12   Me-to-You (continued)

4. After writing something for each comment, reread what you have written, noting your feelings and reactions. Jot these down, too.
5. Write down whatever personal qualities, events, or experiences lead you to know the other person.
6. Imagine yourself with the other person, and speak to him/her about what is foremost in your mind.
7. Read the dialogue aloud, and write down feelings or reactions you have while reading it.
8. Continue with the dialogue until you wish it to end.
9. Read the dialogue to yourself silently.
10. If you will be seeing him/her again, record the actual dialogue as it occurred.

The Exercise:

Write your reactions to the following comments in your journal.

The person I wish to conduct a dialogue with is:

The essence of my relationship with him/her is:

Things that have been positive about the relationship are:

Things that have been negative about the relationship are:

We have passed through the following phases in our relationship:

Box 5–12   Me-to-You (continued)

I am avoiding saying things to him/her about:

My hopes, fears, and thoughts about possibilities for the relationship are:

Now that I have read what I had written above, my feelings and reactions are:

Things I know that make him/her more of a person to me are:

If I were to speak with him/her, the dialogue would proceed in the following way:

If I were to judge the helpfulness of these responses to my understanding of this relationship, I would say:

If I were developing this exercise, I would add/change:

Answer the changes or questions you've added here:

Evaluate the effect of the changes/questions you added here:

Box 5–13 My Work

My Work is an exercise that can be used to evaluate and integrate the "work" of learning.

Objective:

To assist you to evaluate your progress.

Directions:

1. Silently think about your work moment.
2. When you are ready to listen to your inner voice, write down your responses to the comments in the exercise section below.
3. Reread your responses, and write down your feelings while rereading the responses (be careful not to judge your responses; merely note down your feelings while reading them).
4. Pretend that you can talk to your work, and iron out difficulties you are having with it. Write in your journal what you would say and what your work would say if you could talk to it.
5. The next time you are engaged in or with your work, remember this written dialogue, and see whether it can help you in some way.

The Exercise

I decided to become a nurse educator* because:

Difficulties I have encountered in becoming a nurse educator are:

I overcame these difficulties by:

Work seemed to come to a standstill due to:

My expectations for myself as a nurse educator are:

(continues)

Box 5–13 My Work (continued)

> My current feelings about becoming a nurse educator are:
>
> I couldn't stand being a nurse educator if:
>
> I would like to talk to my work and tell it (now write the dialogue you would like to have with your work):
>
> **Evaluation:**
>
> How has this exercise been of help to you?
>
> If you were developing this exercise, what would you add? Add it here:
>
> How has adding this portion enhanced your understanding?
>
> *This exercise could just as well be used for a nurse, learner, staff member, or adult learner.

The Role of the Nurse Educator with Journal Writing

The role of the nurse educator is to provide a sustaining environment for journal writing. If learners choose to read aloud from their journals, the nurse educator can provide time and space.

Learners may be asked to turn in their journals as proof they have completed a journal writing assignment. Because journals are so personal and creative, they are rarely graded, but nurse educators can use them as evidence that a specific self-awareness objective has been met, and then return the journal to the author. Even when not graded, journals can be used as assignments, such as asking learners to "write in your journal about that today" (when learners are stuck, emotionally distraught, in conflict, or when they cannot get a handle on an assignment or situation.)

Journal Writing Suggestions

The following suggestions for journal writing have been culled from years of journal writing with learners (Clark, 2000), and from the words of Cortright (2003) and Bouziden (2003). These suggestions for journal writing can be adapted by nurse educators and provided as one or more handouts for learners.

1. Before beginning, purchase a journal that has personal meaning and a writing instrument that allows for free-flowing writing.
2. Banish the internal editor.
3. Choose either utter silence or soothing music. Experiment with both. When using music, classical or inspirational music works well. Write to the mood of the music.
4. Consider writing in a different location. Go outside, sit on the ground, or by a lake. A change of scenery can add a new perspective.
5. Date each entry with time, place, and any details regarding mood and emotions.
6. Begin by saying: "I'm thinking about _____ (topic)."
7. Write quickly, allowing words to flow. Trust the process.
8. Start at least one journal entry with the title, "Expectations of myself," and use the information to remember how expectations can sabotage or promote growth and learning.
9. Keep writing without erasing or crossing-out any words. Let the original writing stand, but go back frequently to reread entries and add to them as new ideas and memories surface.
10. If writing goes in an unwanted direction, start a new paragraph and make a mark this could signal a sign of an issue that needs attention.
11. When stuck about what to write, record snippets of conversations, facts, feelings, fantasies, descriptions, impressions, quotes, images, and ideas. Write in iambic pentameter or poetry. Draw pictures. Make a collage from a magazine. Try clustering: put the central idea in the center of the page and circle it; without pausing, make associations, placing them in new bubbles and tying them to the main idea, developing a matrix of ideas.
12. Write unsent letters to people you have unresolved relationships with.
13. To clarify issues, write both sides of a dialogue with a nurse educator, another learner, a client, a friend, or family member.
14. Rather than burdening others, release old hurt fears, and low self-esteem.

15. Clarify ideas for an upcoming assignment by journal writing.
16. To prevent censoring what is written, examine feelings about privacy and sharing and how they relate to journal writing.
17. Write about parts of self that have been lost along the way.
18. Go down roads not taken and write down what you see.
19. Write about an ideal day and then make it happen.
20. Explore feelings about self by writing about what parents said or did about themselves.
21. Gain experience in dealing with loss by writing about how to deal with them, and how to say good bye.
22. Write about a relationship you wish to be enhanced; write to that relationship as if it were a person.
23. Choose a wise person and have an imaginary dialogue with that person about a problem; save any ideas that can be incorporated into a daily regime.
24. Ask a colleague to journal about you, providing a look at yourself through another's eyes.
25. Challenge beliefs. To change your life, change thoughts or beliefs. Use journal writing to analyze thoughts and feelings and put them in perspective.
26. When feeling misunderstand—journal.

Poetry Writing

Poetry writing can be used to convey sense perceptions and personal emotions. It is a way of reducing experiences to their essence. Sound devices, rhythm, and compression of statement are used to produce a special effect for the reader.

> Poetry writing conveys sense perceptions and personal emotions, reducing experiences to their essences.

Samantha decided to try poetry writing, but she didn't think she could master the technique, let alone teach the learners in her class. Despite her concerns, she practiced writing a few poems and then introduced the procedure to her class.

■ **Nurse Educator Challenge**

Did Samantha make a good decision? Give a rationale for your answer.

Uses of Poetry Writing

Poetry writing can be used to assist learners in capturing the essence of a teaching/learning experience or a nurse/client relationship. Poetry writing also has the same advantages that other written exercises have: it allows the author to stand back from the experience and examine it from a different perspective (Raingruber, 2004; Hunter, 2002).

Poetry Writing Techniques

Poetry writing requires the use of specific techniques. The length of the lines is part of the visual and auditory form and is used to convey a mood. Non-rhyming devices, such as using words that sound like the object being written about (**onomatopoeia**), or starting several words in a row with the same letter (**alliteration**) yield reader interest.

> Onomatopoeia means using words that sound like the object being written about.

> Alliteration means starting several words in a row with the same letter.

Rhyming devices such as words that do rhyme, use of the same word in different lines, words that have similar (but not the same) sound, and "eye rhymes" or words that look alike but sound different are also used to increase interest and complexity (Phenix, 1975). Usually sound devices are varied to keep reader interest.

Rhyme and meter can be abandoned in favor of free verse. Lines of a poem can be constructed to lengths that will mold the poem into the shape of the object being discussed. Sentence structure is used at times to form a rhythm by using a question-and-answer format.

The poem in Box 5–14 illustrates the question-and-answer format as well as the repeated use of a variation of the last line of each verse. Images can be conveyed by comparing one object with another, by using unexpressed or unique relationships, or by using symbols.

In general, a poem should startle the reader; it should not contain clichés. Conventional language is twisted to form unique combinations. Sweeping generalizations are not used, nor is archaic diction. Poems should indicate some kind of internal struggle that can be conveyed through argument, contrast of feelings or ideas, or exaggeration of common ideas. A poem is meant to have a unity of feeling and a logical sequence. All in all, a poem is meant to have power to move the reader and a vivid meaning (Phenix, 1975).

Because nurse educators and learners are frequently confronted with powerful and moving experiences, poetry would seem to be a useful medium from which to

Box 5–14   School

This poem illustrates the use of the question-and-answer format and repetition.

School

Did you really want me to see what was there?
Or what you wanted me to see?
Some did.
Is there really that much to see?
Or the same many ways said?
Some was.
Were there any who could teach?
Or just some who learned?
Some could.
Is it sitting in class, or sitting alone, or talking with others?
Is it dissecting things, or learning the term, or analyzing,
concretizing, philosophizing?
Some is.
Can you teach it to somebody else?
Some can.
Can you see it as others can see?
Some can.
Can you write it so others will know?
Some can, can you?

Note: Copyright 2007, Carolyn Chambers Clark. Used with permission.

learn about each experience by attempting to express it in poetic form. Confusing and frustrating experiences can take on new meaning for an author when expressed through a poem. For example, the poem "Hers" (see Box 5–15) helped the author work through feelings about a client who died unnecessarily by being given the wrong treatment.

Nurse educators may be uncomfortable with the medium if they are not familiar with its use, and this may lead them to feel that it is a format beyond the competence of most teachers and learners. Youngsters and community residents have produced poetry after listening to examples of others' poetic efforts (Collom and Noethe, 1994).

Box 5–15 Hers

This poem helped its author to work through feelings she had about her relationship with a client.

Hers

Legs were swollen cylinders
Scales of blue and crimson
Welts like hornet stings
My legs? Or hers?

"It's the circulation."
"No. It's from drug addiction."
What? My legs or hers?

Wet and clammy sheets encased me.
I bolted and ran for the light.
Pain? I feel pain.
In my legs, or hers?

Mother used to say, "They went to sleep."
A different kind than Bill beside me had.
Were mine sleeping, or would hers soon be?

Note: Copyright 2007, Carolyn Chambers Clark

The techniques of poetry writing may be of less import than the power, meaning, and feeling expressed through the poem. Learners who have technical expertise in poetic creation might be encouraged to use this medium, but all learners might be exposed to poetry writing as a means of self-expression and self-understanding. They can also be encouraged to use the medium with clients who may be unable to verbalize their feelings or conflicts but can write about them in free verse and symbolic language.

Summary

This chapter has explored the use of values clarification, values hypotheses, perceptual exercises, journal writing, and poetry as learning devices. The next chapter focuses on individualized learning, self-instructional learning, computer instruction, the use of videotape, and how to evaluate hardware and software systems.

EXERCISES FOR NURSE EDUCATORS

1. Identify ways of using values clarification.
Delineate areas in nursing education where values clarification exercises could be used.

2. Invent values clarification exercises.
Choose one of the areas you delineated and develop a values clarification exercise. Consider the following steps or processes for possible inclusion in your exercise:

    a. Prizing and cherishing,
    b. Clearly communicating one's own values and actively listening to others',
    c. Choosing freely,
    d. Choosing thoughtfully between alternatives,
    e. Trying out the value choice,
    f. Developing a pattern of action, and
    g. Value hypotheses.

3. Identify ways to use value hypotheses.

4. Devise a value hypothesis situation for learners.
Refer to this chapter for information and steps to follow.

5. Identify ways of using perceptual exercises.

6. Invent a perceptual exercise.
Choose one of the areas you delineated and develop a perceptual exercise. Consider which of the following purposes you wish to fulfill through the exercise; be sure to choose a format that takes the appropriate component of the experience and the time frame that meets the purpose chosen.

    a. Set an atmosphere of looking at oneself in an unthreatening atmosphere.
    b. Clarify terms, and tie learner knowledge to a conceptual model.
    c. Share perceptual experiences with members of a group.
    d. Become aware of how expectations and past experiences can color present and future nurse/client relationships.
    e. Prepare learners for a new role.

7. Identify ways to use journal writing.

    a. Delineate areas in nursing education where journal writing could be used.
    b. List crossroads, decision points, or transition periods that nursing learners might encounter.
    c. Think about how these might serve as the basis for journal-writing exercises.

8. Devise a journal writing exercise.

Develop a journal writing exercise including the following information:

a. Title,
b. Objectives, and
c. Directions, including built-in feedback.

9. Identify situations when poetry writing can be used.

List specific times or situations that lend themselves to poetry as a self-understanding and self-awareness tool.

10. Create a poem.

Consider the following guidelines and techniques for developing a poem that expresses a meaningful relationship that you hope to clarify with clients or learners:

a. Use length of line to convey meter or to develop a shape that relates to what is being expressed.
b. Use various kinds of rhyme.
c. Use a question-and-answer format.
d. Convey images by comparing one object with another, by using unexpressed or unique relationships, or by using symbols.
e. Attempt to startle the reader with unique combinations of words and images; indicate internal struggle through argument, contrast of feelings or ideas, or exaggeration of familiar ideas.
f. Be sure to create a unity of feeling and a logical sequence.

ADVANCED LEARNING EXPERIENCES

11. Try out

Try out one of the following with at least three learners and write up the results: values clarification, perceptual exercise, journal writing, or poetry writing.

12. Problem Statement

List problem statements for research on value clarification, perceptual exercises, journal writing, and poetry writing.

13. Research Design

Devise a research design for one of the problem statements you listed.

References

Bouziden, D. (2003). *Eight ways to enhance your journaling experience.* Retrieved March 2, 2007 from http://www.journalforyou.com

Clark, C. C. (2000). *Integrating complementary health procedures into practice.* New York: Springer Publishing Company.

Cole, S. W., Kemeny, M. E., Taylor, S. E., & Visscher, B. R. (1996). Elevated physical health risk among gay men who conceal their homosexual identity. *Health Psychology, 15,* 243-251.

Collom, J., & Noethe, S. (1994). *Poetry everywhere: Teaching poetry in school and the community.* New York: Teachers & Writers Collaborative.

Cortright, S. M. (2003). *The art of journaling.* Retrieved March 2, 2007 from http://www.journalforyou.com

DasGupta, S., & Charon, R. (2004). Personal illness narratives: Using reflective writing to teach empathy. *Academic Medicine, 79*(4), 351-356.

Davison, K. P. (1999). Therapeutic writing and immune function. In C. C. Clark (Ed.), *The encyclopedia of complementary health practice.* New York: Springer Publishing Company.

Hall, E. G. (1990). Strategies for using journal writing in counseling gifted students. *The Gifted Child Today, 13*(4), 2-6.

Hunter, L. P. (2002). Integrative literature reviews and meta-analyses: Poetry as an aesthetic expression for nursing: A review. *Journal of Advanced Nursing, 40*(1), 141–148.

Kok, J., & Chabeli, M. M. (2002). Reflective journal writing: How it promotes reflective thinking in clinical nursing education: A students' perspective. *Curationis,* (3), 35–42.

Maslow, A., & Lowry, R. (1998). *Toward a psychology of being (*3rd ed.). New York: John Wiley & Sons.

Mayo, K. (1996). Social responsibility in nursing education. *Journal of Holistic Nursing, 14,* 24-32.

Pennebaker, J. W. (1997). *Opening up: The healing power of expressing emotions.* New York: Guilford Press.

Petranek, C. F., Corey, S., & Black, R. (1992). Three levels of learning in simulations: Participating, debriefing, and journal writing. *Simulation & Gaming, 23*(2), 174–185.

Phenix, P. (1974). *Education and values.* A course given at Teachers College, Columbia University, New York, NY.

Phenix, P. (1975). *Poetic Creation,* Part of a course entitled Invention given at Teachers College, Columbia University, New York, NY.

Raingruber, B. (2004). Using poetry to discover and share significant meanings in child and adolescent mental health nursing. *Child and Adolescent Psychiatric Nursing, 17* (1), 13–20.

Simon, S., Howe, L. W., & Kirschenbaum, H. (1995). *Values clarification.* New York: Warner.

Spera, S. P., Buhrfeind, E. D., & Pennebaker, J. W. (1994). Expressive writing and coping with job loss. *Academy of Management Journal, 37,* 722-733.

SIX

Individualized Learning, Self–Instruction, and Media Use

■ **INSTRUCTIONAL GOALS**

Upon completion of this chapter and the nurse educator's learning experiences, the learner will be able to:

- Discuss the auto-tutorial method and its use
- Evaluate one individualized learning system
- List ways of individualizing learning systems
- Devise a self-instructional learning module
- Evaluate one self-instructional learning module
- Evaluate one programmed instructional unit
- Demonstrate the basics of creating a computer program
- Devise ways of using computer and Web instruction with learners
- Write a script for an audiotape or DVD recording
- Develop a storyboard or script for a five-minute instructional film or videotape
- Evaluate some available hardware and software systems of media forms
- Describe the future of technology use in nursing education

Upon completion of this chapter, the more advanced learner will be able to:

- Compare and contrast findings from the evaluation of an auto-tutorial, individualized unit, and self-instructional unit
- Devise problem statements for a research project in individualized learning, self-instruction learning, programmed instruction, Web instruction, audiotape or DVD, and videotape
- Choose one of the devised problem statements and develop a research design to study the problem

Key Terms

Asynchronous learning

Auto-tutorial learning

Distance education

Individualized instruction

Inquiry

Modules

Programming

Self-instructional learning systems

Stimulated recall interviews

Storyboard

Synchronous learning

Introduction

This chapter presents the basics of auto-tutorial learning, individualized instruction, Web and distance learning, DVDs, audio-taping, videotaping, and film. Suggestions are also provided for using each of these methods with learners. Hints of what nursing education in the future may be are also provided.

Auto-Tutorial Learning

Auto-tutorial learning is a guided approach based on individual learning needs. It provides a variety of learning activities. Learners set the pace, but work together with faculty or staff to maximize their learning. Nurse educators select activities to accomplish specific behavioral objectives and outcomes. Learning can take place in various settings including labs, computer centers, and even at home (SUU Nursing Faculty Handbook, 2005).

> Auto-tutorial learning is a guided modular approach that provides learning activities based on educator-specified learning objectives.

Dolores, a new nurse educator, wanted to develop an auto-tutorial approach for teaching parenting skills. She wasn't quite sure how to start and whether she should use audiotape, videotape, CD/DVDs or computer programs. She talked to a colleague about her dilemma. Her colleague suggested she spend some time specifying learning objectives, which might lead her to the best formats to use.

■ **Nurse Educator Challenge**

Was Dolores' colleague right? Give a rationale for your answer.

Elements of the Auto-Tutorial Approach

The auto-tutorial approach is made up of modules that contain directions needed to complete each skill. Modules can be available on audiotape, videotape, CD/DVD, and/or computer. Learners often are presented with a lab kit of supplies to use for practice and validation of a particular nursing skill.

Modules coordinate study using a variety of media forms; they are sets of instructions that guide the learner in the use of other learning mechanisms to satisfy learning objectives.

> Modules are sets of instructions that coordinate learning using a variety of media forms.

Learners may be assigned a problem to study, or they may be given the option to choose their own problem; learners then sign a learner/educator contract to delineate solutions and learning activities, think out or try out each solution, and decide on the appropriate one. Assigning problems to learners and including the cues and prompts of learning activities and solutions may be most useful early in a nursing program, or with learners at low levels of cognitive complexity.

Asking learners to choose their own enrichment or application activities may be most beneficial later in the nursing program, or with learners at high levels of cognitive complexity. Box 6–1 shows a format that could be used to develop a learning package.

Nurse Educator Tip

A module can be based on a certain aspect, a course unit, or a segment delimited by time constraints (e.g., activities that could be completed in one or two hours), or it could present the material usually presented in a lecture.

Box 6–1   Format for a Teaching/Learning Module

Module title:

Principles, concepts, values, or skills to focus on:

Prerequisite skills or behaviors needed:

Prior to beginning this module, see your instructor for an evaluation of needed skills or behaviors.

Terms and concepts to learn:

Learning objectives:

Given the suggestions in this module, you will be able to:

Learning activities and experiences:

Choose different types of activities and experiences from the list below:

Problems to solve or study:

Use the following activities to solve or study the problem of _____
or
Choose a problem you wish to study, and then fill in the following information.

The problem is:

Learning activities are:

Possible solutions are:

Possible consequences of each solution are:

Decision:

(continues)

Box 6–1   Format for a Teaching/Learning Modules (continued)

Evaluation of learning:

Obtain a copy of the quiz for this module, fill it in, and return it to your instructor.

Evaluation of module:

Which part of the module was least enjoyable?

Which part of the module was most enjoyable? Explain why.

Name the activities that interested you:

How can this module help you in your work?

In terms of this module, what do you think you need to learn more about?

Learning modules may be called by different names—for example, contract activity packages (CAP), learning activity packages (LAP), teaching/learning units (TLU), or self-instructional packages. Whatever they are called, they all contain the same basic information, including:

1. Principles, processes, concepts, and skills to be studied.
2. Behavioral objectives.
3. Diverse activities to reach these objectives.
4. Procedures for evaluating learning and learner reactions to the module.
5. Enrichment or application activities.

Some learning modules contain pretests and/or entry-skill behaviors. Modules are as diverse as the authors who produce them. Some modules are portable, while others are studied in a centralized location. Critical elements for each skill are established and available for learner viewing. Live, televised, DVD, or computer demonstrations are made available for learners so they can compare their performance to a model one.

Auto-tutorials can involve independent study sessions during which learners are given behavioral objectives and auto-tutorial materials to use in meeting the objectives. Auto-tutorial materials are selected to provide multiple sensory stimulation. A nurse educator may prepare an audiotape to direct the learner through a lesson. During the lesson, the learner will be acquainted with the learning objectives and then may look at a series of slides, read parts of a textbook, or examine and/or use equipment pertinent to a nursing procedure.

The senses of hearing, vision, touch, and (even) smell are stimulated. Independent study may be only part of the approach. Learners may also participate in a general assembly session, where guest lectures, examinations, and films are presented, or a small assembly where eight learners and an instructor meet to focus on learning objectives related to the study unit. Usually there is an opportunity to try out new learning approaches and seek answers to difficult problems, an integrated quiz session, and other special projects and written assignments.

Learners are not given clinical laboratory experience in the area under study until they have completed the objectives for the auto-tutorial and general assembly sessions. Nurse educators who produce their own audiotapes and other software, such as films, are encouraged to speak to the learner through the media in a conversational tone. This can give learners the feeling that there is a relationship with educators even though they are not physically present. Although initial lesson planning costs are high, they drop off considerably, and thus the auto-tutorial method is a cost-effective one.

Faculty Responsibilities in Auto-Tutorial Learning

Faculty responsibilities in this method of learning include (SUU Nursing Faculty Handbook, 2005):

- Being available during scheduled learner practice times,
- Posting practice and validation schedules two weeks in advance,
- Assisting learners to submit preparation documents and log clinical lab hours, and
- Validating learner attainment of skills.

Learner responsibilities in an auto-tutorial approach include:

- Working in pairs or groups of three and providing feedback for one another,
- Talking to the model or mannequin and integrating communication skills with physical and emotional responses,

- Not bringing children, food, or friends to the auto-tutorial setting,
- Using mannequins whenever possible for practicing clinical procedures and avoiding performing invasive procedures on other learners except under the direct supervision of a nurse educator,
- Being respectful of equipment and one another,
- Washing their hands prior to each simulation to keep mannequins and equipment clean and to avoid cross-contamination, and
- Developing an increasingly smooth performance of skills by bringing module information, books, or notes to the auto-tutorial and resolving to practice, practice, practice.

Individualized instruction has some elements in common with auto-tutorial methods.

Individualized Instruction

Although similar to auto-tutorial methods, individualized instruction often depends more on learner input. Even objectives may be set by learners or at least devised in collaboration with learners.

Individualized instruction refers to an approach that provides learners with a personalized system of learning consistent with their learning needs, preferences, and styles. Learners control the pace of learning and are free to choose from different modes of learning and to interact with various media forms according to their own learning styles (Gagne, Briggs, and Wager, 1992a). Learners work on their own, using materials geared to their academic level. When a set of materials (or module) is completed, the educator corrects the exercises and hands out more materials (Gagne, Briggs, and Wager, 1992a).

> Individualized instruction provides learners with a personalized system of learning consistent with their learning needs, preferences, and styles.

Research Base for Individualized Instruction

Hal Beder (2005) studied individualized instruction with adult learners. His research team videotaped learners in six classrooms, then reviewed the videos for behaviors of theoretical interest, such as when they engaged, how they engaged, and with whom they engaged. They observed what was said, eye movements, hand movements, and the turning of pages of related materials. The team showed the episodes to the videotaped learners and asked them why they were doing what

In stimulated recall interviews, researchers use videotapes or other materials that stimulate recall and then interview involved parties to obtain information about their thoughts and feelings.

they did, and what they were thinking at the time. This enabled researchers to couple their observations about learner behaviors with the learners' thoughts about them. These are called **stimulated recall interviews.** The same process was repeated with educators. They found very little socialization (indicating high engagement in learning tasks) or grandstanding (indicating participants were not influenced by the researchers' presence).

The Beder research team analyzed the video and stimulated recall data using grounded theory, a method that uses constant comparison. For example, if one educator acted in one way and another educator acted in another way, the researchers tried to determine what might account for the difference. The question became a point of analysis they investigated as data analysis continued.

Adult learners showed high engagement in learning tasks because they were highly motivated. When learners wanted to achieve a goal, achievement of that goal provided motivation. The self-based nature of individualized instruction makes the model learner friendly. It works especially well with learners who tend to fall behind and may feel belittled or worry about falling behind (Beder, 2005).

Other findings of Beder's studies include:

- Learners like individualized instruction because they can pick up where they left off in the materials and not feel as if they missed anything.
- How the educator interacts with learners is an important factor in engagement.
- Educators must systematically encourage learners to support motivation.
- Educators must decide to spend less time helping each learner and reach more learners during a class or give more in-depth help and reach fewer learners, which can result in disengaged learners who have to wait too long for help.
- Educators can help keep learners engaged by encouraging learners to help each other and by providing alternative work learners can do while waiting for assistance.
- Although one argument against individualized instruction is that it does not teach critical thinking and problem solving, Beder believes that learners pick up other valuable skills such as self direction and problem solving as they work through the learning materials.

Developing Individualized Instructional Materials

To develop an individualized learning module to help reduce stress in clients post-MI, Samantha, a nurse educator, worked with a media expert to develop a video-taped interview with a stressed client before and after using the suggestions in the module, an online list of related resources, and a DVD containing relaxation exercises and calming music.

■ **Nurse Educator Challenge**

What principle of individualized learning was Samantha practicing? Give a rationale for your answer.

Educators can use interrelated media presentations, self-instructional learning systems, or educator- or learner-directed learning experiences. This section describes some of the various ways to individualize instruction.

Interrelated Media Presentations

Interrelated media presentations are often built in to individualize learning systems. This is based on the principle that integration of concepts and new skills requires a mix of different learning experiences (Gagne, Briggs, and Wager, 1992b).

Media are used to provide the reinforcement and feedback that are often given by the classroom instructor. When media take over this function, the educator is free to manage and individualize learning experiences.

Self-Instructional Learning Systems

All learners who participate in **self-instructional learning systems** are assisted in learning the same material, yet the pace at which they work may vary; this is in contrast to individualized learning, where learners also work at their own pace, but may use different material. In a self-instructional experience, a class of learners may be given learning objectives, a programmed instructional learning booklet, and an audio- or videotape or DVD; the tape or DVD is frequently used to direct them through the learning

> Self-instructional learning systems allow learners to work at their own pace.

system. A Web-based system can also be used. In this case the instructor develops the learning experiences and places them on the Internet for learners to work at using the pace that suits them.

Individualized instruction differs from self-instruction in that the former is a function of the frequency with which instructional presentation is varied based on the assessment of the individual learner's achievement and learning preferences and styles. Either method may be combined with mastery learning, where learners take a criterion exam (or a version of it) until they succeed in attaining a preset score (Gagne, Briggs, and Wager, 1992a).

Stella, a nurse educator, was just learning about self-instructional and individualized learning. She wasn't sure, but she thought self-instructional learning was a function of how often she had to vary the kind of learning presentation.

■ Nurse Educator Challenge

Was Stella correct? Give a rationale for your answer.

Increasing Learner Control

Learners with high levels of cognitive complexity are often classified as "good learners" by educators, and they do well with any and all types of learning formats. Learners who score low on pretests and who may have lower cognitive complexity levels are often labeled as "bad learners" by educators; they may be able to do well when they are in control of the learning situation (Gagne, Briggs, and Wager, 1992a).

Stella identified five learners who scored low on pretests. She decided to let these learners help to develop their own learning objectives and choose the type of learning formats they used. To her amazement, these learners outperformed many learners who had scored high on pretests.

■ Nurse Educator Challenge

How do you explain why the learners who scored low on pretests did so well? Give a rationale for your answer.

The nurse educator should keep this researched correlation in mind when making decisions regarding individualization of learning experiences. Individualization puts the learner in control of learning.

Other Factors that can be Individualized

Samantha wanted to individualize some of the learning experiences for a course she was developing. She wasn't sure how to begin so she spoke with a more seasoned educator who she knew individualized some portions of her instruction. Her colleague gave her more ideas than she could possibly put into practice.

■ **Nurse Educator Challenge**

If you were Samantha, what things would you individualize in the course? Give a rationale for your answer.

Learning can be individualized along a continuum from the ideal of total individualization (completely learner-directed), to group-oriented and educator-directed choice of learning experiences. Nurse educators may individualize some or all of the following factors:

- Attendance at class,
- Materials for study,
- Method of studying,
- Pace of study,
- Decision making,
- Teaching focus,
- Educator's role(s),
- Teaching method,
- Environment,
- Time structure,
- Evaluation procedures, and
- Purposes of the program.

Class attendance, choice of materials for study, methods for study, and pace of study could be based on individual choice, individual achievement, group achievement or group consensus, or it could be mandatory.

Decision making could range from authoritarian (educator decides), to active (educator directs or guides), to responsive (learner and educator decide together), to permissive (learners decide individually or in a group, but may work with an adviser or counselor).

Teaching focus could range from a more traditional approach to learning content to a more active approach to learning skills and concepts to a teacher/learner focus on process to a learner-centered focus on values. In nursing, where all of these are important foci, the nurse educator may individualize more or less in each area, or try to combine all four in one individualized approach.

Teaching function is related to decision making. According to a more traditional approach, the educator is the center of and directing force for learning; in a less traditional approach the educator presents materials or models skills; in a learner/educator collaborative effort, the educator guides the learner; with a permissive approach, the educator is available or accessible to learners.

Teaching method may range from drill and repetition, to explanation and discussion, to graded discovery where cues and prompts are used to aid problem solving, to unspecified discovery.

The learning environment can be individualized in the sense that all learners sit at their desks, move between desk and resource areas, move between their desks and various parts of the school, or move between their desks and various areas in the community or world, if the Web is used.

Timing can be completely structured by the educator, structured by the learning group or individuals within the group, or fluid, nonstructured, and dependent on learner choice. Evaluation can be based on examinations and class rank, based on quantity of work and criterion references, broadly based, or based on learner evaluation.

Program purposes can range from efficient mastery to understanding to adjustment to development of maturity and independence.

Advantages and Disadvantages of Individualized Learning

The idea of individualizing learning through tutors and apprenticeship programs is not new. The use of simulations, games, programmed instruction, and adaptation of lessons based on diagnosis of individual learner needs is a more recent development.

Wendy, a nurse educator, was trying to introduce individualized instruction into a course she was preparing. When one of her colleagues asked what were the benefits of such an approach, Wendy could not say.

■ **Nurse Educator Challenge**

If you were Wendy, what advantages of individualized learning would you provide?

Both old and new approaches to individualization have advantages and disadvantages. Some advantages of individualized and self-instructional methods found in the literature (Benschoter, Hays, Jackson, and Lindeman, 1991) are that these methods:

1. Encourage learner growth in ability to organize their own learning activities and to learn how to learn.
2. Provide for learner success rather than failure.
3. Build learner self-image.
4. Permit peer interaction.
5. Decrease learner dependency on the educator.
6. Provide problem-solving experiences.
7. Develop internal motivation rather than peer competition.
8. Develop critical analysis abilities.
9. Allow learners to learn through various perceptual structures, learning styles, and routes to learning outcomes.
10. Assist learners in developing individual potentials by recognizing and attending to learner needs.
11. Allow educators time to work with individual learners to diagnose, inspire, motivate, or assist them to learn.
12. Allow educator time to enrich or supplement lessons or to provide remedial work.
13. Encourage educators to provide opportunities for alternative learning experiences.
14. Require fewer faculty members to work with the same number of learners.

Some disadvantages of individualized and self-instructional methods (Benschoter et al., 1991) are that:

1. They require a great amount of initial planning, development, and tryout time.
2. Educators may be unfamiliar with available materials, be financially unable to purchase them, or lack skill in developing their own.
3. Educators may lack commitment to the changeover in attitude and action that is required.
4. Available clinical agencies or educational administrators may exert pressure for learners to attain the same learning level at the same time.
5. Educators may not be able to negotiate release time or extra pay to design learning systems.

6. Educators may be unskilled or lack flexibility in the roles of diagnostician, facilitator, consultant, media specialist, and program designer.
7. Learners may dislike prolonged interaction with media.
8. Educators may continue to stress behavioral objectives that are content-oriented.
9. Educators may not be completely clear regarding the learning that must occur during a course or semester.
10. Learners may require remedial work focused on learning how to pace their learning.
11. Learner/educator interaction may go one way, and thus learners may not be able to interact with the educator to any great extent.
12. Information may be biased to include only one source or framework, thus limiting learner ability to gather many solutions or to problem solve.

The author developed a program at Pace University–Westchester to teach family nurse practitioner learners about group dynamics. Learners were given lists of objectives and tasks to accomplish objectives. Objectives were divided into three levels. Learners who completed level one received a C grade, and were told this at the beginning of the semester. Objectives for this level are shown in Box 6–2.

At this level, learners were provided with specific tasks they must accomplish. At levels two and three, learners had some choice in the method used to attain the goal. Learners had to complete level one objectives prior to leading a group and prior to beginning level two objectives. This approach ensured that all learners developed some basic skills and experiential learning prior to working with actual clients. Although learners could not work on level two prior to completing level one, they could begin work on any objective within that level.

Learners could also opt to work alone, in pairs, or in small groups to complete the tasks. Level two objectives concerned leading a group and identifying and reporting appropriate interventions for basic group problems and processes. Learners who had completed specific tasks in level two could begin to serve as peer supervisors for other learners. Learners who attained level one and two objectives received a B for the course. Level three objectives required that the learner show evidence of being able to intervene in more complicated group problems. Learners who opted to do so could then work on enrichment activities or problems related to group dynamics. Instructor guidance was provided to them individually, or in small groups. Learners who completed levels one, two and three received an A for the course.

Box 6–2 First Level Objectives for a Course in Group Dynamics

First Level Objectives

Each of these objectives must be met prior to your leading your first group meeting.

Objectives	Tasks to Accomplish Objectives	Instructor OK
To identify qualities of an effective group leader.	Read Chapter 1 and clarify unclear portions with instructor or peers.	_____
To list ways of decreasing resistance to leading a group.	Participate in simulations in text "Sharing with Others" and "Perceived Problems of Being in a Group."	_____
To identify a target population for your group experience.	Seek out own group experience. Clear your choice with instructor	_____
To list administrative issues to be dealt with prior to starting a group.	Read Chapter 4 and clarify unclear portions with instructors or peers.	_____
To provide evidence of ability to intervene in administrative issues.	List approaches planned to deal with administrative issues. Discuss results of approaches.	_____
To state how to prepare group members for group experience.	Write one paragraph stating the method you plan to use to prepare group members for group.	_____
To prepare for group leadership.	Participate in simulation in text "Introductions." Participate in guided imagery: "Preparation for Group Leadership."	_____

(continues)

Box 6–2 First Level Objectives for a Course in Group Dynamics (continued)

Objectives	Tasks to Accomplish Objectives	Instructor OK
To identify appropriate group goals.	Read Chapter 4, "Early Group Meetings." Clarify with instructor or peers.	_____
	Take quiz.	_____
To draw up a written group contract with your group.	Present written contract.	_____
	Participate in simulation in text "Stating Purpose."	_____
To identify ways of increasing group cohesiveness.	Present simulated written process recordings and/or present verbally in simulated group with instructor present. Participate in simulations in text "Paraphrasing" and "Nonverbal Communication."	_____
To identify clues to group anxiety and communication skills.	Take quiz.	_____
To identify issues to work through with co-leader.	Read Chapter 5, "Co-leadership." Clarify with instructor or peers.	_____
To provide evidence of working through relationship with co-leader.	Take quiz on co-leadership.	_____
To practice being a peer evaluator.	Correct three quizzes taken by a peer.	_____

Suggestions for Individualizing Instruction

There are some prepared individualized instruction systems available that include objectives, slides, cassettes, games, posttests, and learner guides to learning. Nurse educators may choose to use part or all of a prepared individualized system, or may wish to develop their own systems.

To develop an individualized system, the educator should start with a single classroom and specify behavioral objectives. Hiemstra and Sisco (1990) recommended that the educator begin to individualize a program by allowing learners to determine their own out-of-class assignments, set deadlines for a given set of activities, and participate in group discussion on solutions to classroom problems. A suggestion box can be used, and learners requested to drop in slips of paper, with one problem and one solution per page. Other ways to ease into individualized instruction include:

- Selecting objectives that allow learners to achieve a desired goal.
- Devising ways of rectifying learner errors or misunderstandings.
- Using pretests to determine proper curriculum placement.
- Motivating learners by using reinforcement, contracts, points, or criterion levels.
- Presenting core concepts in depth by planning enrichment or problem-solving activities.
- Devising ways of informing learners what courses or learning will assist them to maintain their present skill level.
- Increasing the number and type of materials available to learners for study.

Delving deeper into individualized instruction, educators can:

1. *Level content*— divide content into four levels and assist learners to work at their own level. The first level is entry skill; at this level learners are helped to resolve learning deficiencies or review previously acquired skills. The second level is the common or essential curriculum or referent situation knowledge. Once learners have completed these two levels, they can progress to the optional-required level where they choose a specified number of units or activities from a selection. Learners who have mastered the other levels may participate in optional enrichment activities that are valuable but not essential, and which are based on learner interest and teacher guidance.

2. *Vary learning objectives*—educators should provide for individual differences by varying the degree of complexity, difficulty, and type of objective

(cognitive, affective, perceptual-motor) and by allowing for reasonable choices in objectives.

3. *Vary time spent on a task*—allow learners to finish early and move on to something else, and allow others to finish later without incurring a penalty.

4. *Provide a number of optional ways of reaching an objective*—build on learning preferences and styles.

5. *Provide more frequent and specific individual feedback*—learners regarding what they need to learn and what they have already mastered.

Additional ways of individualizing instruction include:

1. Allowing learners to select some topics, goals and study habits.
2. Encouraging learners to locate their own sources of information.
3. Providing teacher, peer, or programmed instruction tutorial help to grasp the underlying structure or overview of a concept or process.
4. Encouraging learners having difficulty to try new study or practice methods.

Timothy, a graduate assistant, implemented the following individualized instruction methods. Some of them worked quite well and some didn't. Several learners were very enthusiastic about the classroom changes and one even asked if he had more ideas other than to ask learners to locate their own sources of information, obtain peer feedback about their grasp of concepts, use pretests to determine their knowledge, and vary the pace of their own learning. Timothy thought about it, but couldn't come with any more ideas.

■ Nurse Educator Challenge

Pretend you're Timothy and provide at least five other ways to individualize instruction.

A final consideration in developing individualized instruction is to devise a system for keeping track of each learner. Evaluation forms, progress charts, or work folders may be used, or learners may keep track of their own progress (see Box 6–2). Once a learner has completed a level of objectives, the educator signs the progress sheet and collects it. After a number of learners have used an instructional system, it is time to evaluate it.

Evaluating Individualized or Self-Instructional Learning Systems

One area to be examined when evaluating this kind of learning system is the percent of learner success on various learning objectives. Learning objectives are examined in each area: affective, cognitive, and perceptual-motor.

If learners do not attain 80 or 90 percent on an area, that portion of the system should be redesigned. Another area to examine is the extent to which the system allows learners to progress at their own rate. When some learners complete all modules or systems well before the terminal date, others take up to or past the terminal date, and slower learners repeat quizzes but finally reach criterion level, the educator can infer that this area has been fulfilled because there is marked variability in learning, and self-pacing is possible. If learners all seem to progress through the system in a lockstep fashion, the educator must attempt to build in a greater variety of activities, learning experiences, and learner choice. If slower learners do not improve with repetition, remedial materials are developed to bring them to entry or criterion level.

Another area to consider is the extent to which learners exercise options to choose and complete additional projects. If most learners complete enrichment or self-designed learning experiences, the design may be considered successful in this area. Another indicant of this is the frequent and spontaneous suggestion by learners for new learning experiences or projects.

This is a relatively subjective judgment, but if no learners complete or design enrichment activities and no suggestions are forthcoming, there is something wrong with this design aspect. Most likely reinforcement and feedback aspects as well as increased nurse educator counseling and orienting behaviors are needed.

Another area to consider is learner self-evaluation. Cambra-Fierro and Cambra-Berda (2007) found that self-evaluation may be helpful when evaluating reflective learning. Self-evaluation may also be valuable when learners are engaged in learning nurse-client relationship skills. Kluge, Glick, Engleman, and Hooper, (2007) found that after 35 baccalaureate nursing and allied allied health care learners completed a five week therapeutic communication module that included an innovative computer-based simulation of clinical nurse/client encounters, nursing learners were significantly more likely to report increased confidence and competence using therapeutic communication skills. Based on these findings, the nurse educator should ask whether there might be a benefit to having learners evaluate themselves.

A final aspect to be examined is the extent to which the system provides learners with skills in the design and development of their own learning experiences. Modules that require learners to design their own enrichment experiences or to delineate and solve problems will afford the nurse educator data on this aspect.

Independent learning, responsibility for learning, and learning how to learn are objectives particularly pertinent to nursing education. They can be easily observed when there is individualized and self-instructional learning. Some observations the nurse educator can make about learners in this assessment area are whether they:

1. Start self-assigned or teacher-assigned tasks promptly,
2. Carry out the learning task without reminders,
3. Complete the task despite interference or interruption,
4. Continue beyond the requirements of the task,
5. Make efficient use of media and resources,
6. Plan learning priorities,
7. Complete priority tasks,
8. Work out solutions when faced with unexpected situations,
9. Develop individual approaches to tasks,
10. Demonstrate independent thinking despite verbal opposition to ideas,
11. Ask questions that attempt to relate new material to previous content,
12. Seek additional or remedial learning,
13. Turn in an original project, and
14. Work on a nonrequired task.

Programmed learning principles may also be of value to nurse educators.

Programmed Instruction

Programming is a process of arranging material to be learned in a series of sequential steps (or frames), where the learner is guided from the familiar to more complex

> Programming is a process of arranging material to be learned in a series of sequential steps or frames, guiding the learner from familiar to more complex material.

material. Many different kinds of stimuli can be used to guide the learner including printed matter, films, filmstrips, teaching machines, drawings, and computer printouts. Often very small segments of information are interspersed with required learner responses (Mergel, 2001). In this way learners are continually active as they respond to a question or statement. Feedback is immediate. Learners receive a written, oral, or visual reaction to their responses as a demonstration of the consequence of their performances. Learners either receive confirmation that their performance is appropriate or correct and so proceed to the next step, or receive feedback directing them to (re)take certain steps until they are successful

A program is devised to enable systematic learning. Often learners are asked to read a book to learn what is expected. But books contain little or no predetermined interaction in the form of required response and feedback, unless it is built in through the use of programming techniques. In many programs, small steps are used. There are different meanings assigned to the small-step concept including:

- Only a sentence or two of material is presented before learner response is required.
- The steps or frames are arranged in increments so correct responding is highly probable. Each frame represents an advance toward a learning objective.
- Whenever new concepts or principles are introduced, cues, hints, or prompts aid learners to make the correct response.
- Responses are effortless because the learner is led to the correct ones.
- Less and less prompting is used, until the final frame of a concept is unprompted and serves as a test.
- There is much repetition of new concept, leading to over-learning and an enhanced ability to recall the information after a prolonged period without stimulation (Shiffman, 1995).

Advantages and Disadvantages of Programmed Materials

Written programmed instructional materials have the advantage of being self-instructional and providing immediate feedback, predetermined and systematic learning, retention and recall, a likelihood of success, a permanent record and reference source, and ready access to update of materials. Most are relatively inexpensive, portable, and easy to use.

Some disadvantages of written programs are that they can be boring, are not adaptable to learner preferences and styles, are often weak in providing opportunities to generalize to other situations, and present only one viewpoint. Computer instruction can be programmed, and often is. It is discussed next.

Advantages and Disadvantages of Computer Instruction

Computer instruction is a programmed approach that has the advantages of self-instruction, immediate feedback, systematic learning, and likelihood of success, but not those of low cost, ease of use, or permanent record for learner reference. It can provide an immense variety of stimulus displays, which a written program cannot. Advantages of computer instruction include the following:

1. *Saves time*—a computer can be programmed to store vast amounts of resource material. Learners are able to research topics, saving considerable time that would usually be spent in searching through books and bibliographies or talking with resource librarians.

2. *Telescopes time*—the computer is like a simulation or a simulation game, where a slice of reality can be speeded up and the implications of long-term processes can be grasped in much less time than real life takes. For example, the computer can serve as a client whom the learner interviews for a nursing diagnosis; in real life, clients may omit valuable information, be mistrustful and not share information, not keep appointments, and so on, wasting useful learning time. Possible nursing intervention results can also be presented by the computer in a brief period of time, while real-life nursing intervention might not show results for days, weeks, or even longer. Computer models also allow the learner to grasp the underlying structure or overview of a concept or process. Learners can move through data points so quickly that the essential structure becomes immediately apparent.

3. *Allows for dialogue*—although early computer-assisted instructional (CAI) programs were of the tutor or drill-and-practice variety, there is now the potential for learner-computer dialogues, problem solving, game playing, and enrichment activities. The ELIZA system at MIT demonstrated that a computer could be programmed to "understand" typed learner sentences. Such breakthroughs have led to a flexible adaptive interaction between computer and learner. This can prove especially useful with learners of low cognitive complexity or motivation, who seem to learn more when they are given control over the learning situation (Mergel, 2001). Diagnostic simulations are also examples of dialogues where learners have increased control over the learning situation. Computer games have been widely used in business administration courses and are usually played by two teams of learners who compete to win by making the best possible decisions with regard to action in the simulated environment.

4. *Allows inquiry*—**inquiry** is a kind of computer enrichment experience that is provided when a learner is able to ask questions of a database that represents phenomena in the referent situation. Examples of inquiry use in other disci-

plines are the Standard and Poor stock market tapes and histories of legal cases. In nursing, it is possible to develop similar databases of laboratory results, nursing histories and client records, personnel interactions, or nurse/client, nurse/family, or nurse/group sessions.

> Inquiry is a type of computer enrichment experience that allows learners to ask questions of a database that represents phenomena in the referent situation.

5. *Manages learning*—another advantage of computer use is management of learning. Computers can be used to administer tests, analyze test results, prescribe remedial instruction, identify the most effective paths and modes of instruction for individual learners, identify weaknesses in instructional content and ways of improving the course, schedule learner use of equipment to maximize efficient usage, maintain learner progress records, provide for learner flexibility and accessibility in choice of instructional materials, alert the instructor whenever a learner is identified as having learning problems, and perform clerical tasks such as rote calculation, freeing the learner to focus on more significant learning tasks (Mergel, 2001).

Factors that may mediate against widespread use of computer capability include:

1. *Many CAI programs still require hours of instruction in computer use.* This learning time can cancel out time saved by the computer through telescoped time techniques and literature searches.
2. *Some computers are relatively nonportable and require learners to learn in a centralized location.* This disadvantage can be decreased somewhat by adding terminal inputs into the computer and allowing learners to use portable terminals and/or by sharing computer services among several learning institutions or hospitals. Learners who have laptops do not have this disadvantage.
4. *Faculty may be suspicious of machines.* Educators are often unfamiliar with technology in general, and therefore may distrust computers that can seem formidable to the novice user.

Types of Written Programs

There are two basic types of written computer programs, linear and branching. In the traditional linear program, all learners read and respond to the same frames in the same order. There is a single line or path for all learners, and small amounts of material are presented. The linear program is usually response-centered; the frame is presented to evoke a response and permit reinforcement of each response. Linear programs that present large amounts of information emphasize presentation of material (Mergel, 2001).

There are variations where frames are longer or there are multiple paths to follow. For example, criterion frames can be used to test entering behavior at various points in the program to determine whether the learner should complete the next sequence of frames or move on to a more advanced level, as shown in the example below.

Criterion frame

1 2 3 4 5

$\downarrow$ _ $\uparrow$

The criterion frame is an example of combined linear and branching techniques. Branching programs are stimulus-centered. Learners proceed through frames until they make an error; then they are "branched" to supplementary frames to receive remedial instruction. The example below shows a portion of a branching program.

Error

$1 \rightarrow 2 \rightarrow 3$

$\downarrow$ error

$4 \rightarrow 5\ 8$

$\downarrow \uparrow$

$6 \rightarrow 7$

In branching programs, the learner reads the frame and then selects an alternative from a multiple-choice question. Each choice refers the learner to a different page in the text for remedial work. The correct response is affirmed as correct, and new material is presented. In the example above, the learner gave incorrect responses at questions 3 and 5 and was branched to remedial work. A learner who made no errors would be directed to move from question 3 to question 8.

Neither linear nor branching techniques are superior in themselves. The decision of which type to use must be based on instructional objectives, entering behavior of learners, and whether responses or stimulus learning is important. It is possible to shift from linear to branching to linear throughout one program (Mergel, 2001).

Another method of programming is the "mathetic" approach pioneered by Gilbert. This approach begins with a simple overview of the concept(s) or skill. The first exercise gives learners sufficient instruction to describe for themselves a large section of the material to be learned, ending with the last event or behavior. The second exercise will guide learners through much of the material but will require them to finish on their own. Other exercises follow, until the learner is able to proceed without cues or prompts (Anglin, 1995).

Mager suggests beginning with a demonstration of mastery performance and then asks learners to request information or explanation as they feel they need it. This approach is much more learner-centered than most linear or branching programs. The method is not very efficient, but it allows for individualized learning. In addition, with experience, the programmer soon learns the kind of questions learners ask most often and can narrow down study sequences to popular questions. One way to use this method is to have learners complete pre-programmed short modules of instruction that deal with popular questions and then to have them meet with the instructor to cover questions not anticipated in the module (Mager, 1997). Box 6–3 shows one frame and accompanying exercise from a linear program on hallucinations.

Suggestions for Using Written Programs

Samantha, a nurse educator, did not want to develop a computer programmed learning system, but she did want to know how evaluate available programs. A colleague told her about a system he used, but he did not have any information on how to evaluate its effectiveness. Samantha was unsure what to do next.

■ Nurse Educator Challenge

If you were Samantha's colleague, what would you tell her about how to evaluate a written program?

The development and use of computer programs are beyond the scope of this book, but guidelines for their use appear below. Written programs are especially useful in the following situations:

1. When presenting the same or similar teaching materials to learners.
2. When there is a minimum of teacher supervision required, or when supervision is of a nontechnical, custodial nature.

Box 6–3   One Frame of a Written Program and Its Accompanying Practice Exercise

---

INFORMATION 6

Listed below are the nursing interventions for hallucinations related to social isolation and loneliness.

Intervention	Rationale
1. Provide a "real" person for the client to relate to.	1. The "real" person can be the nurse who provides a more constructive relationship than the one the client has with the hallucinatory figure or voice.
2. Separate yourself from the client's experience.	2. Clients with psychiatric diagnoses or who are disoriented tend to think everyone is experiencing what they are: orientation to who is experiencing what is helpful.
3. Avoid focusing on the hallucinatory content once an assessment of the difficulty has been made.	3. Focusing unduly on hallucinatory content encourages the production of more hallucinatory content and supports socially unacceptable behavior.
4. Focus on the feelings the client is experiencing.	4. Anxiety and loneliness frequently trigger hallucinations.
5. Explore other times the client has had the same feelings.	5. Helping the client to understand his or her experiences is a step toward choosing alternative, more constructive methods of dealing with feelings.

(continues)

Box 6–3   One Frame of a Written Program and Its Accompanying Practice Exercise
(continued)

Practice

Match the nursing interventions with the appropriate rationales by placing the number of the correct rationale in front of the intervention.

Interventions	Rationales
A. Explore other times the client has had hallucinations.	1. The nurse can be the "real" person.
B. Focus on the feelings the client is experiencing.	2. Anxiety and loneliness frequently trigger hallucinatory experiences.
C. Separate yourself from the client's experience.	3. Understanding is a step toward choosing alternative behavior.
D. Avoid focusing unduly on hallucinatory content.	4. When the client is disoriented internally, external orientation can provide structure and clarify perceptions.
E. Provide a "real" person.	5. Focusing unduly on hallucinatory content encourages hallucinations to continue.

---

3. If material is conducive to private study.

4. If a permanent record of learner performance and a reference for learner study is needed.

5. If a predetermined, systematic presentation with immediate feedback and success in learning is required.

6. If some learners require repetition of material and the instructor wishes to move on to new material with other learners.

Deciding Whether to Purchase or Assign Written Programs

When deciding whether to purchase or assign written programs for use, the nurse educator should choose instructional systems that meet all or most of the following criteria:

1. Behavioral objectives that detail what the program will teach are included.
2. The target population for whom the program was developed (including entry characteristics, interest, and grade level) is described.
3. The length of time it will take to complete the program (in average time as well as the range of time for learners) is discussed.
4. The type of program used and whether it provides opportunities to generalize is evaluated.
5. Provisions have been taken to decrease learner potential for cheating and reading answers prior to responding to questions.
6. Evaluation data includes evidence that learners learn from the program, how many learners attained criterion on posttest, what kind of criteria were used on pre- and posttest, how many times the program was tried out and revised, and a sample of the pre- and posttest.
7. Details regarding how to administer the program are included.
8. The program seems to fit within the existing nursing curriculum.
9. There is a low per-unit cost.
10. There is a short training time needed for learners in the use of the program.
11. The program is reusable.

Designing Written Programs

When designing a written program, the nurse educator should follow these steps:

1. *Delineate the target population* (e.g., senior nursing learners).
2. *Select a small content area or skill* that is relevant to the focus of learning.
3. *Make sure the topic is not too wide* and that it has specific facts, concepts, or easily stated skill steps.
4. *Be familiar with the material prior to attempting to program it,* otherwise time will be lost in consultation or reading to learn and digest the essence of the content.
5. *Prepare a content outline* on a segment of material that can be covered in a one-hour lecture.

6. *Define behavioral objectives,* including a description of terminal behaviors. Instructional goals can be stated first, and they can be narrowed and specified to observable behaviors that lead to the accomplishment of each goal.

7. *Develop a pretest* early in program development. The test results will indicate at what level the written program information must begin to match learner entry skills. If considerable variability is noted when the pretest is administered, a branching program may be the most useful type of program to develop. If time makes this step unfeasible, prerequisite learning experiences can be assigned to be completed prior to learners beginning the program itself; this will ensure that all learners have basic skills when beginning the program.

8. *Construct a posttest* of terminal behaviors (DeCecco, 1968).

9. The content outline or list of objectives may need revision now in light of test results.

10. *Construct a flow chart* giving the sequence of essential points to be learned as well as alternative remedial points, as needed.

11. *Begin to write frames.*

    a. Use the first few frames to help the learner understand how programmed instruction works; require the learner to respond to each of the first few frames either by making up an answer or by selecting from a list of possible answers.

    b. Begin a program with something of interest or familiarity, so the learner is immediately motivated either by the novelty or by its familiarity .

    c. Make sure that each frame is clearly written and that sufficient repetition is available.

    d. Construct each frame so the learner is required either to think or to act; a bad frame presents irrelevant information.

    e. Frames should form a continuous dialogue, leading the learner through a learning experience.

    f. Frames should not be too easy or too hard; success should be guaranteed for those who are working well and learning.

    g. Provide confirmation for the learner regarding whether a response is correct or whether the learner needs remedial work.

    h. Use short frames when frequent response and low percentage of learning errors is required.

    i. Use longer frames or a mathetic approach when problem-solving or generalization is needed.

j. Divide long programs into chapters to enable learners to interrupt study between chapters.

k. Use index cards with frames on one side and responses on the other in initial stages of program development.

l. Gradually introduce new material while slowly withdrawing cues or prompts.

m. Use prompts to guide learner responses.

n. Avoid under- and overprompting; an overprompt requires the learner to copy a word that appears in the frame.

o. Prompts may include use of part of a word, dashes to indicate the number of letters missing in a word, or words that call up previously learned associations.

p. Once frames are developed and checked for appropriate sequencing, they are tried out with five or ten learners.

q. Observe learners while they are responding to the written program, or have them work directly from index cards.

r. Revise frames as necessary depending on learner ability to understand wording or respond correctly.

s. Duplicate the program and try it out with 15–40 learners. Their responses will reveal which frames were missed.

t. Make a list of common errors from learner response sheets, and identify ineffective frames. If more than a 10 percent error rate exists on the posttest, those frames should be revised and then tried out. Once the program meets the 10 percent error rate, it can be utilized with the entire class and reevaluated or revised as necessary (Anglin, 1995).

u. Directions to the learner are then prepared and tested out with a representative population.

Directions for a programmed instructional unit on hallucination are shown in Box 6–4.

Prepare an Instructor's Manual

Preparing an instructor's manual should include the following:

- The purpose of the program,
- A description of the target population,
- The intended learning outcomes,
- A copy of the pretest with suggestions for its use,
- Answers to the pretest,

Box 6–4   Directions to the Student for a Written Program on Hallucinations

Directions

When you have finished this booklet successfully, you will be able to:

1. Define five types of hallucinations.
2. List three causal factors for hallucinations.
3. Select three therapeutic nursing interventions in hallucinations related to organic brain syndrome.
4. Select three therapeutic nursing interventions in hallucinations related to sensory deprivation.
5. Select three therapeutic nursing interventions in hallucinations related to sensory overload.
6. Select three therapeutic nursing interventions in hallucinations related to social isolation.
7. State appropriate nursing interventions for clinical situations demonstrating a patient experiencing hallucinations.

If you think you already know the information above, obtain a copy of the pretest from your instructor. If you score 90 or better on the pretest, you need not complete this booklet.

If you do plan to complete this booklet, here is how it's organized. First, you are given a bit of information. Then, you are asked questions about the material through practice activities. At the end of the practice, you are directed where to go for the answers. The answers are found in the sections called Feedback. Begin by turning to page 2.

- A copy of the posttest with suggestions for its use,
- The length of time needed to complete the program,
- How the program was tried out and revised,
- Suggestions for administering the program,
- Instructions for how to use the program within an existing curriculum, and
- A bibliography.

Records are also useful for storing information. The next section discusses audiotape, videotape, and CD recordings.

Audiotape, Videotape, or CD Recordings

Recorders store and retrieve sound and sometimes images. Nurse educators can develop their own materials, or they can purchase prerecorded instructional materials and play them back on a recorder. Instructor-made materials and CDs allow the educator to rearrange the order or eliminate learning segments through editing, and/or to listen for extended time periods.

Although CD-ROMs are more expensive to make than audio- or videotapes, they allow for greater depth of content and may satisfy a broader range of educational needs (Agre, Dougherty, and Pirone, 2002). CAI programs provide an individualized, interactive, and interesting way to learn. They contain visual effects and audio support for written text, and can provide an element of excitement that other methods of learning may not (Castaldini, Saltmarch, Lucky and Sucher, 1998).

To make CDs, the following equipment is needed:

- A CD burner on your computer,
- CD-burning software, and
- Blank CDs.

The equipment allows the user to insert the CD, push one or two buttons on the machine and be ready to proceed. These machines are much lighter than earlier versions and usually have microphones built into them. When recording many speakers and/or conferences, several microphones can be placed strategically and fed into a mixer. Each microphone can be adjusted to the speaker's voice level.

Table microphones should be placed on a layer of books, a soft cloth, or a piece of foam plastic to isolate table vibrations. Masking tape is used to keep the microphone from rolling or moving. When recording, it is important to choose a room where soundproof ceilings and heavy drapes and/or carpets deaden echoes; recording in gymnasiums or large rooms often results in external noise and echoes. The nurse educator who plans to record instructional materials for learners can investigate school resources such as recording studios or special recording rooms where higher-quality recordings can be produced. When recording outside, a wool sock can be cut to fit over the microphone and held on with a rubber band, to eliminate wind noises.

If no recording studio is available, a quiet office or room can be used. A "Do Not Enter" sign is placed on the door to preclude interruptions while recording. The recorder sits at a table or desk covered with a soft material; this eliminates noises from table tops and from shuffled papers. It is important to practice reading the script from typewritten pages until reading and page changes are fluid. Prior to recording, equipment should be tested for sound level and mechanical problems. A portion of the material can be read and then played back to ensure that the machine is recording correctly. Unless the nurse educator usually speaks quite slowly, it is necessary to speak more slowly than normal and to be sure to enunciate words clearly.

> Samantha decided not to purchase a programmed learning system after she heard a colleague was using CDs and videotaping in her class. After examining her budget, Samantha decided she could purchase one or the other, but she wasn't sure which to buy.

■ Nurse Educator Challenge

If you were Samantha, which would you purchase? Give a rationale for your answer.

Advantages and Uses of Making Recordings or CDs

1. Inflection, tone of voice, and verbal emphasis can be used to get the speaker's point across.
2. Tapes can be produced using a conversational tone, allowing learners to feel they are being given a personal lesson.
3. Tapes can be listened to while the learner is at home, traveling, or engaged in another activity.
4. A whole class can be assigned to listen to the same information through headphones at the same (or a different) pace.
5. Learning can be facilitated by using a verbal explanation while the learner looks at a visual aid.
6. Prerecorded lectures by outside experts can be used in the class more easily than by bringing in the actual expert.
7. Short audiotape segments can increase class attention by serving as a change of pace, a teaser for discussion, or a motivational device.
8. Prerecordings of cases or problems can be used to narrate overhead transparencies, slides, or PowerPoint® presentations.

9. Prepared lectures or presentations can be tested and streamlined prior to class and then be used repeatedly for subsequent class presentations.

10. Question-and-answer reviews can be taped for in- or out-of-class use as reinforcement for one-to-one or group learning.

11. Learner-made recordings can be used to record their goals for or evaluation of a course, serve as icebreakers or a forum for issue presentation, assist learners in studying their own verbal communication patterns, and can show the educator and/or class skill improvement.

12. Learners can record interviews or other material prior to class, or they can give the recording to the instructor or to a peer to listen to at their leisure.

13. Makeup and review sessions can be expedited through recording a class session and assigning learners to listen to the tape at a later date.

14. Nurse educators can tape their class sessions and listen to the tapes or CDs at a later date as a method of self-evaluation or peer evaluation.

15. Taped answers to common learner questions can be kept available for learner reference when the instructor is not present and can save time repeating them in class. Learners can go to the study lab or practice lab to listen to the answers.

16. Audio- or videotapes, CDs, or DVDs can be combined with programmed learning booklets or other learning experiences to provide multimedia learning experiences (Mukhopadhy & Parhor, 2001).

Films

Films have long been used by educators. Over time, the standard film gauge has changed; the medium has increased in use due to a decrease in the size of the equipment, which has resulted in greater portability, smaller required storage space, and greater ease of operation.

Advantages of Films

Advantages of films include:

1. Time can be telescoped; for example, a client's course through an illness process can be shown in a much shorter period of time than it could occur in real life.

2. Events that cannot be staged in the classroom can be observed; for example, surgical procedures or interviews with clients who do not wish to be present in class can be shown.
3. Many more auditory and visual stimuli can be presented as a coherent whole.
4. Cost of film use can be reduced through rental.
5. Complex motor skills can be depicted, showing learners the kind of terminal performance expected.
6. Problem solving can be evoked by presenting learners with a clinical dilemma and asking them to predict the outcome.
7. Filmed sequences of events can provide feedback for the learner by confirming predictions about what might occur in a given situation.
8. Individualized instruction can occur when learners view the film at their option and own pace (Kentucky Network, 2007).

Disadvantages of Films

Disadvantages of films include:

1. Most films are devised for continuous presentation, are passive learning experiences, and have minimal response-receiving characteristics.
2. Many films are poorly produced or do not follow principles of effective learning systems.
3. Films for classroom use require specific teacher behaviors such as ordering, previewing, setting up projector and screen, and making sure that electric outlets are convenient.
4. Films are frequently not catalogued in useful order as books are.
5. There is bias in films arising from slanting the content of the film toward a particular point of view.
6. Updating is difficult and costly.

For these reasons, nurse educators may decide to develop their own films. By doing so, principles of effective learning systems can be employed and content that is not available on the commercial market and/or is tailored for a specific curriculum can be developed.

The process of developing and/or reviewing short educational films should focus on principles of learning and effective learning systems, as well as several specific techniques.

Nurse Educator Tip

To enhance critical thinking, develop or use films to:

- Stop after the first five or ten minutes. The soundtrack can direct the viewer to turn the projector off and study programmed materials, conduct a discussion, or write down a list of alternative ways of dealing with a problem or case depicted in the film.
- Pause for the viewer to respond to a question prior to the soundtrack providing feedback about the correct answer.

Steps to Use When Planning or Evaluating Films

Steps for the nurse educator to keep in mind whether planning or evaluating films for classroom use include:

1. Make sure behavioral objectives are stated.
2. Evaluate whether film is the appropriate medium; generally, situations where action is primary to learning, where telescoped time sequences are important, or where clinical dilemmas or procedures that are difficult to expose learners to in real life are depicted present appropriate film subjects. Weigh the advantages of a film versus the time investment.

To produce an end product of 100 feet of usable film that runs 4 minutes, 40 hours or more of faculty time is involved. In addition, technician time for filming and editing may be 10–20 hours; a usable film may not return from the laboratory for between 1 and 6 months.

Part of this decision making includes a thorough search of available films. There may be one already available that will meet course objectives. If none can located, the nurse educator begins to make major decisions about the film.

Samantha and one of her nursing education classes were working with a local community group to develop a film about their health needs to be used as part of a grant application. Samantha had no previous film production experience, but she did know that to be funded, the group had to show a connection between the film and their health education goals.

■ Nurse Educator Challenge

What specific aspects of filming should Samantha be concerned with? Give a rationale for your answer.

The following questions may be useful guides to assist the novice film producer:

1. What is the proposed title of the film?
2. Is a black-and-white or colored film needed?
3. What is the estimated length of the film?
4. What is the estimated cost of the film?
5. Who is the target audience?
6. What are the behavioral objectives for the film?
7. What specific ideas are to be communicated in the film?
8. What overall effect is the completed film to have on the audience?
9. What is the order of major film sequences?
10. What directions need to be given to the cameraperson (cut, fade out, fade in, dissolve, pan, zoom in, zoom out)?
11. Who can serve as curriculum and content consultant to make sure that the film fits within the existing curriculum?
12. How will performers be selected and rehearsed?
13. If clients or minors are used, are there provisions for legal releases to be signed, verifying the use of the film for educational purposes?
14. Where will the filming take place so as to guarantee picture quality and authenticity?
15. Who will edit the film?
16. Will sound be recorded at the time of filming or later?
17. What directions are to be given to the editor regarding sound (fade up, fade down, fade under, mix, pause)?
18. What equipment, materials and props are needed? A technique that is especially useful in planning action media is the **storyboard** (Kentucky Network, 2007). Depending on the production, you may want to develop a one. A storyboard consists of drawings of key scenes with corresponding notes on elements such as dialogue, sound effects, and music (see Box 6–5).

> A storyboard consists of drawings of key scenes with corresponding notes on elements such as dialogue, sound effects, and music.

Box 6–5   Storyboard

Storyboard pages are helpful in preproduction planning for a film. During filming, the storyboard pages can be pinned on a board or wall and revised and used to shoot the sequence of scenes.

A sample of a portion of a storyboard appears below.

Shot Description: Blindfolded man sitting in wheelchair (zoom in slowly)

Music Cut: Background theme under

Narration: What body image changes might this man be experiencing? (Pause for one minute for viewer to respond to the question.)

Steps to Take When Making a Film

When filming actually begins, the following techniques may be of use:

1. Check the camera for film viewfinder adjustment and other factors, as listed on camera instructions.
2. Arrange lights properly and check meter exposure to prevent under- or over-exposure of film.
3. Avoid jerky motions; use a tripod whenever possible to decrease unsteady footage.
4. Do not zoom unnecessarily.
5. Pan (move camera from side to side or up and down) only when following a moving object or person.
6. Vary camera angles and field of view to sustain audience interest and to allow the viewer to get the best learning perspective.
7. Avoid dramatic portrayals with inexperienced actors.
8. Avoid having people talking directly to the audience when lip sync sound is not employed.
9. Shoot more film than deemed necessary, since editing may result in the need for additional footage.
10. Mark each reel with a consecutive code number and the abbreviated film title.

11. Keep narration to a minimum; the action should carry the main thrust of instruction; narration is used to provide explanatory insights, give supplementary information or give problem-solving data.
12. Keep music cuts to a minimum; they require technical and coordinator skills, resulting in time delays.
13. Keep the film simple; novice filmmakers often attempt to convey too much information at once (Kentucky Network, 2007).

For the nurse educator who is not skilled in making films, taking photographs, filmstrips, slides or photos uploaded to the computer may be more feasible. Although action cannot be as realistically portrayed, this medium lends itself to both group class and individualized out-of-class instruction. Once uploaded, DVDs or a series of photos illustrating concepts or theory can be uploaded by individual learners, enabling them to learn at their own pace. It is easy for learners to backtrack or to view entire learning sequences a second time. The content of films can be programmed utilizing the same characteristics as those contained in programmed instruction booklets (Kentucky Network, 2007).

Making Filmstrips

Filmstrips have their own set of rules and procedures:

- Use a copy stand and position the camera to focus on the subject.
- Place lights at a 45-degree angle to minimize glare.
- Read all directions supplied by the camera manufacturer.
- Take pictures or scan in objects of similar size sequentially to minimize the work of readjusting and refocusing the camera.
- Shoot pictures or arrange them in the order they will be used; filmstrip is a continuous band of film. All pictures must face the same way; a filmstrip cannot be turned upside down or sideways in the projector.
- When all photos have been shot, send them to the lab with directions to "process only; do not cut or mount" (Kentucky Network, 2007).

Television

Television is a medium that shares many of the advantages and disadvantages of film (Whittaker, 2006).

Nurse Educator Tip: Learner-Participation Filmstrips

- You can create the filmstrip template (either on computer or by just drawing it). Make copies so you have several pages for the class to use.
- Have learners write their paragraphs on separate paper and type up the copy when finished. Cut out and paste down the copy into the cell block. Have the learner draw the accompanying picture in a cell and go over lines with black marker.
- When your filmstrip section is complete, print a copy of the page on transparency film. Have the learner color in their drawing using vis-à-vis transparency markers (overhead projector markers).
- Cut out your filmstrip segments in groups of three, using thin pieces of clear tape, and join the segments together. Make a sleeve to slide the filmstrip through for viewing on an overhead projector. Take two pieces of cardboard and tape along one long side. Slide the filmstrip in and tuck it down snugly to the taped side. Judge where the filmstrip square falls and mark the size of the square in the center of the long side (so it lines up with the filmstrip). Use a craft knife to cut through the two layers of cardboard, but be sure to remove the filmstrip first before cutting. Use a straight edge to help you cut, and then staple the upper part of the cardboard to hold the two boards secure. Allow enough room to slide the filmstrip through with ease, but keep it lined up with the square.
- You can also display your filmstrip by hanging it in a window.

(Pak, 2006).

Advantages of Television

1. Learners can instantly play back their own or others' performance.
2. A single videotape deck can supply programming to an entire school at once.
3. A television camera recording learner performance can produce considerably more data than can a trained observer taking notes.
4. Learners can more easily learn how to evaluate their own performances, since the impact of the medium forces viewers to be aware of their behavior.

5. Television is flexible and can be presented live, be immediately played back, be broadcast to audiences in distant geographical locations, or store information for later use on videotapes.

6. Television holds the interest of most learners.

7. Learners can work at their own pace, watching television tapes in the privacy of a study carrel or learning laboratory.

8. Cable television can be used to present interactive lectures, where learners talk with the instructor while the program is being taped; subsequent programs include learner questions and the instructor's replies.

9. Editing can occur at the time of shooting by rewinding the tape and taping over the unwanted portion.

10. Microprocessors can be used to allow users easy access to any point on a videotape as well as allow for the programming technique of branching.

Disadvantages of Television

Disadvantages of the television medium and equipment are (Whittaker, 2006):

1. Hardware costs are high, components are fragile, and maintenance costs are high in both monetary and time frames.

2. Tapes made on one system cannot be shown on another, since they are incompatible.

3. Editing of videotapes is difficult, because sound and picture occur in different locations on the tape.

4. Television recorders are can be very sensitive to temperature, humidity, and cigarette smoke. They should be kept in air-conditioned rooms when possible and protected from smoke, and the lens should always be covered when not in use.

Preparing a Videotape

After researching using films and filmstrips, Samantha decided she must inform the community group that producing a videotape might be more in line with their budget and skills. Although she knew her decision was valid, she just was not sure how to proceed.

■ **Nurse Educator Challenge**

If you were Samantha, what would you tell the community group to substantiate your decision? Give a rationale for your answer.

When preparing a videotape presentation to be shown at a later date, the designer considers many of the questions dealt with in the course of producing films, including:

1. What is the main idea to be conveyed?
2. What is the budget?
3. What are the behavioral objectives for the tape?
4. What crew or technical assistance is available?
5. What is the major sequence of action that will convey the main idea?
6. Who will write the script?
7. Should the script be placed on cue cards or a prompter?
8. What visual materials, such as slides, titles or credits, need to be prepared?
9. What arrangements need to be made concerning a shooting location?
10. What directions need to be given to the cameraperson?
11. What actors are needed, and how will they be prepared for their parts and learn common hand signals used in television production?
12. What special items are needed such as lighting, clothing, or materials?
13. When will production start and end?
14. Will editing be done at the time of shooting, afterward, or not at all?

Writing the Script

If the nurse educator plans to write the script, the following guidelines suggested by R. Whittaker at http://www.cybercollege.com/tvp004.htm may be useful:

1. Watch television and observe different camera angles and special effects; try to use what you learn to develop the script. For example:
   a. Conflict can be depicted by placing participants opposite one another at a table.
   b. Placing two actors facing the camera and away from one another can convey indifference, coldness, or lack of awareness of one another.
   c. A V-formation of actors eliminates distance and can convey friendliness.
   d. Physical barriers, such as desks or curtains, produce the effect of distance between actors or can lend authority and formality.

e. Use props to lend authority and credence to a scene as well as to balance a scene or establish a time period, place, mood, or sensation.

f. Elevating the camera to look down on an actor conveys a feeling that he or she is meek or vulnerable and also gives the illusion of a third dimension.

g. Lowering the camera below the actor's head level gives an impression of a powerful, authoritarian, or imposing figure.

2. List the characteristics and scenes needed to advance the objectives or theme.
3. Arrange the scenes in proper sequence.
4. Write a short synopsis of each scene.
5. Use camera terminology appropriate to the medium (see Box 6–6).

Box 6–6 Script

A script format is often used to develop a tape for television audiences; a portion of a script appears below.

Video	Audio	
1. Move from LS of nurse and client.	ANNCR: (VO)	The nurse is interviewing the client about his reason for coming to the clinic. We'll join them now and listen to the interview.
2. Move to CU of nurse and client.	NURSE:	Tell me exactly why you're come to the clinic today.
	CLIENT:	I've been having pains in my back and legs.
	NURSE:	Show me where.
	CLIENT:	(Stands up to point)
	ANNCR: (VO)	Notice how the nurse is eliciting information from the client about his pain.

Key:
CU = Close-up
LS = Long-shot
ANNCR= Announcer or narrator
VO= Voice-over

6. Use a narrator or announcer to establish the opening and to underline important information.

7. When using nonprofessional actors, allow them to ad lib actual words, but provide them with the essence of what is to be portrayed.

8. Try to have some change on the screen every ten seconds; this can be accomplished by a camera movement or a change of scene.

9. Keep the action flowing as naturally as possible.

10. If you want the view to depict the essence of the situation, begin a sequence with a long shot.

11. If problem solving is the purpose of the sequence, use close-ups or special camera angles that provoke the viewer to decide what is happening in the situation.

12. Provide smooth transitions between scenes through the use of action, voice-over, or optical effects.

13. When using more than one camera, label the script and cameras (for example #1, #2, #3, and so on) so actors and camera people will know how the action flows.

In addition to producing a tape to be played at a later date, video can also be used effectively for immediate playback to give learners feedback on their performance. It can be used to tape learners completing practice procedures, interviews, role playing, or simulated situations.

Immediate feedback has the advantage of dramatically increasing the probability of learner success. To achieve this, the following procedure is suggested:

1. Set the recorder at 000, or write down the number registered on the recorder prior to the learner's performance.

2. Check the equipment to make sure that the learners to be taped are in the camera viewfinder, with adequate lighting.

3. Adjust voice levels and other special requirements according to the manufacturer's directions.

4. Turn on the camera and recorder and signal learners to perform the task; it is often useful to model the appropriate performance and allow learners to practice prior to taping them.

5. At the end of the performance, rewind the tape to 000 or the appropriate number where the performance began.

6. Replay the tape, using the pause button to show learners their errors or accomplishments.

7. Make at least one positive comment about the performance.

8. Prior to having learners replay the task or scene, restate one or two points to be concentrated on for this performance; for example, "Be sure to make eye contact with the client and speak more slowly." Do not attempt to correct more than one or two errors, or the learner will become frustrated and confused.

9. Stop the camera from recording whenever the learner does not perform according to the instructor's directions; use prompting such as, "Start again and look into the client's eyes."

10. Start the camera and begin recording again, and proceed until the learner does not perform per instructor's directions or until the task is completed.

11. Rewind the tape to the beginning of the learner performance or to the beginning of the replay; point out the change in learning by using the pause button.

12. Ask the learners to comment on how they felt about their performance, what changes they noticed in their behavior, and what they feel needs further practice.

In addition to providing high motivation and quick feedback, this procedure conveys to learners that their behavior can be changed and that learning can occur quite quickly in small increments.

Media Decisions

There are no clear-cut rules for selecting media. In many situations there will be more than one media option. The trend in media use seems to be toward multimedia, combining programmed instruction with film, audiotape, or filmstrip with a workbook and a game.

Media use can be humanized by providing learners with greater control over their own learning. Multimedia can enhance this effort by providing learners with a variety of models of learning.

One major error nurse educators may make is to purchase equipment (hardware) first, and then purchase films or software to fit the specifications of the hardware. The reverse order is suggested. First the nurse educator compiles a list of objectives and searches for a medium to evoke learning outcomes, and then buys the needed equipment. Unfortunately, most materials are indexed not by learning objectives, but by topic. Unless the nurse educator takes the time and effort to preview the materials, it is not clear whether the materials will meet the planned objectives. Also, many materials have not been pretested with equivalent populations so it is difficult to be sure what learners learn from the materials.

Because Samantha had faculty experience with media, the dean asked her to serve as a consultant for the purchase of additional hardware and software. At first she said no and told the dean she did not believe she had the expertise. With urging, Samantha finally said she would serve as a consultant. When she returned to her office, she became anxious about her decision and wasn't sure what kind of input to give.

■ **Nurse Educator Challenge**

Describe the information Samantha could give the dean about purchasing software and hardware. Give a rationale for your answer.

Decide on the priority of an attribute and then select the media method(s) likely to meet that attribute. Some attributes to consider are: ease of use, cost, availability, an ability to telescope time, structure, sensory or emotional impact on learners, whether it presents new material or individualizes learning, facilities for being monitored by a nonprofessional or a learner, learner control, immediate feedback, manipulation of data, and fast access to data or models.

Once these attributes have been analyzed and prioritized, software can be purchased or developed. Next, hardware is purchased based on the following principles. The nurse educator should:

1. Analyze hardware for multipurpose use; find out whether there is more than one aspect for its use.
2. Choose equipment that is relatively easy to operate.
3. Choose equipment that is appropriate to the size of the learner group.
4. Investigate the possibility of a service contract or plan.
5. Refer to a telephone directory for information concerning supply and repair of hardware.

Once hardware has been purchased, there are storage and assignment factors to consider, including the following as recommended by Educational Technology (1973):

1. Centralization of hardware and software with school library resources.
2. Development of a manual of services and supplies.
3. Development of an assignment and accountability method for use of equipment, making as few people responsible as possible.

4. Provision for instruction of staff members and learners in how to use the equipment.
5. Development of a checklist system of possible replacements or additional equipment that may be needed.
6. Designation of a person to be responsible for repairing and maintaining equipment.

If teaching needs are special or likely to change often, nurse educators will benefit from devising their own multimedia programs. If combination cassettes, games, and written materials are to be developed, it may be to the educator's advantage to consult a media packaging expert prior to developing the program. Some companies will custom-design new products. It is helpful to request catalogs from packaging companies to find out what is available for what price. Some specific packaging ideas available are: durable, custom-made containers for workbooks, slides, tapes, films, and filmstrips in heat-sealed vinyl; corrugated boxes that provide packaging that is less durable, but is also less expensive and takes up less space; imprints on plastic tape that allow for location of a program segment or exercise on an audio-cassette.

Development of multimedia materials takes time and money. It may be wise to canvass a nursing faculty to see whether a consensus exists about the generalized need for mediated instruction. If there is, a funding source may be located to assist with the development of materials. Much of education is moving toward a distance education model. For this reason, it is imperative that nurse educators learn about distance education methods.

Distance Education

Distance education refers to situations when the teacher or the learning institution are separated from the learner by time, place, or both. Distance education could be as simple for the educator as sending a learning course pamphlet or as complex as preparing an entire curriculum taught online. Some of the advantages are that learners learn the content as well as they do in a traditional classroom (a review of 238 studies conducted from 1928 to 1997 found no

> Distance education refers to situations when the educator or learning institution are separated from the learner by time, place, or both.

significant differences in the competencies of learners taught by traditional classroom methods versus distance education), but may also learn how to work as a team, how to seek out information, and how to be self-activated learners as well (American Association of Colleges of Nursing, 2000).

Research on Distance Education versus Traditional Lecture Mode

One of the primary concerns facing distance learning today is to find ways to increase the amount of learner involvement. Without involvement, learners may not maintain an interest in what they are learning (Hirschbuhl, 2007).

When given a choice, learners may prefer a blended mode of delivery over strictly online and regular classroom formats, even if quantitative analysis shows that learners' satisfaction with online and regular courses and online and regular instruction appears equal (Tang, 2007).

Jang, Hwang, Park, Kim, and Kim (2005) examined the effects of a Web-based teaching method (versus a traditional lecture method) on undergraduate nursing learner learning of electrocardiography (ECG). The authors developed the Web-based program and implemented it for four weeks. The sample included 105 senior nursing learners. Fifty-four were assigned to an experimental group (Web course), and 51 were assigned to the control group (lecture). The ability to interpret ECG recordings was significantly higher in the Web-based group.

Nurse educators learn new skills as well when they teach using a Web-based classroom. They spend more time responding to learner e-mail and reviewing online activity in chat rooms when courses use distance education formats. They become facilitators or coaches, urging and assisting learners to be more active in learning and to seek out new sources of information (AACN, 2000). Colleges and universities may benefit because it is more cost-effective to run smaller, more specialized classes, which enhance the quality of learning (AACN, 2000).

Synchronous vs Asynchronous Learning Online

Synchronous learning occurs in real time. Learners use video conferencing or online "live" chat; this type of learning is ideal when interactive group discussion enhances the material. Synchronous learning gives learners a big advantage because they can ask questions and share information as content is being presented.

> Synchronous learning occurs in real time.

Asynchronous learning occurs at a time chosen by the learner and as such is more self-directed. Prepared materials or messages are downloaded at the convenience of the learner, which allows arrangement of coursework around other activities and across multiple time zones and even countries.

> Asynchronous learning occurs at a time chosen by the learner.

Moving from Traditional Classroom Teaching to Online Facilitating

Dr. Whitaker, a seasoned nurse educator, had spent many years teaching in a traditional classroom. She was used to lecturing to her classes and was not ready to give that up. The next month when a new dean took over the program, Dr. Whitaker was forced to consider changing her classroom activities. The dean announced several of her courses were moving to an online status and all faculty were expected to be up to speed.

■ Nurse Educator Challenge

What would be an easy way for Dr. Whitaker to move toward online status?

Nurse educators who have grown used to the lecture method may find the idea of developing an entire online course daunting. Mahoney and colleagues described the design and evaluation of an online module as a beginning step to developing a complete online course over time. Learners in this hybrid class acknowledged that the online segment fostered critical thinking and was superior to traditional classroom learning because it allowed them to analyze and synthesize information, but required more of the learner (Mahoney, Marfurt, daCunha, and Engebretson, 2005).

A gradual movement toward more active learner learning and responsibility can be achieved by developing a module a semester and posting it online. This will serve to get both educator and learner feet wet in the online format. This kind of modular approach will help to socialize learners to more active learning (Kluge et al., 2007), teach them time management skills, and provide experience in the technology-based real world (Mahoney et al., 2005).

Building an Online Course Syllabus

When developing an effective course syllabus for an online course, it is important to reflect on teaching methods and how they must change for Web delivery. Palloff and

Pratt (1999) suggested the nurse educator answer the following questions and then build a syllabus around the answers.

- What do I want this course to accomplish? (e.g., objectives)
- What requirements does the institution require (e.g., office hours)?
- What unique requirements are important for this course?
- Which rules and roles do I want to be non-negotiable, negotiable, and learner-guided?
- How do I want to organize the online segments, given the constraints of the software?
- Will I use traditional testing or papers or do I want to use collaborative assignments, case studies, essays, simulations, and other online exercises as evaluation tools?
- How will I address attendance and participation requirements?
- Will I establish online office hours and when would be the best times to do so?
- Can I offer any face-to-face tutoring, meetings, focus groups and so on, and if so, what are the logistics?

A syllabus for a distance learning course focuses on learning objectives and provides a group discussion theme centered around a related reading for each week. Clear guidelines for what is acceptable class participation need to be written in unambiguous language and include grading guidelines. Examples could include:

1. *30 percent of the grade*—each learner will be responsible for facilitating a reading-related discussion for two weeks during the quarter; all learners are responsible for completing assigned readings every week and participating in online discussions that stay focused on each week's assigned topic.

2. *30 percent of grade*—each learner will participate in experiential exercises and case studies.

3. *40 percent of grade*—each learner will write a paper that integrates readings, discussions, and class exercises into a paper on a topic chosen from the list of available topics generated by the instructor. There will be one learner per topic, so the instructor should be contacted once you have selected a topic. The remaining available topics will be posted weekly. If a learner wishes to write a paper on an additional topic, the instructor should be contacted to discuss your rationale for doing so. Paper topics must be chosen by the end of the fourth week of class.

Constructing Online Course Sites

When designing an online course, the following questions should be asked (Porter, 1997):

1. How can I make the online course site look current, interesting, and accurate by using sounds, pictures, color, music, or graphics?
2. What do viewers need to know first?
3. How much information needs to be on the home page? On other pages?
4. What types of materials will be included—background information about the course, links to assignments, sample documents, graphics, simulations, interactive quizzes and tests, e-mail correspondence, and so on?
5. How should material be linked—external links, hypertext links, hypermedia links, navigational links to pull-down or pop-up menus, icons, mailto:?
6. How often do links need to be checked for accuracy?
7. How will learners work with documents—read them, view examples and manipulate them, take interactive quizzes, send e-mail to the instructor?
8. What other types of communication with learners will be needed—mailing lists, discussion groups, newsgroups, videoconferencing?
9. How often does the Web site need to be updated?

The online course site provides an organizational structure for learners to interact with each other and find and use resource materials. Regardless of the software application being used, online sites usually include:

- A welcome area for important announcements, guidelines, and questions,
- A community area for learners to meet, support one another, and share information about the course,
- Course content areas, including learning links, arranged to match course guidelines,
- An area for learners to post assignments and take exams,
- A course evaluation area, and
- An area for learners and instructors to post reflections on the learning process (Palloff & Pratt, 1999).

Dr. Whitaker took the plunge and put a learning module online. When that worked well, she decided to develop a course syllabus and plan for an online course. She knew she wanted to build an online community area for the learners to discuss topics among themselves and provide support for each other. She also wanted to require a final paper as part of the grading process and to establish office hours, but she wasn't sure if they should be online or offline.

> ### ■ Nurse Educator Challenge
>
> What elements has Dr. Whitaker overlooked, and in addition to those elements, what advice would you have for her about the items she's already chosen? Give a rationale for each of your points.

Online Discussion Groups

A common method of promoting critical thinking and group discussion is the online discussion group. Clegg and Heap (2006) provided some useful reflections on teaching evidence-based practice, and some suggestions for responding to learner online comments. The nurse educator serves as a combination facilitator, source of support, and tutor in this kind of situation. Some comments that might be helpful in this type of situation are shown in the Nurse Educator Tip on the next page.

As Dr. Whitaker's online course began to take shape, she realized she needed some rules and guidelines for the course. They would have to be somewhat different from her face-to-face courses, but she wasn't exactly sure how different they must be. For example, how was she going to make sure learners were involved in the course and were doing the assigned readings?

> ### ■ Nurse Educator Challenge
>
> What kind of advice would you give Dr. Whitaker about learner rules and guidelines for online behavior? Give a rationale for your choices.

Online Course Guidelines for Learners

Learners need specific guidelines for how to operate when online. Some guidelines suggested by Palloff and Pratt (1999) include:

1. Learners must log in and post a minimum of twice a week.
2. All posts must be substantive, take a position on a topic, or add significantly to the discussion; writing "I agree" or repeating someone else's comments is not sufficient.

Nurse Educator Tip for Responding to Online Comments

Some examples of helpful nurse educator comments to learners include:

- "Well done. You've shown how your answer is linked to the recommended text and one of the assigned articles."
- "You mentioned an important concept: randomization. You could expand your answer by discussing types of samples, representatives, and bias."
- "You've raised an interesting issue about the effect of the nurse's self-care practices on teaching clients to be involved in self-care efforts. You might want to check the research and see if anyone has studied this issue."

3. All assignments, case studies, and papers must be posted online. Each learner must make at least one constructive comment about each other learner's assignments (e.g., "I love the title of your paper and the topics you covered, but I think adding more up to date references would enhance your assignment.")
4. If any problems arise, deal with them directly with the person via e-mail or phone.
5. Use good "netiquette":
   a. Stay on subject when you post.
   b. Use pertinent subject titles and respond to only one issue per post.
   c. Use upper- and lowercase only; putting any words in all capitals is like shouting.
   d. Read your post prior to sending it into cyberspace and make sure it is positive and correct.
   e. Avoid forwarding anyone else's messages without obtaining permission.
   f. Cite all quotes, references, and sources.
   g. Use humor and criticism carefully; use emoticons such as :) to indicate you are being humorous.

Sharing Responsibility for Facilitating the Course

Active learning is a desired outcome of online courses. Although the nurse educator may begin the course by serving as facilitator, as the weeks proceed, it is important to assign learners responsibility for leading a portion of the discussion. This can be done based on learner interest, extra credit, random assignment, or some other method. Some of the possible roles learners can take include:

- Facilitator of discussions
- Process observer, commenting on group dynamics
- Content commentator, summarizing group learning since last week
- Team leader who evaluates peers' work
- Presenter on a particular topic, book, or area of interest (Palloff and Pratt, 1999)

Using Groups Online

Collaborative learning is often a big part of Web-based courses. The following questions can assist the nurse educator in the development of collaborative learning.

1. Which parts of this course lend themselves to small-group learning activities?
2. What small-group goals should be developed?
3. What size groups should be developed to achieve goals?
4. Who should form these groups? The nurse educator? Learners?
5. What should determine the composition of groups? Interests? Strengths?
6. Should the composition remain the same for the quarter/semester or should it change?
7. How should groups be structured to enhance participation?
8. How should roles be assigned?
9. How can rewards/motivation be built into the groups?
10. How will accountability be built in?
11. How will the learners, instructor, and group performance be evaluated and by whom?
12. How can feedback to learners be built into the course?

Course and Time Management Techniques

Problems can arise with online courses that may not be evident in traditionally led courses. Paloff and Pratt (1999) provided suggestions for the nurse educator in dealing with specific course and time management issues online:

- Minimal participation due to information overload.
  1. E-mail learners to determine the cause.
  2. Suggest setting a daily logon time to read others' comments and become familiar with an online approach.

3. Assist in managing outside reading for the course; assign readings in smaller, manageable chunks.

4. Suggest some possible online responses.

5. Encourage discussion group and forum participation and ask learners to request assistance from peers.

- Communication anxiety

  1. Make personal e-mail contact with learners.

  2. Give supportive comments every time learners post until anxiety is reduced.

  3. Ensure learners are comfortable with the technology involved; refer them to helpful technicians or workshops.

- Lack of participation due to technical difficulties

  1. Contact learners via e-mail.

  2. Contact systems administrators to resolve technical problems.

  3. Make sure technical assistance is available for learners.

- Lack of participation due to privacy and exposure concerns

  1. E-mail learners to determine the nature of their concern.

  2. Offer support to learners.

  3. Encourage learners to share only what they feel comfortable sharing.

  4. Work with systems administrators to plug any security leaks and change passwords if necessary.

- Excessive posting

  1. E-mail learners to provide feedback on participation and provide support.

  2. Suggest learners log in only once daily.

  3. Limit posts for all learners to two per week and no more than 500 words/login.

- Feeling pressured about responding

  1. Print out messages so they can be read when time is available.

  2. Write responses into a file; revise as necessary and then copy and paste to course site.

Nursing Education: The Future

The future of learning is technology-based. In fact, some futurists proclaim the classroom will soon be obsolete (Downes, 1998). In the future, personal access devices (or PADs) may become the dominant tool for learning, especially for online education. The PAD combines the function of book, notebook, and pen. It is a lightweight computer with touch-screen functions and high-speed wireless Internet access. It will look like a contemporary clipboard and will weigh about as much. Its high-resolution screen will deliver easy-to-read text, video, and multimedia. The PAD will accept voice commands, recognize the owner's handwriting, and accept input via touch-screen access (Downes, 1998).

Educational software of the future will include features present in video games and more. This software will do more than present a stream of information. It will place the learner in an environment where all information needed for success will be available at a touch of the screen. Some of these predictions have already come to pass. Mohide, Matthew-Maich, and Cross (2006) reported using electronic gaming to promote evidence-based practice in nursing. A problem-based learning case study under investigation was posted online and learners defined the research question, then searched for, retrieved, and interpreted the research findings.

Virtual reality and simulations will move far beyond what is available today. Without entering the emergency room, nurse learners will have a vivid idea of what a client in the emergency room says and does, what it feels like to be treated, what the nurses and doctors say and do, and what role the learner can play (Downes, 1998).

Asynchronous conferencing online will include full multimedia ability. Learners will be able to embed images, videos, and sound into their messages (Downes, 1998).

Education will become more personalized. Classes will no longer be time-based, with learners starting at the same time, studying the same materials at the same pace, and ending together. This model is heavily dependent on the teacher. Education in the future will be more topic-based and much less class-based. The menu of available courses for learners will be dependent on prior learning. According to Downes (1998), selecting a course will be like selecting a channel on television. This quest model is already available in gaming environments and will soon be available for college learners.

As learners progress through a course, they will be able to select from a library of background information on the topic, which may be presented with a discourse from Florence Nightingale on a topic related to their quest, or may be presented by the nurse educator when additional information is requested by the learner (Downes, 1998).

This kind of learning will occur because it is more efficient, not because learning results are better (although they often are), or learners prefer it (although many do). As mentioned earlier in this book, lecture is not a very effective or efficient method of learning. Educators often spend too much reviewing material that only a few learners need, boring the rest of the class, or they do not spend enough time on new material that may not be absorbed by half the class. The time spent answering learner questions (that only relate to one or a few learners), or providing directions (which could just as well be found in a handout) will be eliminated through personalized education (Downes, 1998).

Learning styles will be tailored to learning systems. Nursing educators will know preferred learner learning styles and provide appropriate learning materials. For example, learners who learn best by exploring will be presented with a variety of options to pursue, those who learn best in a linear fashion will be provided with a video stream of materials, and those who learn best visually will be shown graphic representations of concepts (Downes, 1998).

Much learning will be constructed by learners. They will have input into the usefulness of resource materials, the types of experiences needed to be effective in clinical sites, and the feedback needed from nurse educators.

Learning will be online-based and schools and colleges will shrink in size as place of education will not be as important. Nurse educators will take the lead in providing learning resources, but in the community, facilitators who provide individual support and help in the form of peer support groups will be hired by institutions. Face-to-face learning will still occur, but it may not be at the college level. Learners may live in Europe, but attend a U.S. school. The person who provides connection for most learning will be an Internet nurse educator, but learners will find support from community facilitators who work for their college or university.

Grading procedures will also change. A computer will assist nursing educators to track learner interactions online that show how individual learners used concepts or theory during the course of study. Results from learner work with simulations can be fed directly into the learner's course database (Downes, 1998).

EXERCISES FOR NURSE EDUCATORS

1. Evaluating individualized learning systems.
Choose one of the individualized learning systems mentioned in the text, or locate another one. Evaluate the system in terms of its individualization of the following factors:
   a. Class attendance,
   b. Materials for study,
   c. Method of study,

d. Pace of study,
e. Decision-making,
f. Teaching focus,
g. Teacher role,
h. Teaching method,
i. Environmental structure,
j. Time structure,
k. Evaluation procedures, and
l. Program purposes.

2. Individualizing learning

List specific ways in which you would individualize a specific course. If possible, develop and test your ideas.

3. Devising a self-instructional module

Use Box 6–1 or develop your own format to devise a teaching/learning module for one or more principles, concepts, values, or skills. Try out the module as part of the developmental process. Revise it based on tryout.

4. Evaluating a self-instructional learning system

Locate a self-instructional learning system, or use the one you developed, and try it out with a group of learners; then evaluate it in term of the following factors:
a. Percentage of learner success with each learning objective,
b. Ability for learners to progress at their own rate,
c. Extent to which learners exercise options to choose and achieve options, and
d. Extent to which learners are provided with skills to design and develop their own learning experiences.

5. Evaluating a programmed instructional unit

Locate a programmed instructional unit and evaluate it, using the list below to ensure that each is included:
a. Behavioral objectives,
b. Target population for whom the program was developed,
c. Average and range of time needed to complete the program,
d. Type of program used and its ability to provide opportunities for learners to generalize what is studied,
e. Cheat-proofing,
f. Evaluation data,
g. Directions for administering the program,
h. Fit within an existing curriculum,
i. Cost per unit,

    j. Training time needed to prepare the learner to use the program, and

    k. Reusability of the program.

After having evaluated the unit, devise ways you would strengthen it based on its inability to meet the above criteria.

6. Designing a written program

Design a written program using the following procedure:

    a. Choose a small topic with which you are familiar.

    b. Delineate the target population.

    c. Devise a pretest, and give it to the target population.

    d. Assign prerequisite learning experiences if necessary.

    e. Construct a posttest.

    f. Revise objectives if necessary.

    g. Construct a flow sheet with the essential points to be learned and remedial points as needed.

    h. Begin to write frames, using the guidelines for developing a program in this chapter.

7. Evaluating some available hardware and software systems

Peruse catalogs or examine available hardware and software systems according to the following criteria and decide on those most likely to meet behavioral objectives for the area of nursing you are most interested in:

    a. Cost,

    b. Instructional advantages and disadvantages,

    c. Space limitations,

    d. Ease of use,

    e. Personnel needs and skills,

    f. Fit with existing curriculum,

    g. Availability,

    h. Ability to telescope time,

    i. Ability to structure time,

    j. Ability to have a sensory or emotional impact,

    k. Ability to present new material,

    l. Degree of individualization,

    m. Degree of learner control,

    n. Degree of feedback provided,

    o. Ability to allow learner access to data,

    p. Multipurpose uses, and

    q. Ease of obtaining service and repair.

8. Optional experience

Devise the following procedures to use with the hardware and software systems you have chosen:

a. Centralization with school library,
b. Manual of services and supplies,
c. Assignment and accountability method,
d. Instructions for staff members and learners regarding the use of hardware and software,
e. Checklist of replaceable or additional equipment, and
f. Designation of a person responsible for repair and maintenance of equipment.

9. Autotutorial Exercise

Compare and contrast findings from the evaluation of an auto-tutorial, individualized, and self-instructional unit.

ADVANCED LEARNING EXPERIENCES

10. Problem Statement

Devise problem statements for a research project in three of the following areas:

a. Individualized learning,
b. Self-instructional learning,
c. Programmed instruction,
d. Web instruction,
e. Audiotape or DVD, and
f. Videotape.

11. Research Study

Choose one of the devised problem statements and develop a research design to study the problem.

12. Issues/Situations

Choose one of the issues/situations from the future of nursing education section and develop a:

a. Proposal,
b. Problem statement for study,
c. Research design, and
d. Paper to guide you in the next phase of your career.

References

American Association of Colleges of Nursing. (2000). Distance learning is changing and challenging nursing education. *AACN Issue Bulletin* (January). Retrieved November 15, 2006 from http://www.aacn.nche.edu/publications/issues/jan2000.htm

Agre, P., Dougherty, J., & Pirone, J. (2002). Creating a CD-ROM program for cancer-related patient education. *Oncology Nursing Forum, 29*(3), 573–580.

Anglin, G. J. (Ed.) (1995). *Instructional technology: Past, present and future* (2nd ed.). Englewood, CO: Libraries Unlimited, Inc.

Beder, H. (2005). Research on factors that shape engagement. *Focus on Basics:Connecting Research and Practice, 7*(March), 1-7.

Benschoter, R. A., Hays, B. J., Jackson, B. J., & Lindeman, M. G. (1991). Adapting an established curriculum to the self-instructional format: Rationale and process. *Journal of Continuing Education in Health Professions, 11*(1), 43–52.

Cambra-Fierro, J., & Cambra-Berdan, J. (2007). Students' self-evaluation and reflection (part 1): "Measurement." *Education and Training, 49*(1), 36-44.

Castaldini, M., Saltmarch, M., Luck, S., & Sucher, K. (1998). The development and pilot testing of a multimedia CD-ROM for diabetes education. *Diabetes Education, 24*(3), 286–286, 295–296.

Clegg, P., & Heap, J. (2006). Facing the challenge of e-learning: Reflections on teaching evidence-based practice through online discussion groups. *Innovate 2*(6), article 290. Retrieved November 17, 2006 from http://www.innovateonline.info/index.php?view=article&id=290

Dececco, J. P. (1968). *The Psychology of Learning and Instruction.* Englewood Cliffs, NJ: Prentice-Hall.

Downes, S. (1998). The future of online learning. *Online Journal of Distance Learning Administration, 1*(3). Retrieved November 12, 2006 from http:www.westga.edu/~distance/downes13.html.

Educational Technology: A reference of hardware and software. (1973). Columbus, OH: Ohio State Nurses' Association.

Gagne, R. M., Briggs, L. J., & Wager, W. W. (1992a). *The conditions of learning* (2nd ed.). New York: Holt, Rinehart & Winston.

Gagne, R. M., Briggs, L. J., & Wager, W. W. (1992b). *Principles of instructional design* (4th ed.). Fort Worth, TX: Harcourt Brace Jovanovich.

Hiemstra, R. & Sisco, B. (1990). *Individualizing instruction: Making learning personal, empowering and successful.* San Francisco: Jossey-Bass.

Hirschbuh, J. J. (2007). Designing, developing, and implementing an interactive learning system. *Journal of Computing in Higher Education, 19*(1), 1–115.

Jang, K. S., Hwang, S. Y., Park, S. J., Kim, Y. M., & Kim, M. J. (2005). Effects of a web-based teaching method on undergraduate nursing learners' learning of electrocardiography. *Journal of Nursing Education, 44*(1), 35–39.

Kentucky Network. (2007). *How to make creative and inexpensive movies.* Retrieved March 14, 2007 from http://www.ket.org/cgi-bin/itv/marc_menu.pl?marc_id=1236

Kluge, M. A., Glick, L. K., Engleman, L. L., & Hooper, J. S. (2007). Teaching nursing and allied health care students how to "communicate care" to older adults. *Educational Gerontology, 33*(3), 187-207.

Mager, R. (1997). *Measuring instructional results* (3rd ed.). Atlanta, GA: Center for Effective Performance.

Mahoney, J. S., Marfurt, S., daCunha, M., & Engebretson, J. (2005). Design and evaluation of an online teaching strategy in an undergraduate psychiatric nursing course. *Archives of Psychiatric Nursing, 19*(6), 264–272.

Mergel, B. (2001). *Instructional design and learning theory: Learning theories and the practice of instructional design.* Saskatoon, Canada: University of Saskatchewan.

Mohide, E. A., Matthew-Maich, N., & Cross, H. (2006). Using electronic gaming to promote evidence-based practice in nursing education. *Journal of Nursing Education, 45*(9), 384.

Mukhopadhy, M., & Parhor, M. (2001). Instructional design in multi-channel learning systems. *British Journal of Educational Technology, 32*(5), 543-556.

Pak, A. (2006). *The civil war filmstrip report.* Retrieved April 1, 2007 from http://home.rochester.rr.com/inwoods/civilwar-filmstrip.htm

Palloff, R. M., & Pratt, K. (1999). *Building learning communities in cyberspace: Effective strategies for the online classroom.* San Francisco: Jossey-Bass.

Porter, L. R. (1997). *Virtual classroom: Distance learning with the Internet.* New York: John Wiley & Sons.

Schiffman, S. S. (1995). Instructional systems design: Five views of the field. In G. J. Anglin (Ed.), *Instructional technology: Past, present and future,* 2nd ed. (pp. 131-142). Englewood CO: Libraries Unlimited, Inc.

SUU Nursing Faculty Handbook. (2005). *Auto-tutorial learning modules general policies and procedures.* Retrieved November 18, 2006 from http://www.suu.edu/sci/nursing/facbook/appendix-c.html

Tang, M. (2007). Regular versus online versus blended: A qualitative description of the advantages of the electronic modes and a quantitative evaluation. *International Journal of E-Learning, 5*(2), 257-266.

Whittaker, R. (2006). *The production sequence.* Retrieved April 1, 2007 from http://www.cybercollege.com/tvp004.htm

INDEX

A

academic rigor and learner-centered environments, 32

accommodative learning
creativity, 163
flexibility, 163
reading books, 163
self-expression, 163

active case simulation, 183

active learning
accommodative learning, 163
assimilative learning, 163
cognitive complexity, 163
evidence-based learning, 97
forces working against, 26
rationale for, 163
teaching procedures, 99,

administrative barriers and learner-centered environments, 32

adult learning
activating prior knowledge, 22
active learning and, 22
as an egalitarian process, 22
constructivist school and, 22
Knowles's theory of andragogy, 22
problem-solving, 22
self-direction and self-responsibility, 22
the need to know and, 22

affective components
of behavioral objectives, 15
of learning, 15

affective domain
feeling, 23–24
learning strategies, 23–24

affective learning objectives
internalizing values, 107

G

Gagne's Learning Theory
  assessing performance, 133
  coaching and, 133
  cognitive strategies and, 128
  eliciting a performance, 132
  encoding information, 131
  enhancing retention and transfer, 133
  Events of Instruction, 128
  explaining and demonstrating, 130
  facilitating retention of material, 134
  gaining attention, 128–129
  identifying current knowledge, 130
  information processing model, 128
  informing learners of the objectives, 129
  intellectual skills, 128
  motivation, 130
  motor skills, 128
  music or multimedia program, 129
  praising, 131
  presenting new content, 130
  pretesting learners, 130
  providing feedback, 132
  providing learning guidance, 131
  repeating a task to criterion, 133
  stimulating recall of learning, 130
  using prompts, 132
  using questioning, 133
  verbal information, 128
Generation X learners, 31
Generation Y learners, 31
Gilligan's moral development stages
  conventional stage, 70
  postconventional stage, 70
  preconventional stage, 70
  transitional stages, 70
grading
  criterion-referenced, 136–137, 149
  nurse educator tips, 136, 149
  obtaining objectives, 149
  on the curve, 149

graduate nursing education
  accountability, 9
  competency, 9
  independent thinking, 9
  interdisciplinary approach, 9
  leadership, 9
Grasha-Reichmann Learning Styles
  avoidant, 61
  collaborative, 61
  competitive, 61
  dependent, 61
  independent, 61
  participant, 61
group leadership, defined, 233
group learning
  disadvantages, 234–235
  disagreements and arguing, 234–235
  monopolizing and scapegoating, 235
  monopolizing vignette, 235
  pressures within groups, 234
  problem solving or solution
    finding, 235
  vignette, 234
  warm-ups and, 236–237
group methods, and
  active learning, 230
  advantages, 233
  constructivist school of learning, 230
  focus, 13
  learner enthusiasm, 232–233
  narrative pedagogy, 232
  peer learning, 229–284
guilt, and nurse educator, 18

H

health care shifts and learning
  acute to chronic health care, 99
  curing to caring, 99
  lifestyle in health promotion, 99
  nurses nurture themselves, 99